David M. Aronstein, MSW
Bruce J. Thompson, PhD
Editors

HIV and Social Work
A Practitioner's Guide

Pre-publication
REVIEWS,
COMMENTARIES,
EVALUATIONS . . .

"**S**ome of the most salient aspects of working with people living with HIV are threaded together under this cover to provide a bigger picture of the challenging AIDS service context. The lens from which the work is described is that of those on the front lines, making it both relevant and useful. This is an invaluable primer for social workers, case managers, and other providers of health and social services."

John Auerbach, MBA
Massachusetts State AIDS Director,
Department of Public Health,
Boston, MA

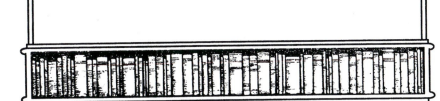

"*HIV and Social Work: A Practitioner's Guide* is a unique and comprehensive resource that deserves a prominent place in the libraries of all medical and mental health professionals actively involved in the care of people living with HIV infection. The contributors represent a wide array of well-recognized, highly proficient human service professionals and the text is thorough in delineating all the potential contexts in which social workers may be involved in the care and case management of HIV-infected people.

What is most impressive about this excellent text is the sense of understanding of the myriad potential barriers that people living with HIV may face. Thus, chapters that deal with housing, economic supports, working with the schools, and working with couples all flow together very clearly, given the excellent editing and the underlying philosophy that the purpose of social workers in the care of people living with HIV is to facilitate their ability to live full and productive lives. This holistic approach makes the text an extremely engaging one to read and the provision of references at the end of each chapter makes this text highly useful for social work and other mental health professional training students.

It has been edifying in recent years to see the advances made in HIV therapeutics, but as this retroviral disease becomes a chronic immunosuppressive infection, the need for well-trained social workers will only grow. This well-edited and extremely worthwhile text will be of great benefit to educators and students in social services for years to come, because of its ability to provide a well-integrated and thoughtful foundation for social service and mental health professionals to organize their work with HIV-infected individuals in the appropriate social/cultural and operational contexts."

Kenneth H. Mayer, MD
*Director, Brown University
AIDS Program;
Professor of Medicine
and Community Health,
Brown University,
Providence, RI*

The Harrington Park Press
An Imprint of The Haworth Press, Inc.

HIV and Social Work
A Practitioner's Guide

HAWORTH
Psychosocial Issues of HIV/AIDS
R. Dennis Shelby, PhD
Senior Editor

HIV and Social Work: A Practitioner's Guide edited by David M. Aronstein and Bruce J. Thompson

HIV/AIDS and the Drug Culture: Shattered Lives by Elizabeth Hagan and Joan Gormley

HIV and Social Work
A Practitioner's Guide

David M. Aronstein, MSW
Bruce J. Thompson, PhD
Editors

The Harrington Park Press
An Imprint of The Haworth Press, Inc.
New York • London

Published by

The Harrington Park Press, an imprint of The Haworth Press, Inc., 10 Alice Street, Binghamton, NY
13904-1580

Cover design: Sametz Blackstone Associates, Boston.

The Library of Congress has cataloged the hardcover edition of this book as:

HIV and social work : a practitioner's guide / [edited by] David M. Aronstein, Bruce J. Thompson.
    p. cm.
  Includes bibliographical references and index.
  ISBN 0-7890-0180-2
    1. AIDS (Disease)—Social aspects—United States. 2. Social service—United States. I.
Aronstein, David M. II. Thompson, Bruce J.
RA644.A25H5788 1997
362.1'969792'00973—dc21
                                          97-21867
                                          CIP

ISBN 1-56023-906-9 (pbk.)

To
Bill Kreidler
and
David Meltzer

CONTENTS

SECTION III: PEOPLE IN SPECIAL CIRCUMSTANCES

SECTION IV: ECONOMIC SUPPORTS AND HOUSING

SECTION V: CARING FOR THE PROFESSIONAL CAREGIVER

ABOUT THE EDITORS

David M. Aronstein, MSW, is the founder of The ACS Group in Boston where he consults with health, education, and human service groups on issues of planning, program design, and organization development. He was a founding member of the senior management of the AIDS Action Committee of Massachusetts, where he served as its first Director of Client Services and as Director of Policy, Education, and Planning. He was a member of the National Association of Social Workers' HIV Task Force and the Boston AIDS Consortium. He is president of the Board of Directors of the Community Research Initiative of New England, which conducts research on promising HIV therapies.

Bruce J. Thompson, MSW, MS, PhD, is a professor and chair of the Social and Health Services Program at Roger Williams University. He is also a visiting professor at Smith College School for Social Work where he organized and taught a course on social work treatment issues related to AIDS. He received an MSW from Syracuse University, MS in Health Services Administration from Harvard School of Public Health, and a PhD in Social Work from Smith College. He maintains a private psychotherapy practice in Providence, Rhode Island, and has written and lectured extensively on the impact of AIDS on gay men and their families and on AIDS case management.

Contributors

Gregory Anderson, MSW, has worked for many years in the field of gay and lesbian gerontology. As supervisor of Individual Services at SAGE (Senior Action in a Gay Environment) in New York City, he provided direct services to the gay and lesbian elderly community and coordinated a program for AIDS and the Elderly. He is a former co-chair of the HIV/AIDS and Aging Task Force of New York and is currently HIV patient coordinator with Schenectady Family Health Services in Schenectady, New York.

Jeffrey S. Austin was born in Columbus, Ohio, and escaped to New York City at his earliest opportunity. His activities there, and later in Boston, resulted in an infection with HIV sometime between 1979 and 1981. Testing positive in 1986, Austin, by now residing in Rhode Island, cast off an unsatisfying career in advertising and film production, and in 1990, became the founding Executive Director of Sunrise Community housing, Inc., which has received national and local recognition as an AIDS service organization.

Judith Hanson Babcock, MSW, has been an HIV/AIDS social worker at Deaconess Beth Israel Hospital in Boston since 1986. She brings to her work rich experiences from rural hospitals in Jamaica and Northern New England where she learned the importance of identifying both traditional and nontraditional sources of support. She has developed innovative approaches for providing support to caregivers and families of HIV/AIDS patients as well as for people living with HIV/AIDS.

Robert J. Battjes, DSW, is the Deputy Director of the Division of Clinical and Services Research, National Institute on Drug Abuse. He has worked at NIDA since 1977 in program planning and research administration. Current areas of responsibility include research on drug abuse treatment, health services, and medical consequences of drug abuse. His principle area of research and publication is monitoring trends in HIV infection and risk behaviors among injecting drug users.

Fred F. Boykin, MSW, LCSW-C, is a senior social worker for the National Institutes of Health in Bethesda, Maryland. He is also in private practice with Counseling and Psychotherapy Services in Washington, DC. He has written numerous articles and spoken nationally on issues of social work and HIV/AIDS. He lives with his life partner, Jack Killen, and his two cats, Garth and Biff.

David J. Brennan, MSW, has been involved in AIDS care since 1983 from hotline volunteer and buddy with the AIDS Action Committee in Boston, Massachusetts, to his present position as the AIDS program coordinator at Hospice Care, Inc., Boston. He has been a case manager, advocate, supervisor, and clinical social worker. He is the former social work and bereavement coordinator at the Hospice at Mission Hill. He has a private practice specializing in HIV bereavement. He is a member of the National Hospice Organization's AIDS Resource Committee, as well as the Massachusetts Hospice Federation's AIDS Task Force.

Stephan L. Buckingham, MSSW, developed one of the first comprehensive psychosocial programs for persons diagnosed with HIV/AIDS at the UCLA Medical Center in Los Angeles. He has directed HIV programs at Hollywood Community Hospital and Sherman Oaks Community Hospital and AIDS Project Los Angeles and served as director of psychological services at Pacific Oaks Medical Group where he developed a model program for neuropsychological screening and assessment in conjunction with the UCLA Neuropsychiatric Institute. Currently, Mr. Buckingham is Vice President at Kallir, Philips, Ross, Inc., a healthcare communications firm in New York. He has written extensively on HIV and neuropsychology and is editing the book *A Mental Health Practitioner's Guide to the Neuropsychiatric Complications of HIV/AIDS.*

Steven A. Cadwell, PhD, has done research on burnout, empathy, and countertransference in clinical work with gay men with HIV. He provides consultation to agencies, clinics, and hospital staffs who work with people with HIV. He has led support groups for both patients and professionals affected by HIV and has been involved in treatment and service development for these individuals for the past twelve years. He is currently in private practice in Boston, Massachusetts.

Amy Curell, MSW, University of California, Berkeley, 1987, BA in psychology, Williams College, 1983. She studied at the Family Institute of Cambridge in 1989. Ms. Curell has worked in the field of HIV/AIDS for the past seven years. She is currently the clinical coordinator of Family Life Resource Center, an adjunct faculty member at Roger Williams University, and has a private practice in Providence, Rhode Island.

Peter J. Delany, DSW, is currently a senior social science analyst in the Division of Clinical Services Research at the National Institute on Drug

Abuse. Prior to joining NIDA, Dr. Delany taught at both The Catholic University of America, where he received his doctorate, and at The University of North Carolina. He is a licensed clinical social worker and a member of the Academy of Certified Social Workers and has twelve years of experience in the fields of addictions and mental health.

Lee W. Ellenberg, MSW, BCD, is the Associate Director of Mental Health at Fenway Community Health Center in Boston. He began his work with HIV and mental health issues on the Mental Health Subcommittee of the AIDS Action Committee of Massachusetts in 1984. Over the past 12 years, he has given numerous presentations on HIV and gay and lesbian issues throughout New England. Mr. Ellenberg also maintains a psychotherapy practice in Brookline, Massachusetts.

Susan M. Gallego, MSSW, LMSW-ACP, has over fifteen years experience in service provision, program management, supervision, and training. For the past seven years, she has been the director of client services at AIDS Services of Austin, where she supervises case management, nursing, food bank, and financial assistance programs. She has extensive experience in client advocacy issues, women's health, child abuse, medical social work, substance abuse, and childhood development. She has over seven years experience in community health working with adolescent pregnancy, reproductive rights, and women's issues. She has served as consultant and trainer on cultural competency issues. Ms. Gallego is an adjunct faculty member at the University of Texas-Austin's and the Southwest Texas State University's Schools of Social Work. She is currently on the advisory board for the NASW HIV and Mental Health Training Project.

Larry M. Gant, CSW, PhD, has created, implemented, and evaluated programs in the area of HIV primary prevention and harm reduction for sexual minorities, people of color, and injection drug users since 1985. He is currently an associate professor of social work at the School of Social Work, University of Michigan. He has conducted program evaluations on case management systems for persons living with HIV/AIDS, both in Michigan and nationally. Dr. Gant has published numerous works related to HIV and community-based harm-reduction initiatives and on the development and ownership transfer of community-based interventions. He serves on numerous national boards including the National AIDS Fund and the National Hemophilia Foundation. He was a member of the HIV/AIDS Task Force of the National Association of Social Workers.

Patricia U. Giulino, MSW, LICSW, Smith College School for Social Work. She was the coordinator of mental health at the AIDS Action Committee of Massachusetts and was co-chair of the Mental Health Task Force of the Boston AIDS Consortium. Currently, she is on staff at the Andrews Unit in the Department of Outpatient Psychiatry at the Massachusetts General Hospital and maintains a private practice with individuals and couples in Boston.

Lana Ka'opua, MSW, ACSW, is a licensed clinical social worker in a community-based mental health center in urban Honolulu. She is also a doctoral candidate at the University of Hawaii and has an interest in minority health issues. Under the auspices of the John A. Burns School of Medicine, University of Hawaii, she developed a curriculum on cultural competency and HIV, which has received widespread usage. She currently serves as advisory board member and trainer with the NASW HIV Spectrum Disease and Mental Health Training Project.

Jay Laudato, MSW, previously served as the coordinator of financial advocacy at the Gay Men's Health Crisis in New York City. He is currently the assistant director for Behavioral Health, HIV, and Special Needs at the New York City Health and Hospitals Corporation where he works on HIV/AIDS policy and program development in the public hospital system. Jay is also the co-chair of the Board of Directors for the People with AIDS Coalition, New York.

Emily Leavitt, MSW/LCSW, is currently the supervisor of the Psychiatric Consultation Service of the University of California-San Francisco AIDS Health Project. Ms. Leavitt has worked in HIV mental health for six years. She also mothers two girls and a small dog.

S. Michelle Martin, MSW, LMSW-AP, is the former executive director of a nonprofit organization. She has worked in the nonprofit world for many years with various populations including the elderly, school-age children, women, trauma survivors, and people living with AIDS. She holds a Masters degree in social work with an emphasis on administration and planning. Ms. Martin is a Texas-based consultant to nonprofit organizations.

Jane K. O'Rourke, MSW/LICSW, received her MSW from Smith College School for Social Work in 1991. She worked at Maine Medical Center as the clinical social worker on the AIDS Consultation Service's interdisciplinary team. She then became the director of Support Services at the AIDS Project in Portland, serving southern Maine's HIV population.

Susan S. Patania, RN, MSW, has been a social worker for people with HIV since 1988. She worked for the AIDS team of the Visiting Nurses Association in Houston, and then as the mental health coordinator and social work director at the AIDS Foundation, Houston. She was nurse manager for Baylor College of Medicine's outpatient psychiatry service at the Harris County Thomas Street HIV Clinic. Since 1993, she has taught "HIV/AIDS Clinical Social Work Responses" at Smith College School for Social Work. She is a PhD candidate at Johns Hopkins School of Public Health and is a therapist and researcher at the Moore (HIV) Clinic Psychiatry Department of the Johns Hopkins Hospital.

Avi Rose, LCSW, has been doing HIV work in a variety of communities and settings since 1985. He is currently the HIV Services Manager and Assistant Director of Tri-City Health Center in Fremont, CA. He is also a psychotherapist in private practice in Oakland, CA.

Kitsy Schoen, MSW, LCSW, was an original member of the internationally renown AIDS Homecare and Hospice Program in San Francisco where she worked for seven years as a hospice social worker and the coordinator of Bereavement Services. For the past six years Kitsy has been writing, speaking and consulting with hospice, HIV and health care organizations on issues of staff support and grief and loss in the workplace.

R. Dennis Shelby, MSW, PhD, is a member of the Core Faculty of the Institute for Clinical Social Work and a Candidate at the Chicago Institute for Psychoanalysis. He is the author of *If a Partner Has AIDS* and *People with HIV and Those Who Help Them* and many papers on clinical work with HIV-related problems and psychotherapy with gay men. He is the senior editor of The Haworth Press book program, "Psychosocial Issues in HIV/AIDS" and maintains a psychotherapy and consultation practice in Chicago, Illinois.

Thomas F. Sheridan, MSW, is the president of The Sheridan Group, a Washington, DC–based government and public relations firm. As a political aide to Vice President Walter Mondale, Tom Sheridan campaigned in nine states and served on the national staff of Mondale's 1984 presidential campaign. Mr. Sheridan is recognized as an expert and leader on domestic policy issues through his work for the National Association of Social Workers, as the assistant deputy director of the Child Welfare League of America, and as the director of public policy for AIDS Action Council. He was the principal lobbyist and architect of the Ryan White CARE Act of 1991 and one of the leaders of the movement to pass the Americans with Disabilities Act. He completed his undergraduate degree at Dominican College and earned his MSW from The Catholic University of America.

Michael Shernoff, CSW, ACSW, is in private practice in Manhattan and is an adjunct faculty member at Hunter College Graduate School of Social Work. Author of more than fifty articles and brochures on HIV/AIDS and mental health issues of lesbians and gay men, he has also edited five books. Currently, he is a board member of the National Social Work AIDS Network.

Margaret Smith, MSW, UCLA, has been involved in HIV-related work since 1985. She was the original clinical director of Sunrise House, the first AIDS residence in Rhode Island. In 1991, she was named Rhode Island Social Worker of the Year for her work with people with HIV. She co-authored (with Ian Stulberg), "The Psychosocial Impact of the AIDS Epidemic on the Lives of Gay Men," published in *Social Work* in 1988. She is currently working at The Miriam Hospital, Providence, Rhode Island.

Jack B. Stein, MSW, LCSW, is a senior project director involved in a number of professional training and research programs on drug abuse and HIV-related issues. For the National Institute on Drug Abuse, he oversees the development of educational materials based on scientific research for the general public, policymakers, and health care providers. He has published numerous chapters on HIV and substance abuse and was chairperson of the National Association of Social Workers' Task Force on HIV.

Ian Stulberg, MSW, LCSW, has worked professionally with HIV/AIDS patients for more than ten years, initially as a clinical social worker on immune-suppressed units in Los Angeles area hospitals, and, since 1991, as the manager of the Mental Health Program at the AIDS Service Center in Pasadena, California. He is a guest lecturer at UCLA's Department of Social Welfare and is on the board of directors of the Lesbian and Gay Psychotherapy Association of Southern California.

Mary Beth Sunenblick, MEd, MSW, worked as a clinical social worker with children, adolescents, and families for twenty-five years, doing both inpatient and outpatient work within the Department of Child Psychiatry at the Maine Medical Center, Portland. She taught for three years in the Counselor Education program at the University of Southern Maine. She is a member of the Maine Clinical Social Work Society and is a Board-Certified Diplomat in Clinical Social Work.

Perry S. Sutherland, MSSW, is the coordinator of community programs at Community Counseling Center in Portland, Maine. He received his MSSW from the University of Tennessee, Knoxville, with a clinical focus on cognitive behavioral treatment, as well as services to sexual minorities. He was the director of The AIDS Project in Portland, and has provided clinical and administrative social work services since 1982.

Susan Taylor-Brown, MSW, PhD, MPH, is the chair of the Health Care Concentration at Syracuse University. She has done AIDS work since

1986 including cofacilitating groups, supervision, legislative advocacy, teaching, and research. The major focus of her work is women and their families, which includes permanency planning. She holds numerous leadership positions including social work consultant with the Community Health Network, is a member of National Planning Committee for HIV/ AIDS Leadership Summits, chair of the American Public Health Association, and the NASW AIDS Liaison.

Jay R. Warren, MSW, is a senior clinical social worker in Health Care Associates, a primary care practice at Beth Israel Deaconess Medical Center in Boston, Massachusetts. He also maintains a private practice in Boston.

Lori S. Wiener, PhD, MSW, ACSW, has been working on the frontline of this disease since 1982. Originally from New York City, Dr. Wiener accepted a position at the National Institutes of Health in 1986 to help incorporate the treatment of pediatric HIV disease into the pediatric oncology program. Dr. Wiener has conducted numerous studies examining parental needs and coping, children's coping, and interventions to meet both parents' and children's needs. Perhaps her most important publication has been the book *Be a Friend: Children Who Live with HIV Speak,* which reveals the inner thoughts, fears, and hopes of HIV-infected children and their siblings.

Foreword

The first cases of AIDS were identified in 1981. In the intervening sixteen years, we have witnessed the explosion of a worldwide epidemic. By the end of 1981, there were 257 identified cases in the United States. This number grew to 2,000 by the end of 1983 and to 360,000 a decade later.

These have been years of pain and loss, of tragedy and prejudice, and of neglect. The medical and helping professions were slow to respond to the epidemic; they seemed almost immobilized, like deer caught in the headlights of an oncoming car. However, with the heroic activism of the gay community and the efforts of a few pioneering professionals, denial and avoidance began to be overcome and HIV was recognized as a major threat to the health of this nation and of the world. Service and research efforts multiplied and knowledge began to accumulate about the nature of the disease and the needs of those suffering from it.

Social workers have had a long experience working in the delivery of health care services, working with ill people and their families on what Cobot and Cannon, founders of medical social work, termed "the social frontiers of medicine." Social workers who work with people suffering from acute, chronic, and life-threatening illnesses, and with their families could be of assistance in serving the HIV/AIDS population. HIV/AIDS shares many of the characteristics of other life-threatening conditions. However, HIV/AIDS was also very different, thus calling for the development of new knowledge, skills, and strategies.

This difference arose because a second and parallel epidemic developed along with HIV/AIDS, an epidemic of stigma, fear, ignorance, and discrimination. This second epidemic shapes the lives of those infected, the social world in which they live, the kinds of care they receive, and the attitudes and behaviors of helping professionals. People infected with HIV face social isolation; disruption of social and sexual relationships; lack of needed services; loss of jobs, insurance, and housing; and alienation from family and friends.

The social frontiers of HIV/AIDS demand intense attention. Not only does the quality of life of an infected person depend on the healing of the social fabric, but the process of the disease itself is related to the availability of needed treatment and services, the reduction of stress, and the existence of a supportive and caring human network.

An effective response to HIV thus requires a range of skills: flexibility, creativity, and a willingness to follow the problem wherever it might lead. Thus, social workers have much to bring to this field of practice. Our traditional broad psychosocial perspective encourages social workers to be sensitive to all of the factors that impact the life of a person with HIV. Social workers are prepared to work with individuals, couples, families, groups, and communities. They call upon multiple roles depending on the situation: counselor, psychotherapist, social broker, organizer, advocate, program and policy developer, and social change agent. This is the flexibility, the breadth of vision, and the multiple service roles that responding to HIV/AIDS requires.

This volume brings us the results of social workers' work in this area of practice. Presented here is neither theory nor distancing analysis, but the practice wisdom and useful knowledge and skills that have arisen from the lived experience of practitioners out there in the trenches. This is a rich and useful book for people entering HIV/AIDS work who want guidance, for experienced people who want to sharpen their skills, and for all social workers who, no matter where they work, are going to find people with HIV or their family members in need of help.

As devastating as the illness is, the work in this volume brings hope and optimism by demonstrating that there are things that can be done. Very specific kinds of help can make an enormous difference in the lives of people with HIV/AIDS and those who love and care for them.

Ann Hartman, DSW

Preface

In October 1996 in Washington DC, ACT UP, the AIDS social action coalition, held a "political funeral march" from the Capitol Building to the White House. The march culminated with the ashes of people who had died of AIDS being spread on the lawn of the White House. As the march proceeded, the cry rang out, "What do you want?" The response from the crowd: "A cure for AIDS." Then, "When do you want it?" The response, "Now!"

This book, written by social workers on the front line of AIDS work in the United States, echoes the emotional outrage, grief, and hope of the millions of Americans affected by the epidemic. Intended as a guide—a practice handbook—for social workers new to the field and/or new to AIDS work and for those who wish to learn more about social work practice with people with HIV/AIDS, this book is organized accordingly. The appearance of a practice handbook in 1998 raises the frequently asked practice question, "Why now?" To many, the past year in the AIDS pandemic, at least in the United States, has been a time of optimism generated by an overall lower rate of infection and hope that new anti-HIV therapies will result in AIDS becoming a manageable chronic condition. AIDS seems to be, at last, on its way to being under control. While some optimism is warranted, it is now more important than ever that social workers renew their commitment to those disenfranchised groups who are still at higher risk of infection. These are the poor, minorities, and young people—adolescents who are gay and/or IV drug users. These groups are not only at higher risk of infection, but they also may be least likely to benefit from new therapies due to underinsurance or no insurance and late disease-stage entry into the medical care system when new therapies are least helpful.

Some basic demographic dimensions of HIV/AIDS are as true now as they were in the early days of the epidemic. Minorities of color are tremendously overrepresented in the infected population; this is particularly true for women and children of color who comprise nearly 80 percent of women and children with HIV/AIDS. Most people who are infected do not know they are HIV positive because they have not been tested. Many people who know they are infected in the United States do not have access to new anti-HIV therapies; most of the developing world has no access to anti-HIV therapy. In the United States, gay men still represent the largest single group of the infected population. Though the percentage of infected gay men has steadily declined over the years, an alarming increase in infection has occurred in some subsets of gay men, particularly in younger gay men. Finally, a cure for AIDS still does not exist.

Social workers have been very actively involved in the HIV epidemic from the beginning. They have responded with their clinical skills to help individuals, couples, and families deal with the trauma of learning about the infection, with the "roller coaster" of disease progression, and frequently with confronting the final stages of disease and death. They have responded with their organizational and political skills, helping with the founding and implementation of community-based organizations to educate and advocate on behalf of people with HIV/AIDS. Social workers have also responded with their research skills to help demonstrate "what works" in interventions aimed at helping people with HIV/AIDS and their loved ones. Indeed, it is striking that AIDS emerged in the late twentieth century at a time that coincided with the maturity of the social work profession—that a new medical, social, psychological, and political phenomenon which disproportionately effects members of society who have been traditionally marginalized and stigmatized has challenged the social work profession "in its stride." AIDS has placed demands and expectations on the profession to remember its core values such as self-determination, the dignity and worth of the individual, distributive justice, and commitment to the poor and the vulnerable. As a result, local, regional, national, and even international conferences and continuing education programs on HIV/AIDS for social workers have been developed. Some schools of social work have initiated separate courses on HIV/AIDS; many have incorporated AIDS-related material throughout the curriculum. The National Association of Social Workers has adopted a policy statement on HIV/AIDS. Additionally, many individual social workers, just as those who have contributed to this book, have developed specialization and practice wisdom through their work with people with HIV/AIDS.

So, it is appropriate to now have a volume by social workers for social workers on HIV/AIDS—as it provides an opportunity to share the knowledge (practice wisdom) gained over the past fifteen years and, perhaps, to pass it along to new generations of social workers who will still be dealing with the AIDS pandemic in one form or another for many years to come.

While acknowledging that the horror of the HIV epidemic has affected so much of the world, we are aware of some of the extraordinary gifts that our work in the epidemic has given us. Contrary to the intuitive thought that social work in this epidemic is relentlessly depressing, draining, and sad, working in this epidemic has had a profound personal and professional impact on us. We wanted to see if our colleagues shared this perspective; therefore, we asked each contributing author to tell us something about what he or she had learned while working with people affected by HIV. As Larry Gant from Michigan noted, "There's something a little off-center in discussing personal transformations resulting from the greatest plague of the last half of the twentieth century." Yet we found that remarkably similar spiritual, intellectual, and emotional transformations had occurred in the social workers who wrote this book.

All of the contributors discuss their work related to HIV/AIDS as compelling and "transformative" in one way or another. For some gay men and lesbians, the work has coincided with (and provided a vehicle for) coming out professionally and giving something back to their communities. For most people, the work has challenged them with fundamental, existential questions related to meaning, anxiety, freedom, responsibility, and death. For some the work has resulted in a recognition of limitations, a new tolerance for uncertainty and ambiguity, a need to demand that systems of heath care and human service stretch to meet new needs—and finally, a need to be self-protective against fatigue and burnout.

Six themes emerged from the authors' responses:

1. Learning to Live Life More Fully

It is ironic that in the face of sadness, illness, and sometimes death, social workers feel they have learned to celebrate their own lives more fully. Judith Babcock from Boston states, "I've learned from my clients how to celebrate life more fully," and Susan Taylor-Brown from Syracuse adds that, "HIV demands a focus on the here and now—the importance of doing what you want in your life. My world is richer, my love and pain are deeper, and my laughter is louder." Stephan Buckingham from New York says that, "HIV/AIDS has taught me that life is right now, not sometime in the future, but right now!" Perry Sutherland from Maine has learned "the importance of honoring and cherishing the spirits in my life, those before me and those who have passed on." Michael

Shernoff from New York told a moving story about the death of his lover, Lee:

> I was able to hold him fifteen minutes before he died, tell him how much I loved him and how much I'd always treasure the years we shared . . . After reassuring him that though I'd miss him terrible, I'd be all right, he peacefully left this earth. I honestly don't believe that I could have been there for Lee as completely on the variety of ways that were necessary had I not been working in this field.

2. Learning Not to Make Assumptions

Many people discussed how their work has challenged their thinking, assumptions, and paradigms. Susan Gallego from Texas says that her work "has meant stretching, bending, turning, growing, moving, and changing everything I knew, learned, and believed." Beth Sunenblick from Maine talks about being "more elastic" and "suspending judgment." Judith Babcock has learned the following: "Entering a situation from a position of 'not knowing' all the answers (or even any answers) allows me to join people in their attempts to chart the unknown territory they've entered, to help them become clearer about what they want for their lives."

3. Learning to Listen to Our Clients

Consistently, social workers realized how much their clients had to teach them, if only they would listen. Jane O'Rourke from Boston writes, "The heart of the matter is being with each soul as you can, stretching in the moment—as it is profound and temporal." Fred Boykin from Washington, DC, noted, "Listening to clients gives me the strength to grow professionally and to pass on their wisdom to the newly diagnosed and their loved ones." Lana Ka'opua from Honolulu adds, "I forget that there is always more to learn, that there is no substitute for slowing down and listening to the person who is across from me, learning from them, and most of all—learning that I am not alone and do not have to do it all myself." Beth Sunenblick from Maine stresses how difficult it is to listen sometimes: "I know that my clients will instruct me if I only listen, but I have to be prepared not always to understand their directions. My primary debt is to my clients who, with extraordinary courage and forbearance, have persevered in teaching me how to work with them." For many authors, writing their contributions for this book was a way to share what they had learned. "I thank each of them [clients] for teaching me these lessons and for allowing me to share them with others," explains Lori Wiener of Maryland.

4. Learning About Courage

Through their work with people with HIV and their families, social workers talked about the courage they have seen and the courage they have found in themselves. David Brennan from Massachusetts spoke about "the tremendous courage that people with AIDS and their families exhibit on a daily basis . . . Courage to wake up and face each new day and challenge with integrity, grace, and humor." He adds that his work over the past twelve years has convinced him of the following:

> All human being have an inherent greatness. For some, it may take more time to see, but it is there. And I will always want to look for it and celebrate it. This is the courage I have gotten from those for whom I have cared and loved and truly miss.

Susan Taylor-Brown is "inspired by the courage and capacity to grow of the PWAs" she works with, and Lori Wiener adds, "There is not a day where I am not moved by the strength, courage, and wisdom that the children I work with express in their own unique way."

5. Learning One's Own Limitations

Not surprisingly, many authors learned about their own limitations, their expectations of themselves, and how to measure progress differently. Susan Taylor-Brown states that she is "more aware of and strives to be more accepting of [her] own limitations." Ian Stulberg of Southern California wrote of an experience clearing overgrown vines in his backyard:

> One Saturday afternoon, I found myself standing shirtless in the backyard, sweating profusely as I attacked the vine, which had almost—but not quite—smothered a small lemon tree. I was determined that I would kill this vine before it was able to kill the lemon tree or any other living shrub in my backyard. In the midst of the battle, I suddenly stopped and, as I panted furiously trying to catch my breath, I thought, "Hmmm, I don't think this is about landscaping!" I realized that I was responding to my perceived impotence at the hospital to prevent my patients from dying, by doing battle with

a plumbago vine in my backyard. But I have realized subsequently that even if my work in this field can't necessarily prevent PWHIVs from dying, it can make a difference in the quality of their lives. And making a difference in the quality of other people's lives has made the difference in the quality of my own.

6. Learning to Take Care of Oneself

In spite of the inspiration that this work has brought to many social workers, it remains very difficult work, and many authors emphasized the importance of self-care. Susan Taylor-Brown explains the "importance of taking care of of myself as I care for others. I play and nurture myself as hard as I work. I make the time to be with my children, family, and friends. I stay centered by remembering to love and care for my children before reaching out to other people's children." In the final analysis, people had a realistic view of the joys and pains for social workers in the HIV epidemic. Lori Wiener stated that for her, "this work is incredibly intense, profound, existentially seductive, and sad," but she also stressed that "there is a fine line between being sad and being depressed." Confronted with the enormity of the work, Lana Ka'opua adds, "I forget that there is always more to learn, that there is no substitute for slowing down and listening to the person who is across from me, learning from them, and most of all—learning that I am not alone and do not have to do it all myself."

HOW TO USE THIS BOOK

The dilemma we faced in compiling this book was to give readers easy access to sufficient information about different aspects of HIV and social workers' roles in effectively engaging their clients without overwhelming them with so much information that they would be afraid to dive in. The result is that while we have tried to address a broad range of issues that social workers face, this is not a comprehensive, in-depth encyclopedia of all HIV and social work–related knowledge. Each section is designed to give the reader some of the essential facts, issues to consider, and numerous examples of how issues arise and ways that social workers might intervene. While not all sections are organized exactly the same way, many of them follow a simple outline:

- Why Do This? Statement of the Problem/Issues
- Facts the Social Worker Needs to Know Before Proceeding
- Examples of How the Issue May Present

- Key Questions to Ask the Client
- Cultural Competency Considerations
- Action Steps for Successful Intervention
- Potential Barriers to Successful Intervention
- What the Client Should Know Before Taking Action
- Policy Implications and Related Actions
- Conclusion
- Recommended Readings

Recognizing that there are increasing demands on the time and attention of social workers in all settings, we have organized this book so that readers can use sections in an "as needed" approach to learning. Each section includes suggestions for further reading in that particular area.

The chapter "Essential Facts Every Social Worker Needs to Know" is recommended as foundation reading for anyone who has never worked with HIV/AIDS clients and as an update for social workers who may need a quick review. "Getting Started: Basic Skills for Effective Social Work with People with HIV" gives a broad view of different aspects of practicing social work in the HIV epidemic by a veteran practitioner, Michael Shernoff. He reminds us of the importance and challenge of returning to our fundamental social work skills, thus using our thoughts and feelings with intelligence and consideration in the best interests of the client. While all sections address issues of ethnic, racial, gender, and sexual orientation differences, "Multicultural Competence" highlights three primary competencies that are necessary in this increasingly complex and diverse epidemic, regardless of the practice setting.

The core of this book is Section II, "Practice Settings," in which practitioners skillfully outline the essential questions and issues confronting practitioners in many different settings. Part A, "Services in Health Settings," discusses acute care, hospice care, home care, and some special considerations concerning access to clinical trials and practical issues such as health care proxies and living wills. Nonetheless, we recognize that people's lives and workers' practices do not neatly fall into these categories. Similarly, Part B, "Services in Mental Health Settings," discusses individual, group, couples, and family clinical issues, recognizing fully that most professionals' practices combine a mixture of clinical approaches. This section also includes techniques on addressing clients' risk behaviors when they arise in the clinical setting and some of the ethical issues that present themselves. The challenges of treating people with HIV in private practice are considered, and an introduction to identifying and treating HIV-associated dementia is presented, which is useful for any practitioner, regardless of the setting. The mental health section concludes with some practical advice on organizing support groups and working with people with HIV who have chronic mental illnesses.

Given the epidemiology of HIV, Section III, "People in Special Circumstances," looks at practice issues from a "demographic" perspective rather than from a treatment modalities perspective. There is a section specific to substance abuse issues and HIV although these issues and clinical anecdotes of clients with substance abuse histories are included in numerous other sections. Recognizing that many social work practitioners focus on children, families, and adolescents, there are sections devoted to the particularly complicated issues that arise when different generations of family are infected with HIV. Similarly, some practitioners focus primarily on services to gay men, women, the elderly, people in rural areas, and people in prison. HIV presents unique challenges to practitioners working with these populations, and such challenges need to be thought about carefully.

Because HIV is not "merely" a physical or emotional illness, but also one with devastating economic and social implications, the chapters "Economic Supports and Advocacy" and "Housing" address such issues faced by people with HIV. Many of these people have complex psychosocial histories and experiences with the social welfare systems, and neither the systems nor the individual clients and workers have been well prepared to deal with these issues.

All of these issues and populations present very difficult personal and professional emotional challenges for social workers. Often, social workers are asked to "care" for the emotional needs of their medical colleagues who may be less prepared for the emotional vicissitudes of treating people with HIV. However, without paying close attention to one's own emotional needs, one's effectiveness lessens. The chapter "Meeting the Emotional Needs of Health Care Providers" addresses both these issues.

Finally, because social work's knowledge base and values are rooted in the view of people as part of complex psychosocial systems, the chapter "Changing the System: Don't Mourn . . . Organize!" is on macro approaches to systems change with practical advise that any social worker can use, regardless of setting.

We have struggled with what to include and exclude and have tried to strike a balance that will be useful to a broad range of social workers. Our aim is to challenge the specialist readers without confusing the generalists. We have tried to minimize the use of jargon and build on the core skills and values that form the foundation of social work practice in the age of AIDS. Our hope is that this book will encourage readers to become allies with their fellow social workers in the battle against HIV.

Acknowledgments

It would be impossible to write a book of this size and complexity alone. The authors in this volume have written their sections in the belief that the lessons they have learned and the practice wisdom they have acquired need to be shared with their social work colleagues. We appreciate their willingness to tolerate our editorial suggestions and criticism with humor and gentleness. This "contributed work" is truly theirs.

The initial idea for this book came from the National Association of Social Workers Press who approached the NASW HIV Task Force to write it. We would like to thank the members of the Task Force, Jack Stein, Rebecca Ashery, Susan Gallego, Larry Gant, Sandra Lew, Nathan Linsk, and Jim Brennan of the NASW staff. Their guidance and encouragement to undertake this project was invaluable in making an idea become reality. While the final book is very different from the initial concept, it continues to reflect the Task Force's belief in the important role social work can and should play in fighting the HIV epidemic. It also reflects our mutual belief that social workers need to have good resources to improve their practices and that the best resources for social workers are created by social workers.

We would like to thank John B. Smith for his assistance in helping us deal with every word-processing program known to humankind. We are proud to initiate The Haworth Press's book program on Psychosocial Issues of HIV/AIDS and want to thank Dennis Shelby, the editor of this program, for his help and encouragement.

David Aronstein would also like to thank his former colleagues from the AIDS Action Committee of Massachusetts from whom he learned so much: Michael Connolly, Larry Killian, Larry Kessler, Anne Marie Silvia, Bob Rimer, Louise Rice, Tom McNaught, Robert Greenwald, and Dianne Perlmutter. In addition, he thanks Gary Raymond, whose consistent professional and personal support has shown him the best in social work and friendship.

Bruce Thompson would like to thank three Deans who have supported his work: Katherine Gabel and Ann Hartman of Smith College School for Social Work and John Stout of Roger Williams University. He would also like to thank clients and students who have taught him more than he ever knew he did not know, and his family, particularly his brother Brian, for their courage and love.

Finally, we want to acknowledge our social work colleagues who have lived with HIV and from whom we have learned so much. In particular, we want to thank Diego Lopez and Tony Candeloro, both of whom were early social work and HIV pioneers who died much too soon. Their work and passion continue to inspire us.

SECTION I:
INTRODUCTION

Essential Facts Every
Social Worker Needs to Know

Larry M. Gant

INTRODUCTION

The literature on HIV/AIDS is incredibly extensive and is growing annually. Each year, new information about the pathogenesis and treatment issues of HIV/AIDS extends, changes, and modifies prior information. This brief chapter outlines essential facts about HIV/AIDS for social workers. It is not intended to be a comprehensive overview of the pandemic; for that, the reader is referred to Lloyd (1995) and Stine (1996). Still, the current chapter serves as an initial point of information and departure.

LEARNING THE LANGUAGE OF HIV DISEASE

A basic understanding of medical terminology has application both for understanding physical health in general and HIV/AIDS-related issues in particular. In this chapter's Appendix, the reader is provided with basic terminology that can be used to establish a basic foundation for understanding health terms and HIV/AIDS terms. Social workers can further enhance their knowledge of medical jargon by purchasing a medical dictionary.

Basic HIV/AIDS Terminology

HIV/AIDS terminology constantly changes. The following information is current as of April 1996. Readers are urged to confirm the information presented with other sources, including health care providers, HIV/AIDS service organizations, the Red Cross, and the Centers for Disease Control (CDC).

3

AIDS: Acronym for acquired immune deficiency syndrome; a progressive weakening of the immune system with primary cause of infection identified as HIV. According to the 1993 CDC definition, an HIV-positive person has AIDS when CD-4 count falls below 200 or when diagnosed with one of twenty-three specific illnesses.

alternative treatments: Any substance or procedures a person chooses to use other than FDA-approved medications.

antibody: A protein that identifies, kills, or neutralizes antigens such as bacteria, viruses, or fungi.

antigen: Any substance that the body reacts to by mounting an immune response, including forming antibodies.

antiretroviral: A drug used to treat infections with a retrovirus. HIV is a retrovirus; AZT, ddI, ddC, and 3TC are antiretrovirals used to treat HIV infection.

CD-4 cells: A type of blood cell important to the immune system. HIV results in a loss of CD-4 cells, reducing the immune system's ability to fight infection. Also called T4 cells and CD-4 lymphocytes.

CD-4 count: Also known as CD-4 lymphocyte count or T4-cell count. A measurement of CD-4 cells (number of CD-4 cells per cubic millimeter of blood). Usually HIV progression is associated with a decrease in the number of CD-44 cells.

drug trials: Also called clinical trials; enable researchers to determine proper dose, benefits, and risks of drug or treatment.

ELISA Test: Acronym for enzyme-linked immunosorbent assay. A blood test most often used to screen for HIV infection. ELISA detects HIV antibodies—not HIV. A positive ELISA test must be confirmed by a more specific test, the Western blot.

HIV: Acronym for human immunodeficiency virus, the retrovirus that leads to AIDS.

invasive cervical cancer: AIDS-defining condition that occurs among HIV-positive women.

Kaposi's sarcoma (KS): The most common tumor associated with HIV, particularly in gay men; characterized by abnormal growth of blood vessels, which develop into purplish or brown lesions.

neuropathy: General term for any disease of peripheral nerves—those that control muscles and sensation.

nosocomial: Hospital-related; usually refers to illnesses acquired in hospitals.

opportunistic infection (OI): When the immune system is damaged, infections take advantage of the opportunity and flourish.

pathogen: Any agent that causes a disease, such as viruses and bacteria.

pathogensis: Progression of a disease from initial to end stages.

Pneumocystis carinii pneumonia (PCP): The most common infection in people with AIDS; often the first defining AIDS illness for many infected persons.

protease: An enzyme that HIV uses to make new copies of itself inside infected cells.

protease inhibitors: A drug that stops protease from making new copies of HIV that can infect other cells.

retrovirus: A type of virus that replicates mutant strains.

risk behaviors: Actions that put people at risk for HIV infection such as unprotected sex and sharing needles with injection drug users.

safe sex: Any sexual activity in which there is no exposure to another person's body fluids.

safer sex: Sexual activities that reduce but do not eliminate risk of HIV transmission.

seroconversion: Occurs when people exposed to an infectious agent (such as HIV) develop antibodies to that agent. In HIV disease, seroconversion ordinarily takes place within weeks to a few months after the initial infection.

thrush: Yeast infection occurring in the mouth.

universal precautions: An established set of techniques and barriers to control the transmission of pathogens. In the case of HIV, this refers to the use of barrier methods to prevent HIV transmission between providers and patients.

wasting syndrome: A loss of 10 percent or more of body weight with no explanation other than HIV infection.

Western blot: A test for detecting specific antibodies to a particular pathogen, such as a virus or bacterium; used to confirm a positive ELISA blood test.

EPIDEMIOLOGY OF HIV IN THE UNITED STATES

As of April 1996, almost 500,000 people in the United States have died from HIV-related illnesses. Approximately 170,000 people in the United

States are currently living with AIDS, and nearly one million more people are HIV-positive.

In the United States, male-to-male sex is cited as the most frequent route of transmission. Since 1992, however, injection drug use has replaced male-to-male sex as the most frequent cause of new infections. HIV cases due to heterosexual transmission have increased 1,200 percent between 1986 and 1993 (Gant, 1995; Blake, 1993).

In the early years of the pandemic, the overwhelming majority of AIDS cases were gay white males. As the pandemic has spread to other populations, the majority of AIDS cases are found among African Americans, Latinos, and women. As of January 1995, African Americans and Latinos comprised 50 percent (33 percent and 17 percent, respectively) of all U.S. AIDS cases. Women are the fastest-growing group of people with AIDS, and nearly 80 percent of women AIDS cases are either African American or Latina (CDC, 1995).

HIV TRANSMISSION AND PREVENTION

Types of HIV Transmission

As a transmissible and progressive disease, HIV can be transmitted in the three following ways:

1. Sexual transmission
2. Blood transmission
3. Mother-to-child transmission

There have been reports of other modes of infection; however, those reports are disputed and, to date, unreconcilable. HIV is not spread through casual contact (e.g., sneezing, coughing, sharing utensils, or using common toilets or swimming pools). Like some other viruses, HIV is inactivated outside a human host; it cannot survive in open air or in water. In short, *HIV is infectious, not contagious.*

Sexual Transmission

The earliest reports of HIV linked the virus with the sexual behaviors associated with gay men. Years later, it became apparent that HIV infection was not associated with any particular sexual orientation, preference, or identity. Rather, the sexual transmission of HIV infection was and is associated with sexual behaviors and activities. Table 1 summarizes common sexual behaviors grouped by probable risk of HIV infection.

TABLE 1. Sex Behaviors and Probable Risk of HIV

Safest sex practices	Dry kissing
	Oral sex with a condom or latex barrier
	Mutual masturbation
	Toys with condom
	Finger play with latex glove
	Abstinence
Safer sex practices	Oral sex without a condom and having a healthy (no sores, no bleeding) mouth
	Vaginal or anal sex with a condom
	Finger play without a condom
Risky sex practices	Vaginal or anal sex without a condom
	Unprotected oral sex with mouth sores

Blood Transmission

The second most frequent transmission route is the most efficient. When infected blood is transfused, the risk of acquiring HIV is extremely high, ranging from 90 to 100 percent (Lifson, 1992; WHO/GPA,1990). Blood transmission of HIV occurs in two ways: (1) transfusion of contaminated blood or blood products and (2) use of contaminated (dirty) needles and syringes.

Transfusion of contaminated blood or blood products. Prior to 1985, blood and blood products were not screened for HIV. This led to the infection of some 10,000 persons with hemophilia in the United States, in addition to hundreds infected by HIV through blood transfusion. In 1985, the U.S. blood industry implemented serological screening of HIV, excluding blood donors assessed to have engaged in risky drug or sex behaviors or who were HIV positive, endorsing the use of autologous transfusion (patient banks his or her own blood for future personal use), and heat treatment of blood products used by hemophiliacs and persons with other hereditary bleeding disorders. The U.S. blood supply and blood-screening protocols are now generally considered quite safe. The American Red Cross has repeatedly emphasized that blood donors cannot become HIV-infected. It is important to note that blood-screening programs are not consistently available or used throughout industrial or developing countries in the world (Lloyd, 1995).

Use of contaminated (dirty) needles and syringes. Transmission of HIV can also occur when dirty or unsterile instruments are use for skin puncture (e.g., tattooing), injection, drawing blood, or ceremonial genital mutilation or scarring. In the United States, injection drug use (IDU) of heroin, cocaine, amphetamines, and steroids is the most common risk behavior related to blood transmission of HIV, and the second highest risk factor for overall HIV infection. Most HIV infection among women is a direct result of sex with partners who are HIV-infected injection drug users (Peterson, 1995). The primary transmission of HIV through the use of unsterile needles and syringes is through the exchange of blood that remains in the syringe or needle and is transferred from one person to another (Gant, 1995).

Communitywide initiatives such as needle-exchange programs and "bleach and teach" projects that teach IDUs correct ways to clean and sterilize needles, syringes, and their "works" (cookers, cotton balls, etc.) have demonstrated success in reducing HIV infection among heroin-using IDU (Gant, 1995; Lloyd, 1995). Needle-exchange programs and other community initiatives are more effective when integrated within continuums of care that provide drug treatment, health care, and HIV-related pre- and posttest counseling (Newmeyer, 1994).

Mother-to-Child Transmission

Fifteen years of epidemiological data and studies indicate that there is *about a 25 percent chance that a child born to an HIV-infected mother will be infected* (Lloyd, 1995; Dabis et al, 1993, Newell and Peckham, 1993). It is estimated that about half of HIV-infected infants will develop severe illnesses during the first year of life. Infected infants surviving the first year will be at risk for AIDS or AIDS-related illnesses for the rest of their lives.

This mode of HIV transmission brings together a source of HIV (in the bloodstream of an HIV-infected woman), a potential target (bloodstream of a developing fetus), and a protected environment (mother's body). Typically, maternal and fetal blood systems are separated by the placenta, which prevents the exchange of blood cells but not nutrients. During the final trimester of pregnancy, small tears can sometimes occur in the placenta, and this can lead to the entry of blood cells from the mother's bloodstream to the fetus's bloodstream. In addition, during the birth process, the child often comes into close contact with the mother's blood due to the bleeding that accompanies delivery.

Detecting HIV in infants is difficult because infants can continue to express maternal antibodies for up to two years. Such infants may receive a diagnosis of "Indeterminate HIV." Recent detection advancements such as PCR (polymerase chain reaction) that test for HIV DNA in infected cells allow for immediate assessment of neonates. The availability of such tests, however, is limited and expensive.

For some HIV-infected women, pregnancy may accelerate the progression of HIV infection to AIDS, and may increase the likelihood of miscarriage or stillbirth. HIV has been found in breast milk, and there are reports of infant HIV infection through breast-feeding (Van De Perre et al., 1991). Because the risk of HIV transmission through breast-feeding depends on many factors (e.g., long-standing vs. newly acquired infection), the infection rates are quite variable. The most currently accepted range of infection rates for babies with infected mothers through breast feedings is between 14 to 25 percent (Newell and Peckham, 1993) *over and above transmission in utero or during delivery.*

The 076 controversy and mandatory mother and infant screening. The results of the 076 AIDS clinical trial group unleashed a heated exchange between and within the public health, medical, and service provision communities. One of the first trials to study the impact of retrovirals on women of childbearing age, this study (1) corroborated the finding of HIV infection in 25 percent of babies born to mothers with HIV, and (2) showed that pregnant women who took AZT reduced the chances of transmitting HIV to their infants from 25 percent to 8 percent.

These findings were used as the rationale for city, state, and national mandatory HIV tests for both all pregnant women and all babies born in the United States. A storm of controversy ensued, as many argued that this public health decision severely compromised the rights to privacy of mothers. Further, many local reports documented increasing numbers of women refusing to seek prenatal care, of abortion rates, and of women delivering babies outside hospital settings. In the summer of 1995, the Centers for Disease Control requested that Congress halt the ten million dollar newborn HIV survey, claiming it was time to determine whether or not the funds could be better spent. The CDC declared the newborn testing unnecessary and instead requested that pregnant mothers continue to be voluntarily tested for HIV.

Patterns of HIV Transmission: Initial and Contemporary Global Geographies of HIV/AIDS

While the three modes of HIV transmission are basically the same around the world, personal and social risk factors in different countries have influenced both the frequency and manifestations of these modes of transmission. Until 1990, worldwide patterns of HIV transmission were clustered into three general but useful patterns of HIV infection (Patterns I, II, and III). While the presentation of these patterns persists in contemporary HIV/AIDS education and information, inherent limitations have prompted others such as Jonathan Mann to articulate a new model of worldwide HIV/AIDS transmission—that is, a new global geography of HIV/AIDS.

Initial Global Geography of HIV/AIDS: Patterns I, II, and III

In Pattern I areas, HIV began its spread during the mid- to late 1970s. The sexual transmission of HIV occurred first and primarily among homosexual and bisexual men; heterosexual transmission also occurred and was rapidly increasing. Blood transmission of HIV primarily involved persons with injection drug behavior, and secondarily those who had undergone a blood transfusion and those with hereditary bleeding disorders who had received blood products. Perinatal transmission was initially uncommon (as few women had been infected) but has increased as heterosexual transmission increased. *Pattern I areas include the United States, Canada, Western Europe, urban Latin America, Australia, and New Zealand.*

In Pattern II areas, HIV also began spreading during the mid to late 1970s. In these areas, however, sexual transmission was primarily heterosexual. Blood transmission of HIV frequently occurred at the many places where HIV screening of blood was not routine. While injection drug use was rare in these areas, the use of dirty, unsterile needles, syringes, and other skin-piercing instruments substantially contributed to the spread of HIV. Perinatal transmission of HIV was and continues to be a major problem in these areas. *Pattern II areas include sub-Saharan Africa, rural Latin America, and the Caribbean.*

In Pattern III areas, HIV began an extensive spread during the 1980s. While early AIDS cases were generally associated with contact with Pattern I and II areas or via imported blood or blood products, indigenous transmission began to occur via sexual transmission (commercial sex workers) and blood transmission (drug injection behavior). *Pattern III areas include Eastern Europe, countries of the former Soviet Union, the Middle East, North Africa, and most Asian Pacific Rim countries.*

Strengths and limitations of the initial geographic model. The simplicity and general utility of the three-pattern model make this model an attractive framework for use by HIV/AIDS trainers and educators. Indeed, it is quite common to see this model presented in contemporary "AIDS 101" classes in college, community, and professional settings.

However, it is also important to understand that the patterns are neither immutable nor inviolable. HIV epidemiology is rapidly changing. For instance, the predominance of gay males and bisexuals among HIV-infected persons in the Caribbean in the early 1980s (typical of Pattern I) was followed by a shift toward heterosexual transmission (typical of Pattern II). Countries such as Thailand are recording increased heterosexual transmissions (characteristics of Pattern II), and in the United States, HIV infection is rapidly increasing among women via sexual transmission (typical of Pattern II).

Given the unstable and volatile nature of the HIV/AIDS pandemic, other researchers have concluded that the three-pattern model of HIV/AIDS transmission is easier to understand, but is essentially simplistic, does not reflect current and changing trends and rates of transmission, and is therefore of limited use in future years. Frustrations with the limitations of the three-pattern model led to the development of ten Geographic Areas of Affinity (GAA). While this model has been slow to gain acceptance in the United States, other industrialized nations generally accept and recognize the GAA model as an appropriate new global geography of HIV/AIDS (Mann, Tarantola, and Netter, 1992).

Geographic Areas of Affinity (GAA)—Contemporary Geographies of HIV/AIDS

Table 2 divides the world into ten GAAs. GAAs were identified by considering the following factors: (1) changing epidemiology of HIV/AIDS in each country, (2) operational and programmatic response to the pandemic, and (3) societal factors, e.g., societal vulnerability to future spread of HIV and other identified geographical realities. While this model is more comprehensive than the three-pattern model, problematic assumptions do exist. For instance, Japan is included with other Northeast Asian countries despite its low HIV prevalence, low rate of heterosexual transmission, and high economic development. All Latin American countries were grouped together in GAA 4 despite divergent trends in primary infection modes in Mexico, Brazil, Argentina, and Central American countries (WHO/PAHO, 1990). With the goal of better understanding local, national, and regional aspects of the pandemic, the GAA model is considered an encouraging but interim classification.

UNIVERSAL PRECAUTIONS

Since the normal course of social worker–client contact does not involve sexual or blood transmission activities, there is no risk of infection transmission for either person. Frankly, an HIV-infected client with a

TABLE 2. Indicators for Geographic Areas of Affinity (GAAs)

Factors	1 North America	2 Western Europe	3 Oceania	4 Latin America	5 Sub-Saharan Africa	6 Caribbean	7 Eastern Europe	8 Southeast Mediterranean	9 Northeast Asia	10 Southeast Asia
Epidemiological										
Year of HIV spread	1978	1978	1979	1978-79	1977-78	1979	1982-83	1982	1982-84	1983-84
Year first AIDS[a] case diagnosed	E80	E80	M80	E80	M80	E80	E80	L80	E80	M80
Availability of HIV/AIDS data	H	H	H	M	H	M	L	L	L	M
Major modes of HIV transmission:[b]										
blood/blood products	L	L	L	M	M/L	L	L	L	L	M
gay/bisexual men	M	M	M/H	M	L	L	H	L	L	L
injection drug use	H	H	L	M	L	M	M/L	M/H	M/H	H
heterosexual	M/L	M/L	L	M	H	H	L	L	M/L	M/H
Urban:rural ratio	3.2:1	5:1	7:1	4:1	1:1	1.5:1	10:1	5:1	5:1	2:1
Prevalence of HIV in general population[c]	.005-3.0	.007-2.8	.03-.2	.0007-.8	.9-7.3	.5-2.0	.0001-.003	.0001-.05	.0001-.002	.01-.29
Gender ratio (male:female) in populations infected with HIV	8:1	5:1	7:1	4:1	1:1	1.5:1	10:1	5:1	5:1	2:1
Operational/Programmatic										
Year of first national response[d]	82	86	84	86	86	87	89	87	86.5	87.5
Level of AIDS program financing	L	L	L	L	H	L	L	L	L	M/H

Societal										
Mean Human Development Index[e]	.98	.97	.97	.82	.26	.62	.90	.38	.83	.51
Mean total female score[f]	81.5	76.3	79.5	63.2	37.0	55.8	76.5	35.0	63.5	50.5
Mean Human Freedom Index[g]	H	H	H	M	M/L	M	L	L	L	M
Urban population annual growth rate (1990-2000)[h]	1.0	.6	1.0	2.5	5.3	2.5	1.4	3.9	4.0	4.1

Source: Mann, J., D.J.M. Tarantola, and T.W. Netter (Eds.). (1992). *AIDS in the world: The global AIDS policy coalition*. Cambridge, MA: Harvard University Press. Copyright © 1992 by the President and Fellows of Harvard College. Reprinted by permission of Harvard University Press.

[a]Because reporting of AIDS cases to the World Health Organization did not begin until 1985 and 1986, dates of diagnosis are approximate. E80=before 1985; M80=1985 to 1987; L80=after 1987.

[b]Estimated HIV prevalence rates in 1990 were obtained for each mode of transmission from a modified Delphi Survey.

[c]The rates represent a range for 1991 from the lowest estimates for rural areas to high estimates for urban areas.

[d]The year of first response to the AIDS epidemic reflects the first occurrence of two variables: the year of a national leader's address on AIDS or the year in which a national AIDS program was created.

[e]The Human Development Index (HDI) combines annual income per capita, life expectancy, adult literacy, and mean years of schooling. Scoring ranges from 0-1.00, with 1.00 being the highest HDI.

[f]The total female score combines several indicators to measure the overall condition of women in individual countries. Of the maximum score of 100, 75 points are based on women's status and 25 points reflect the gender gap.

[g]The Freedom Tax Index is comprised of forty separate indicators, including freedom from arbitrary rule, illegal arrest, and unwarranted attack on person or property; right to life, liberty, security, ethnic and gender equality, and role of law; freedom of assembly, movement, thought, religion, and speech; right to work, free choice of jobs, and adequate standard of living; right to participate in community life and organize opposition parties or trade union groups. 1=1-10; M=11-30; H=31-40.

[h]The annual urban population growth rate should be interpreted as a surrogate indicator for urban migration.

weakened or compromised immune system is at much greater risk for acquiring illnesses from the social worker, such as colds, flus, and other airborne illnesses and pathogens. Typically, therefore, social workers do not use universal precautions in their encounters with HIV-infected persons or clients.

There are approximately 5.3 million health care workers at 620,000 work sites in the United States who routinely come into contact with blood in their daily work, and therefore who are exposed to the possibility of HIV infection. There are another 700,000 workers who routinely come in contact with blood as part of their job (such as people in corrections, education, firefighting and rescue, law enforcement, lab research, and the funeral industry). As a routine course of their work, a substantial number of workers are exposed to HIV/AIDS. The risk of HIV infection due to exposure to contaminated blood is low, estimated at 1 in 200 (.005 percent). This probability, while low, still translates into a substantial number of possible infections (26,500 health care workers, and 3,500 other workers).

In response to the concerns about the risk of contracting HIV disease, two sets of infection-control procedures have been developed. The first set is referred to as universal precautions. The second set is called blood and body substance isolation (Stine, 1995, 1996).

Universal precautions (UP) refer to a set of infection-control practices (e.g., using protective eyewear, facemasks, gloves, and gowns) developed by the Centers for Disease Control and Prevention (CDC) between 1976 and 1991. UP were first recommended as barrier techniques for the prevention of hepatitis B infection (1976). The CDC's *Guidelines for Isolation Precautions in Hospitals* (1983) recommended specific practices to be used when a patient was either known or suspected to be infected with blood-borne pathogens. It was not until 1987 that these specific infection-control practices became known as UP. In 1987, the CDC published the *Recommendations for Prevention of HIV Transmission in Health-Care Settings*. Among the recommendations was one that all blood and body fluid precautions be followed for any and all patients regardless of their blood-borne infection status. This extension of precautions to all patients in all situations is referred to as universal precautions. In 1991, the CDC published another set of recommendations. These recommendations prevent the transmission of HIV and other blood-borne pathogens from infected workers to patients during routine procedures.

Workers observe these precautions on the job to protect themselves from infection or injury. These precautions and actions are called "universal" because they are used in all situations—even if there appears to be no risk involved. UP include the use of barrier protection such as gloves, gowns, masks, and eyewear and careful handling of needles and other sharp instruments. Under UP, blood and certain body fluids (such as semen and vaginal secretions[1]) are considered potentially infectious for HIV, hepatitis B and C viruses, and other blood-borne diseases.

Blood Body Substance Isolation (BBSI) is an alternative approach to the CDC's system of UP. BBSIs are frequently used in communities or areas with high HIV prevalence and incidence. The actual practices of BBSI and UP are very similar. Philosophically, BBSI and UP differ in the following ways:

- UP emphasizes avoiding blood-borne infection; BBSI requires barrier precautions for all body substances and "moist membranes" (such as mucous membranes and open wounds).
- UP reduces the risk of transmission of blood-borne pathogens; BBSI reduces the risk of all nosocomial pathogens.
- UP is used when exposure to identified blood and body fluids is anticipated; BSSI is used for any anticipated contact with blood, body fluids, mucous membranes, nonintact skin (cuts, laceration, abrasions), and moist body substances.
- UP is used with any routine procedure; BBSI use is based on the degree of contact with the blood, body fluids, or tissues of each patient that a specific procedure requires; under BBSI, there are procedures that require minimal to no barrier use.

COURSE OF ILLNESS AND GENERAL TREATMENT ISSUES

Course of Illness

Primary Infection Phase

During the phase of primary infection, only extremely sophisticated tests[2] can detect its presence for the first two to four weeks. At this time, white blood cell counts decrease dramatically, and flulike symptoms (fever, nausea, sweats) occur. The immune system manifests a response to HIV, trapping HIV in lymph nodes and lymphatic tissue. The illness symptoms dissipate, prompting many individuals to believe the illness has passed. In fact, this is the beginning of clinical latency; the person feels stronger, and the immune system continues to eliminate HIV in the bloodstream. During this clinical latency phase, the infected person's system begins producing antibodies to HIV, which blood tests, such as ELISA and the Western blot, can detect.

Clinical Latency Phase

During the clinical latency phase (approximately two weeks to six months postinfection), the amount of HIV in the bloodstream drops to nearly zero. However, undetected HIV in the lymph nodes continues to replicate at extremely rapid rates.

HIV Asymptomatic Phase

During the asymptomatic phase (two to seven years postinfection), HIV disrupts the immune system and the antibody cell count slowly declines. As the cell-mediated response weakens, HIV eventually migrates from lymph nodes through the bloodstream. Eventually, the virus attacks vital organs and the brain.

HIV Symptomatic Phase

In the symptomatic phase (eight to ten years postinfection), HIV replication is extremely rapid and may lead HIV to mutate into different and more powerful strains. Early warning signs of disease progression develop, such as night sweats, weight loss, skin rashes, persistent fevers, diarrhea, fatigue, or oral thrush. In the end-stage phase, lymph nodes collapse and the immune system loses the ability to regenerate. Cell counts diminish rapidly. Opportunistic infections, such as lymphoma, Kaposi's sarcoma, and invasive cervical cancer (among women) occur.

AIDS Diagnosis

During the HIV symptomatic phase, a cell count of less than 200 (cells per cubic millimeter of blood) or the presence of one or more of twenty-three AIDS-defining illnesses result in a person's medical diagnosis of AIDS. Once diagnosed with AIDS, death usually occurs in one to two years; infants usually die more rapidly. Approximately 90 percent of those infected with HIV will progress to AIDS; currently, AIDS is always fatal.

Social workers should understand that the progression of HIV to AIDS reflects the natural history of AIDS as identified by collective observations of many HIV-infected persons over a fifteen-year period. It is not uncommon for individuals to progress at different rates. Social workers should also understand that most of the natural history information about HIV/AIDS has been taken from infected men. There is comparatively little information about the natural history of AIDS among women. In fact, it was not until 1995 that the first national natural history study of AIDS among women was initiated (Thornton, 1996).

About 13 percent of persons infected with HIV will be long-term survivors, remaining free of disease for more than twenty years. "Long-term survivors" are operationally defined as people having gradually declining immune markers and no use of antiretrovirals such as AZT. This group should be distinguished from a smaller (6 percent) group of people identified as "chronic nonprogressors," operationally defined as those who are HIV positive, having stable immune markers, with no progression from early to end-stage HIV. While research is currently underway to understand precisely what makes these individuals "long-term survivors" and "chronic nonprogressors," there is currently no definitive knowledge or information to that end.

General Treatment Issues

Currently, there is neither a vaccine to prevent HIV infection nor is there a cure for HIV. The current treatment regimen consists of combination therapies of antivirals (such as AZT, ddI, ddC, 3TC) and protease inhibitors with drugs to treat and prevent opportunistic infections (such as pentamidine for PCP, ganciclovir for cytomegalovirus, and acyclovir for herpes simplex virus). Early in the epidemic, single antiviral therapy (e.g., AZT) was prescribed; now combinations of antivirals are most commonly prescribed. However, costs for combination therapies are expensive, ranging from $12,000 to $18,000.

Increasingly, HIV-infected persons are incorporating alternative and complementary medications and therapies with their medical regimen. Such alternative approaches include dietary regimens; goldenseal and echinacea, which purportedly enhance immune function; therapeutic massage, which is claimed to modestly increase white cell replication; and acupuncture or accupressure for pain management. While claims of effectiveness are disputed, increasing numbers of physicians urge the study of these treatments, and the recently established (1993) Institute for Alternative Medicine in the National Institute of Health routinely receives far more research proposals than can be possibly funded.

LEGAL AND CIVIL RIGHTS OF PEOPLE WITH HIV, INCLUDING RELEVANCE OF THE AMERICANS WITH DISABILITIES ACT

With the exception of The Americans with Disabilities Act of 1990, most of the legal and legislative activities concerning HIV/AIDS has been generated at the state level. Since 1990, over two hundred bills have been enacted upon HIV/AIDS issues such as testing, confidentiality, housing availability and discrimination, imprisonment, counseling, and medication programs (Stine, 1995; Rothstein, 1989; Gostin, 1990a,b).

HIV/AIDS law changes rapidly and unexpectedly. Currently, the most updated resource regarding legal issues and legal resources for PLWA (persons living with AIDS) is provided in *The Directory of Legal Resources for People with AIDS and HIV* (1993), a 368-page reference published by the American Bar Association's AIDS Coordination Project. For information on the AIDS Coordination Project or to obtain copies of the directory, contact the ABA AIDS Coordination Project, 1800 M. Street N.W., Washington, DC 20036, (202) 331-2248.

The Americans with Disabilities Act of 1990

The Americans with Disabilities Act of 1990 (ADA) is recognized by some as the most comprehensive piece of civil rights legislation since 1964. Basically, the ADA provides legal protection for persons with disabilities—including persons with HIV/AIDS—in the workplace, public accommodations (e.g., hotels, hospitals, doctors' offices), and state and local government programs. The goal of ADA is to remove barriers to work, travel, shopping, and entertainment for forty-three million disabled persons in the United States.

Implemented in four phases (January 1992, July 1992, July 1993, and July 1995), the ADA will apply to all employers with at least fifteen employees and will apply to over five million public facilities in the United States.

While the ADA is not a legal panacea for PLWA, it has provided an important "legal net" of support for PLWA in at least three critical ways: (1) HIV and AIDS are included as handicaps covered by ADA; (2) the ADA provides specific examples of "reasonable accommodation"; and (3) except for drug testing, the ADA will prohibit employers from using preemployment medical exams as screening devices

Other Legal Issues

Generally speaking, many scholars view the current status of HIV/AIDS law with mixed feelings. On one hand, states have worked hard to generate legal protections for PLWA from stigma and irrational discrimination and prejudice. Many states accept research that demonstrates the effectiveness of targeted counseling and education strategies. Many states provide legal guarantees of antidiscrimination, confidentiality, and equal treatment under the law.

However, many state laws reflect the moral view that people who become infected with HIV as a result of risky sex and drug practices are immoral, deviant, and corrupt (Stine, 1995; Conrad and Schneider, 1992). By focusing on minimizing or eliminating recreational drug use and extra-marital sex behavior, legislators ignore the reality that these behaviors have persisted throughout recorded history.

Legislators may succumb to the pressures to exercise coercive and punitive state powers to respond to HIV/AIDS. Despite the evidence to the contrary (National Research Council, 1993), legislation for mandatory screening, quarantine, and criminalization inexorably continues. Gerald Stine has observed that "[t]he use of coercive powers, far from impeding the epidemic, may well fuel it" (1995, p. 342).

CONFIDENTIALITY ISSUES FOR SOCIAL WORKERS

HIV/AIDS raises many ethical issues for social workers, including how ethical codes, moral obligations, and legal duties affect worker responsi-bility to treat patients who pose a risk of transmitting a potentially lethal infection. For social workers, the issue of confidentiality versus the obligation to inform and protect third parties is particularly important.

While the ethics of a "duty to warn" have been determined for physi-cians, other health care personnel, and psychologists (Reamer, 1991; Lloyd, 1995), the extent to which social workers have an ethical "duty to warn" and inform partners when the infected person refuses to do so has not been determined. While the *Tarasoff v. Regents of the University of California* (1976) decision has been used to delimit confidentiality and duty to warn for other professions, neither the *Tarasoff* nor social work code of ethics can be used to establish clear guidelines for breaching confidentiality and invoking a duty to warn.

One of the principal dilemmas is the comparison between the threat infecting an unnamed person at an unspecified future time and the threat-ened act of violence against a specific person. Some theorists believe the threat to another person, identified or not, is sufficient grounds for invok-ing *Tarasoff* as a precedent while others strongly disagree with this analy-sis (Reamer, 1991, 1996; Lloyd, 1995). Ultimately, guidelines will likely be established in the courts. Until that time occurs, *social workers are strongly urged to familiarize themselves with city and state duty to warn legislation, and urge their employers and state social work associations to review these issues with HIV/AIDS legal advocacy offices in their locali-*

ties, cities, and communities. Social workers may also contact the ABA AIDS Coordination project mentioned previously.

CONCLUSION

Paraphrasing Harvey Gochros, "HIV/AIDS continues to be quintessential social work" (1992). As other chronic health issues such as venereal disease and polio partially defined a generation and its human service responses, so HIV/AIDS does in the 1980s and 1990s. No one knows when the pandemic of HIV/AIDS will end although Fan, Conner, and Villarreal (1994) offer the cautious optimism that "time is on our side." In the meantime, millions will die and millions more will be affected for decades to come.

HIV/AIDS will dominate the lives of many populations served by social workers. The profession of social work may well be judged by future generations in part by its collective response to the pandemic. Whether or not social workers and the profession realize it, the professional legacy is being written as social workers currently respond to the pandemic. It remains to be seen whether the profession responds to the suffering and death of millions with a legacy of benign diffidence and ambivalence, or one of advocacy; effective leadership in policy, practice, and research; and community empowerment.

NOTES

1. Blood, semen, vaginal secretions, and any fluids containing visible blood have been shown to transmit HIV. Other fluids such as cerebrospinal, amniotic, synovial, pleural, peritoneal, and pericardial fluids have a theoretical risk (Stine, 1995).

2. These techniques include polymerase chain reaction (PCR), brand DNA (bDNA), immunofolescent antibody assays, latex agglutination tests, and passive hemaglutination assays. See Stine (1996) for extended discussion of these and other techniques.

REFERENCES

American Bar Association AIDS Coordination Project (1993). *The directory of legal resources for people with AIDS and HIV.* Washington, DC: American Bar Association.

Blake, D. (1993). AIDS: Epidemiology and the international response. *Tropical Medicine and Parasitology 44:* 130-134.

Centers for Disease Control (1983) *Guidelines for isolation precautions in hospitals.* Atlanta, GA: U.S. Dept. of Health and Human Services, Public Health Service, Centers for Disease Control, Office of the Deputy Director (HIV).

Centers for Disease Control (1987). *Recommendations for prevention of HIV transmission in health-care settings.* Atlanta, GA: U.S. Dept. of Health and Human Services, Public Health Service, Centers for Disease Control, Office of the Deputy Director (HIV).

Centers for Disease Control (1995). *Facts about HIV Type 2.* Atlanta: Author.

Conrad, P., and Schneider, J. (1992). *Deviance and medicalization: From badness to sickness,* expanded edition. Philadelphia: Temple University Press.

Dabis, F., Msellati, P., Dunn, D., Lepage, P., Newell, M.L., Peckham, C., Van De Perre, P., and the Working Group on Mother-to-child transmission of HIV (1993). "Estimating the rate of mother-to-child transmission of HIV." Report of a workshop on methodological issues in Ghent (Belgium, February 17-20, 1992). *AIDS 7:* 279-280.

Elgin, S.H. (1994). *Staying well with the gentle art of verbal self-defense.* Englewood Cliffs, NJ: Prentice-Hall.

Fan, H., Conner, R., and Villarreal, L. (1994). *The biology of AIDS,* third edition. Boston: Jones and Bartlett.

Gant, L.M. (1995). HIV/AIDS: Men. In *Encyclopedia of social work,* nineteenth edition (pp. 1306-1314). Washington, DC: NASW Press.

Gochros, H.L. (1992). The sexuality of gay men with HIV Infection. *Social Work 37*(2): 105-109.

Gostin, L.O. (1990a). The AIDS litigation project: A national review of court and human rights commission decisions. Part I: The social impact of AIDS. *Journal of the American Medical Association 263:* 1961-1970.

Gostin, L.O. (1990b). The AIDS litigation project. Part II: Discrimination. *Journal of the American Medical Association 263:* 2086-2093.

Lifson, A.R. (1992). Transmission of the human immunodeficiency virus. In V.T. Devita, S. Hellman, and S.A. Rosenberg (Eds.), *The global impact of AIDS* (pp. 183-190). New York: Alan R. Liss.

Lloyd, G. (1995). HIV/AIDS. In *Encyclopedia of social work* nineteenth edition. (pp. 1257-1283). Washington, DC: NASW Press.

Mann, J., Tarantola, D.J.M., and Netter, T.W. (Eds.) (1992). *AIDS in the world: The global AIDS policy coalition.* Cambridge, MA: Harvard University Press.

National Research Council (1993). *The social impact of AIDS in the United States.* Washington, DC: National Academy Press.

Newell, M.L., and Peckham, C. (1993). Risk factors for vertical transmission of HIV-1 and early markers of HIV-1 infection in children. *AIDS 92/93:* S91-S98.

Newmeyer, J. (1994, May 17). "HIV and drug users: Prevention on the cheap in San Francisco." Presentation at Wayne State University, Detroit, Michigan.

Peterson, K.J. (1995). HIV/AIDS: Women. In *Encyclopedia of social work* nineteenth edition. (pp. 1325-1330). Washington, DC: NASW Press.

Reamer, F. (1991). *AIDS and ethics.* New York: Columbia University Press.

Rothstein, M.A. (1989). Medical screening: AIDS, rights, and health care costs. *National Forum 99:* 7-10.

Stine, G.L. (1996). *Acquired immune deficiency syndrome: Biological, medical, social and legal issues* second edition. Englewood Cliffs, NJ: Prentice-Hall.

Stine, G. (1995). *AIDS Update: 1994-1995.* Englewood Cliffs, NJ: Prentice-Hall.

Tarasoff v. Regents of the University of California, *17 Cal. 3d 425, 551 P.2d 334, 131 Cal. Rptr 14 (1976).*

Thornton, R. L. (1996, April 26). "Living with AIDS." Presentation at the 1996 Michigan Conference on AIDS, Ypsilanti, Michigan.

Van De Perre, P., Simonon, A., Msellati, P., Hitamana, D.G., Vaira, D., Bazuba-gira, A., Van Gosthem, C., Stevens, A.M., Karita, E., Sonday-Thull, D., Dabis, F., and Lepage, P. (1991). Postnatal transmission of human immunodeficiency virus type I from mother to infant. *New England Journal of Medicine 325*(9): 593-598.

World Health Organization, Global Programme on AIDS (WHO/GPA) (1990). *Guidelines for counseling people about human immunodeficiency virus (HIV).* Geneva: Author.

Appendix

A. Basic medical terminology. In learning medical jargon, Haden (in Elgin, 1994) proposes four questions for organizing information:

  a. Which body part is being referred to in the term or phrase?
  b. Where is it?
  c. What is wrong with it?
  d. What are the doctors proposing to do to it?

  a. Which body part is being referred to in the term or phrase?

HUMAN BODY

Extra Terms: Inside the Body

gastro	stomach
hepato	liver
nephro	kidney
spleen	spleen
cholcyst	gallbladder
enter, ili, ile	intestines
hyster	uterus
oophor	ovary
colpo	vagina
orchiio	testicle
cysto, vesic	bladder
procto	rectum/anus
colo	colon

Source: Based on Elgin, 1994, p. 205.

b. Where is it?

If the Problem is Located . . .	Look for this Prefix:
inside	endo, eso, intra
outside	ecto, exo
on, above, or over	epi, supra
under, below	infra, sub
between	inter
beside, around	para
behind	retro
away from	ab
near	ad
through, across	dia
beyond	meta
with, together	syn, sym, syl, sys
against	anti, contra

Source: Based on Elgin, 1994, pp. 204-208.

c. What is wrong with it?

It hurts.	algia, dynia
It's inflamed and/or infected.	itis
It's got a tumor, or swelling.	oma
It's hardening.	scler
It's bleeding or pouring out.	rhage, rhagia, rhea
It's growing, maybe too much.	plasia
It's developing wrong.	trophy
It's too (X).	hyper
It's not (X) enough.	hypo
It's not (X) at all, or without (X).	a, an, in
It's big.	macro, mega

It's small.	micro
It's bad or wrong.	mal
It's phony.	pseudo
It's fast.	tachy
It's slow.	brady
There's more than one of it, or a lot of it.	poly, multi
It's double.	ambi, amphi
There's only half of it, or only half is relevant.	hemi
It's changing.	meta
It's red.	eryth
It's white.	alb, leuko, leuco
It's blue.	cya
It's falling or drooping.	ptosis
It's difficult.	dys

Source: Based on Elgin, 1994, pp. 208-209.

d. What are the doctors proposing to do to it?

Remove it.	ectomy
Look inside it.	oscopy
Make an opening in it.	ostomy
Free it up.	lysis
Fuse it.	desis
Fix it, or sew it up.	pexy
Make it, or reconstruct it.	plasty

Source: Based on Elgin, 1994, pp. 209.

Getting Started:
Basic Skills for Effective
Social Work with People
with HIV and AIDS

Michael Shernoff

WHY DO THIS?
STATEMENT OF THE PROBLEM AND ISSUES

In the second decade of the AIDS epidemic, social workers in practice in large urban centers expect to encounter clients who either have AIDS themselves or have a loved one or family member living with HIV/AIDS; thus, they have begun to develop the knowledge and skills necessary to work effectively with these populations. Even as the epidemic rages on and shows no indications of abating, some social workers believe there is no need to prepare themselves to work with clients whose lives have been impacted by HIV/AIDS. For workers in small cities away from the coasts, in rural areas, or in specialized settings (e.g., Christian counseling centers or agencies that serve Orthodox Jewish families), all too often the assumption has been the following: "AIDS is not a problem in this community so why should I learn about it?"

Current demographics demonstrate that even in rural areas without a well-defined gay or drug-using subculture, cases of AIDS are on the rise. Increasingly, people with AIDS (PWAs) are leaving the large urban centers where they have contracted the illness and are returning home to live out their final days with their families of origin. In *My Own Country* (1994) Abraham Verghese describes his experience providing primary medical care and becoming the local AIDS expert in a remote area of rural Tennessee. He is honest about how his own preconceptions of who his patients were going to be were quickly challenged by the variety of men and women who sought out his services.

AIDS WORK IS THE CUTTING EDGE
OF CONTEMPORARY PRACTICE

Ostrow and Wren (1991) state the following:

> Mental health care providers are increasingly instrumental in efforts to control the AIDS epidemic. AIDS is as much a behavioral as an infectious disease problem. This is evident by the manner of its transmission, its effects on the central nervous system, its stigmatic nature, and its often lethal outcome. Specialists in mental health care and behavioral change are indispensable in controlling the epidemic through education, prevention, treatment, and research. Mental health caregivers can help people overcome the biases that impede rational responses to the disease and fears that characterize the AIDS epidemic by providing compassionate care and by suggesting innovative methods of prevention and research.

Serving people with AIDS encompasses the traditional social work role of advocate for an underserved client population and poses professional challenges as well as satisfaction for all workers. If in-service training on working with PWA for agency or hospital staff has not occurred, then an excellent starting place is to locate an expert who can conduct an introductory training about AIDS for the staff—*even if no clients have presented with HIV or AIDS issues.* If a social agency waits until it is faced with its first client with HIV or AIDS to become familiar with the practical and psychosocial issues relevant to providing good quality care, it has waited too long, and the services to the client will suffer out of ignorance or fear. Therefore, all social workers need to arm themselves with the basic knowledge about assessing risk behavior, finding local resources, and honing appropriate intervention skills in order to be prepared to best serve the vulnerable client. Such a client will surely not be in any condition to educate the worker; however, clients with HIV and AIDS frequently do educate social workers, physicians, and other health care professionals.

This chapter serves as an introductory overview to direct social work practice with people affected by HIV and AIDS. Mental health and casework issues for both the individual who is infected or ill, as well as his or her loved ones will be discussed. I begin by addressing how to integrate HIV risk assessment and prevention into routine interviews with a variety of clients of all sexual orientations and drug-using statuses. Next, the issues involved with helping clients decide whether or not to be tested for HIV and what social workers need to know to be prepared for working with HIV-positive clients is discussed. I then address how workers can be helpful to people actually living with AIDS. The chapter concludes with a detailed discussion of counseling end-stage AIDS patients, their families, and other loved ones as death approaches. While this chapter is intended to be instructive and stand on its own, like all of the other chapters in this book, it can best be complemented by your attending training sessions about HIV and AIDS.

ASSESSING CLIENTS' RISKS OF EXPOSURE TO HIV

Before the development in 1985 of an accurate test to determine the presence of HIV in blood products, people who received transfusions or clotting factors were at risk of contracting HIV through blood they were given. Currently, the vast majority of new HIV infections occur either through sexual exposure or sharing intravenous-drug-using apparatus. In attempting to assess whether a client is at risk for AIDS, a social worker must ascertain both the client's current sexual practices as well as what they were in past. Simply asking "Are you gay?" is not sufficient. Health care professionals cannot assume that a client who is not openly gay has not engaged in sex with other men. Once a man labels himself as gay, this is a good indication that his identity is largely affiliated with his preference for loving men, having male sexual partners, and making choices in his life in order to integrate these desires with a satisfying emotional and social life. Some men who regularly engage in sex with other men never think of themselves as gay or even as homosexual, and they never seek to affiliate with the gay community.

The distinction between men who simply have sex with other men and men who have a gay identity is especially relevant when working with nonwhite and/or non-middle-class men. For example, contemporary African-American culture widely condemns homosexuality, and homosexual identification is widely denied, even though male-male sex is widely practiced. According to a recent survey of 65,000 HIV-positive men, blacks are twice as likely as whites to practice bisexuality, and among black drug users, many of whom turn to prostitution to support their habit, the incidence of bisexuality is four times as high as reported in non–African Americans (Cargill, 1995). Some men who actively engage in sex with other men do not view themselves as homosexual or gay because they are doing the penetrating. For example, a married man with numerous symptoms of progressive HIV infection who had never received a transfusion or blood products, who reported no history of shared needle use or other risk factors for exposure to HIV, and who stated he was definitely not gay, baffled his physician. However, when the man was questioned in an extremely nonjudgmental way by a social worker as to whether he had ever had sex with other men, the client readily stated that he had a long history of sexual activity with men.

In attempting to do a risk assessment for high-risk behavior, the social worker needs to ask questions regarding drug use and sexual practices in an accepting, nonjudgmental, matter-of-fact, gentle way that does not incorporate the use of labels. Springer (1991) suggests that in order to be able to engage chemically dependent individuals in AIDS prevention and treatment, social workers need to learn how to talk to drug users honestly and completely about their drug use. Some examples of these questions are as follows:

- "Have you ever used drugs, and if so, which ones, and how have you taken them?"
- "As an adult have you ever had any sexual contact with another man?" If the answer is "Yes," then ask, "When was the last time?" or "Could you tell me exactly what you did?"

The answers to these questions can provide useful and pertinent information about the client's risk potential. Prior to initiating these discussions, the social worker must offer assurances and guarantees about the confidentiality of the information being elicited. Consistent with social work ethics, workers in all settings must be extra vigilant not to gossip about their clients, who may also be their neighbors. In addition, social workers can reduce their discomfort about asking questions about sexuality and drug use by routinely incorporating them into initial interviews with all clients.

EXAMPLES OF HOW THE ISSUE MAY PRESENT

Social workers working with people who do not self-identify as gay or bisexual, or who report no history of drug use may assume that their clients are not at risk for becoming infected with HIV. It is true that sexually exclusive monogamy will protect people from HIV infection if both partners are already HIV negative. However, the research of Kinsey, Pomeroy, and Martin (1948) and Hunt (1974) suggests that more than 50 percent of heterosexual couples in the United States have more than one sexual partner during the course of their marriage. Even couples who are currently sexually exclusive are not protected from the consequences of risk behaviors in which they or their partner may have engaged prior to their relationship.

Regardless of sexual orientation, people cannot be absolutely certain about the drug use or sexual history of their sexual partners. Because the time from initial infection until the appearance of first symptoms is usually several years, people may unknowingly transmit or expose themselves to HIV, while erroneously believing that they are not at risk because they are currently in a stable, exclusive relationship. In interpreting data from the studies of Kinsey, Pomeroy, and Martin (1948) and Hunt (1974), Hyde (1982) found that only 2 percent of American men are behaviorally exclusively homosexual during their lifetime and that 25 percent are behaviorally bisexual at some point. These data suggest that the majority of U.S. men who are or have been homosexually active may not identify themselves as gay. Many of these men remain in heterosexual marriages, possibly hiding their homosexuality from their wives. Thus, many women falsely assume that they are safe from the risk of contracting AIDS.

AIDS WITHIN HETEROSEXUAL MARRIAGE

Social workers need to be aware of a variety of cultural or dynamic situations that contribute to the likelihood of heterosexually married individuals presenting as HIV positive or with symptoms of AIDS. Societal homophobia powerfully influences many men of diverse ethnicities to hide their homosexual activity within a heterosexual marriage. A husband's or wife's past or current drug use also places unsuspecting spouses at risk for HIV or AIDS. The following cases illustrate a variety of ways that social workers may encounter this facet of AIDS.

A woman client learned in one day that her husband of fifteen years had AIDS, that her marriage had not been a sexually exclusive relationship, and that her husband's relationships outside of the marriage had been with men. The crisis was compounded by the need to decide what to tell their fourteen-year-old son regarding his father's illness and the worry that she herself might have been exposed to HIV.

A social worker runs a group for nondrug-using Latina women with AIDS, all of whom were monogamous but were infected by their husbands who had either contracted HIV from drug use or sexual liaisons outside of the marriage. Issues of betrayal and rage are paramount for these women along with adjusting to living with a life-threatening illness and the stigma of having AIDS within their community.

Social workers on staff at prenatal clinics daily counsel monogamous, heterosexually married, pregnant women who discover that they have been infected with HIV by their husbands.

Two days a week, a social worker sees clients in his private practice in Borough Park, Brooklyn. All the clients are ultraorthodox Jewish Hasidic men who have sought out counseling because they identify as gay and regularly have sex with other men. Each of the men is either already engaged or married to a woman.

AIDS PREVENTION: DRUG USE

Newmeyer (1989) notes that use of alcohol and illegal substances increases a person's vulnerability to HIV in three ways.

1. A person who shares hypodermic needles or other drug paraphernalia—such as "cookers" (the container in which the drug is dissolved in water) or "cotton" (the material used to strain the drug solution as it is drawn up into the syringe)—with someone infected with HIV is at risk of becoming infected.
2. A person who becomes intoxicated or high may lose inhibitions against risky practices, e.g., neglecting the use of a condom during a drunken or stoned sexual encounter.
3. A number of substances, such as alcohol, cannabis, amphetamines, inhaled nitrates, and cocaine, may suppress one's immune system. Heavy use of an immunosuppressive substance by HIV-infected individuals can accelerate the collapse of "helper" T-cell activity.

In describing the "harm reduction" model of working with drug users, Springer (1991) suggests that placing abstinence from drugs as the highest treatment priority unless the client is truly committed to achieving abstinence will only alienate the client or cause him or her to begin a dishonest relationship with the social worker. Thus, social workers attempting to engage chemically dependent clients in treatment must not confuse the goals of providing AIDS education and risk reduction with the goals of helping clients stop using drugs. One way of helping clients accomplish this is by clearly counseling them as follows:

- If you do not want to contract AIDS, the best way to avoid it is by not using drugs. I can refer you to an agency or program that can help you to stop using drugs.
- If you must use drugs, do not share paraphernalia such as needles or cookers. Remember that people can look healthy and still carry the AIDS virus.
- If you must share paraphernalia, flush the needle, syringe, and cooker with bleach, and rinse well with water—or boil for fifteen minutes.

- To reduce the risk of contracting AIDS through sexual contact, use condoms, avoid contact with semen or blood, and learn safe sexual practices.

Taking such an approach in sessions with actively drug-using clients does not condone drug use, but it does acknowledge the reality that people who still actively use drugs are in desperate need of AIDS education services so as not to transmit HIV to drug-using or sexual partners or their children.

SEXUAL PRACTICES

Unfortunately, the vast majority of social workers complete their graduate education and even postgraduate training with little or no education in how to talk with clients about sex and sexuality, and no training in how to take a sexual history. Discussing sexual issues can cause discomfort even for the most sophisticated worker. This is especially true if the discussion involves sexual practices that the clinician believes are immoral, distasteful, repugnant, or representative of a lifestyle or behavior with which the clinician is totally unfamiliar. The potential for countertransferential blunders is enormous when clients disclose marital infidelities or exotic or nonconformist sexual practices or beliefs.

I believe that it is the moral and ethical responsibility of every clinical social worker to introduce the issue of sexual practices in relation to AIDS prevention with each individual:

- who is already sexually active;
- who is contemplating becoming sexually active;
- who is not absolutely certain that he or she has been in a sexually exclusive relationship for at least the past ten to fifteen years; or
- who is not absolutely certain that his or her partner has not used drugs intravenously or been the recipient of whole blood or blood products prior to the screening of the blood supply in 1985.

Some salient points to consider are as follows:

- The highest risk of contracting HIV involves exposure to blood that is already infected. Thus, sharing drug-injecting paraphernalia or engaging in unprotected sex that results in exposure to blood or semen pose the highest risks.
- Unprotected anal sex is the next highest risk behavior, followed by unprotected vaginal sex.

- There is controversy about whether or not fellatio without a condom is high risk. There is a growing body of evidence that suggests it is at least a potentially risky behavior, though not as high risk as either unprotected anal or vaginal intercourse.

The ambiguity regarding the risks of unprotected fellatio is very hard for most gay male clients and others to deal with because they want definitive answers about what is risky and what is not. Many AIDS educators introduce the concept of a risk continuum from lowest risk (mutual masturbation without any penetration) to highest risk. In discussing the relative risks of various sexual acts with clients, social workers must be prepared to have clients get angry at them for not being able to provide definite "dos and don'ts."

HIV RISK REDUCTION AND SOCIAL WORK PRACTICE WITH DIVERSE CLIENTS

Social workers who see adolescent individuals in sexually nonexclusive relationships; newly separated, divorced, or widowed adults; and any person contemplating having sex with a gay or bisexual man, current or former IV drug user, or transfusion recipient needs to learn about safer sexual practices. The current epidemics of all sexually transmitted diseases, including but not limited to hepatitis, herpes, AIDS, and treatment-resistant gonorrhea, has made it appropriate, and in fact, essential for clinical social workers to ask clients effective questions about sexual practices. Some key questions to ask clients are as follows:

- How did you feel when you first heard that you might have to change your sexual behaviors in order not to contract AIDS or other sexually transmitted diseases?
- How do you feel about the fact that AIDS is sexually transmitted?
- Are you concerned about the possibility of contracting HIV?
- When you think about safer sex, what thoughts and feelings do you have?
- What is your definition of safer sex?
- What are you doing to protect yourself and your sexual partners from AIDS?

SAFER SEX COUNSELING IN PRACTICE

Social workers should have understandable concerns about introducing these topics. The issue of whether sexual content becomes experienced as overstimulating or "inappropriately eroticized" must be assessed on a case-by-case basis. Understandably, many clients do not feel comfortable discussing sexual practices and may feel intruded upon or angered by explorations of these issues. However questions concerning sexual behavior outside of marriage or the client's sexuality may raise profound feelings of relief as well as anger.

Anger may occur because any discussion of AIDS shatters the client's ability to deny that the disease can affect him or her. The anger may also reflect how vulnerable and powerless the client feels in seeking social services, and in addition may be a defense in response to having been treated in insensitive or even humiliating ways in prior interactions with social service agencies or workers. If the client's expressions of anger are encouraged, explored, and not judged by the worker, a climate of increased trust and safety often develops between the client and social worker, thus allowing further discussions of highly charged issues. Once clients realize that the social worker welcomes and encourages expressions of all feelings, including negative ones about him or her, clients often express relief that they have a venue for safely discussing such personal and highly charged issues.

It is natural and appropriate for a client to test a worker's responses by gauging how he or she responds when attacked or criticized. Frequently, I have had clients tell me that they would never have felt safe enough to open up and share vulnerable personal issues with me if I had not previously handled their expressed anger or disappointment in a manner with which the client was comfortable.

HIV TESTING

The social worker needs to know where anonymous and confidential HIV testing is available in his or her community in order to make a referral when appropriate. One of the most commonly endorsed protections against HIV-related discrimination is the use of anonymous testing (Marks and Goldblum, 1989). Since even in the second decade of AIDS considerable stigma is attached to an HIV-positive diagnosis, the client needs and deserves assurances of the confidentiality of his or her test results. It is also useful to have developed a relationship with a specific individual at the test site to whom you can refer a client with confidence. Another excellent idea is to know about any existing AIDS service organization and other local HIV/AIDS resources in the community, and which physicians, hospitals, and medical centers are most experienced in treating people with

HIV/AIDS. Social workers should also educate themselves about the stages of the illness and how its progression may present.

Being informed about the disease is especially important in regard to the neuropsychiatric manifestations of the illness since bizarre or non-cooperative responses from clients in the advanced stages of AIDS may be misinterpreted as resistance or hostility as opposed to a symptom of disease-related organicity. If one is going to be working with clients who have HIV or AIDS, it is essential to have a close working relationship with a psychiatrist/psychopharmacologist who is experienced in diagnosing and treating AIDS-related dementia.

There are a number of situations in which a social worker clearly needs to raise the issue of a client's being tested for HIV.

- The client mentions that he or she has recently had or feared he/she has had a sexually transmitted disease.
- A client shares that he or she has discovered that her/his husband/wife/partner has been sexually unfaithful.
- A client has been sexually assaulted or raped.
- A client's partner or spouse is a hemophiliac or has received a transfusion prior to the screening of the blood supply in 1985.
- A client reports high-risk sexual or drug-taking activities, such as sharing paraphernalia.

The worker must remember that no matter how appropriate it may be that the client be tested for HIV, the final decision about whether or not to be tested must always be the client's. Raising the issue of HIV testing will understandably raise the client's anxiety. Even when the client raises the issue of being tested, the worker must spend time exploring salient issues, including why he or she has decided to be tested at this time. If the client has not raised the issue of being tested for HIV it is crucial that the worker inquires how he or she feels about the issue having been raised. In this situation the worker must prepare him/herself for a variety of possible reactions by the client. Many clients react with shock and anger as this suggestion confronts any denial they might still have about possibly being at risk.

COUNSELING BEFORE AND AFTER THE HIV TEST

Each individual planning to take the HIV test needs to receive counseling pre- and posttest regardless of whether he or she tests negative or positive. After introducing the topic of being tested for HIV, but prior to actually taking the test, all clients need to explore the following issues:

- How do they feel they will handle learning that they are HIV positive or HIV negative?
- How will whatever the results are change their life?
- With whom do they want to share this information?
- How do they feel a positive test result will impact their relationships?

The period of time while one is waiting for test results is almost always one of heightened anxiety, which often includes somatic symptoms and sleeplessness. If a client is newly in recovery from alcohol or drug abuse, or in the midst of other interpersonal or intrapsychic crises, it is generally inadvisable to counsel him or her to take the test at that time. Positive test results can be emotionally devastating, sometimes resulting in a psychiatric decompensation or relapse into active use of alcohol or drugs. If a physician feels there are urgent medical reasons indicating HIV testing, then counseling needs to address this and support the medical advice. For individuals who are newly in recovery from chemical dependency, and for whom there is no medical urgency, but only a desire to learn their HIV status, it is advisable they wait until they have at least a year's sobriety to take the HIV test. Posttest counseling must include information on safer sex no matter what the results are, and referrals to medical and mental health services if the client tests positive.

Once a client has learned that he or she has been exposed to HIV, the social worker has a number of crucial tasks in order to help him or her adjust to living with a life-threatening illness. First and foremost, the worker needs to become well-educated about HIV disease and AIDS. The worker should establish a relationship with a knowledgeable medical professional who can explain various symptoms, treatments, and options to the worker so that the client is not spending his or her time educating the worker about the medical issues of the illness. Although AIDS is almost always a terminal illness, it is most often premature for clients to begin preparing for death upon learning that they have just tested positive. Clients need to hear that there is usually a period that increasingly lasts up to ten or more years where people remain asymptomatic and are only HIV positive. (People have full-blown AIDS when their CD-4 cells fall below the 200 mark or they come down with one of the AIDS-related opportunistic infections.) Only when other serological tests indicate that the immune system is severely damaged or the client is seriously ill with one of the major AIDS-related opportunistic infections may the client simultaneously be learning that he or she has been exposed to HIV and is at risk of dying from a serious AIDS-related complication.

Research has demonstrated that women with full-blown AIDS die quicker than men with AIDS (Kolata, 1987). One reason for this is that inner-city people do not generally have a primary care physician, and usually do not go to clinics or doctors for regular or preventative visits. The poor, women, children, and addicts are more apt to use the hospital emergency room for primary medical care, arriving there in run-down conditions with severe HIV symptoms or in advanced stages of one of the opportunistic infections associated with a diagnosis of full-blown AIDS. With this in mind, all social workers with socially disadvantaged clients must use every opportunity to teach these individuals the concept of primary medical care and urge them to seek regular contact with physicians for themselves and their children. In addition, upon hearing of instances in which clinics or physicians have not responded with appropriate sensitivity or urgency, the social worker should immediately use his or her status and professional expertise to advocate with the health care setting on the client's behalf.

ETHICAL, LEGAL ISSUES, AND CONFIDENTIALITY RELATED TO HIV ANTIBODY STATUS

Social workers may find themselves in a situation in which a conflict between loyalty to one's client regarding confidentiality and other ethical concerns occurs.

Case Example

A heterosexually married man sought counseling after learning that a regular male sexual partner had been hospitalized for an AIDS-related condition. These men had never practiced safer sex, and my client was in a panic that he might be infected and that he might have infected his wife, with whom he was still sexually active. After testing positive for HIV antibodies, he was unwilling to share this information with his wife. I was insistent that he let her know what the situation was, especially since she needed to be tested to ascertain what her health status was. After refusing to tell his wife that he was HIV positive for two months, I gave him the following ultimatum. If he did not tell his wife within one month and bring her to sessions so I could be certain that he had indeed told her about his HIV status and her possible risk, I would call her myself and tell her. I made this decision after consulting with my attorney. Based on an interpretation of the *Tarasof* ruling in California, she felt that she could defend my potential breach of client-therapist confidentiality since there was a potentially life-threatening situation involving the wife. Eventually, he reluctantly agreed to tell her that he had been tested for HIV after having visited a female prostitute on a business trip and discovered that he had been exposed to HIV.

This case illustrates several points regarding legal, ethical, and clinical questions of HIV testing in social work practice. Except in cases of suspected or observed child abuse, the confidentiality of a client's discussions with a social worker is an important foundation of the professional relationship. In the previous case, I faced an ethical dilemma not encountered in my previous twenty years of practice. Since this client was in a relationship with a partner who was unsuspecting of the fact that she might have been placed in a life-threatening situation, I felt that his wife's need to be informed about her potential health risk outweighed his need for self-protection. Since my client was not reporting any physical symptoms of HIV disease, there was no medical immediacy for determining his antibody status. Had he been single, I would not have pushed him to have been tested as quickly even though there was a good chance he had been infected. Ordinarily, counseling would have focused on eliciting his feelings regarding learning that his partner was ill, his own fears, and information on how to protect himself and all future sexual partners from spreading the virus.

UNIVERSALITY OF THE ISSUES AFFECTING PEOPLE LIVING WITH HIV/AIDS

It is virtually impossible not to be personally affected by working professionally with people who are seriously ill and dying. When social workers become educated about the relevant issues of people living with HIV and AIDS, they become better prepared to help any client face a life catastrophe. As Gaies and Knox (1991) point out, "By confronting with dying clients the fragility of life and the value of each day, social workers begin to confront the vulnerability of their own lives and to acquire a deeper appreciation of living." Even deeply religious people question why bad things happen to them or to the people they love, and they can greatly benefit from the intervention of a skilled social worker who can help them work through all the accompanying issues and feelings. An additional benefit of doing this work is that it demystifies death and dying. Asking clients questions about why they make the choice to begin or discontinue a particular treatment and what the ramifications of those choices are helps them examine their life values. Working with people who have life-threatening illnesses and their loved ones, and engaging in conversations about sexuality, spirituality, dying, and death, which are all inherent in AIDS work, are invaluable clinical skills that are relevant to all aspects of social work practice with any client population.

FACTS THE SOCIAL WORKER
NEEDS TO KNOW BEFORE PROCEEDING

Living with HIV/AIDS versus Dying from AIDS

When a social worker first encounters a person with HIV/AIDS or a member of his or her family or support system, one of the worker's tasks is to help the client balance a realistic sense of hope with practical issues inherent in learning to live with HIV and AIDS. Increasing numbers of people have been labeled "nonprogressors" because they have a documented exposure to HIV for ten or more years and have remained completely asymptomatic, leading healthy, productive, and full lives despite their HIV status. "Long-term survivors" are individuals who have had an AIDS-related opportunistic infection, recovered from the acute phase of illness, and remained reasonably healthy for at least three years following the diagnosis of the AIDS-related complication.

Therefore, sharing this information with newly diagnosed patients and their loved ones helps them internalize some hope in adjusting to an HIV or AIDS diagnosis. Hearing from a professional that the diagnosis is most often not an immediate death sentence is a very empowering experience. It is usually beneficial to articulate for clients that they or their loved ones are currently living with HIV or AIDS, as opposed to dying from AIDS. Much of the practical concrete—as well as clinical—work will be helping the client adjust emotionally and practically to the state of living with this condition. Nonclinical social workers need to understand this reality and reflect it back to clients. The belief system that "I'm going to die very soon" should be challenged when offered as a rationalization for acting self-destructively, e.g., resuming drug or alcohol use or not following up on referrals that will help improve the client's quality of life.

Supportive Denial

With this in mind, the worker needs to understand the concept of "supportive denial," which can help clients manage living with this condition.

Supportive denial means that the client will not keep an awareness of his or her condition in the forefront of his or her thoughts at all times. This is easier if people are not seriously ill, and are in the early phase of infection, prior to becoming increasingly symptomatic and debilitated. Denial itself is neither bad nor good. If the client's denial is so pervasive and intense that it impairs the individual's reality testing, then the worker needs to challenge such denial. An example of maladaptive and inappropriate denial is a client in the early phase of HIV illness who refuses to undergo a basic treatment for a treatable opportunistic infection stating either that nothing is seriously wrong or "What's the use since I'm just going to die anyway?"

Another maladaptive example of denial is when an individual denies that he or she is, in fact, at risk for contracting or transmitting HIV and therefore refuses to change either sexual or drug-taking behaviors in order to protect his or herself or others. Denial must be assessed regarding its function. If the denial contributes to an adaptive mode of living with the illness, then the worker should not challenge it. One way that supportive denial manifests itself is when a client regularly sees his or her physician, has begun long-term planning for the illness, but does not necessarily feel any need to discuss AIDS during sessions with the social worker.

Casework with People with AIDS

Social workers employed in social service, childcare, or public assistance agencies, drug treatment facilities, or hospitals will all face the daunting reality of trying to help economically disadvantaged individuals or families with AIDS obtain or maintain a variety of benefits and entitlements. The work will be even more difficult in situations in which extensive concrete and social services for people with AIDS do not already exist. The social worker may find him or herself having to wrestle with already overwhelmed social service agencies faced with dwindling resources. As Walker (1995) notes, "effective service delivery to infected persons requires the creation of productive partnerships between health care and social service professionals as well as families and community groups."

Social workers must learn how to help families negotiate with care providers in order to receive accurate information about medical care, treatment options, nutrition, and social services. Walker (1995) goes on to point out that social workers employed in service organizations may regard families with AIDS as requiring an inordinate amount of services, and the worker is at risk of becoming dismayed by what they perceive to be the lack of change on the part of the family despite intensive efforts to help the members. As a result, social workers—like the families themselves—feel overwhelmed by the myriad problems presented by the families, and may regard these clients as burdensome and unrewarding. The social worker's frustration is further exacerbated when he or she tries, often futilely, to negotiate for the families' welfare, disability, and housing benefits through complex mazes of bureaucracy.

Preparing for Serious Illness

As people develop symptoms of more advanced AIDS, they increasingly lose control over their bodies and lives. One task for the social worker is to help people living with HIV and AIDS recognize what they can control. One of the most important areas is being partners in their health care with the physicians, determining which treatments they want to begin or discontinue. Rabkin, Remien, and Wilson (1994) point out the following:

> For many clients, the concept of developing relationships with medical providers and becoming an active member of the medical team is a foreign one. This is especially true for poor people who typically receive care at emergency rooms and clinics where frequent staff rotations and institutional insensitivity is common. Social workers can teach clients how to assert themselves more effectively without being considered abrasive. Role playing is a useful technique for helping clients develop these skills. (p. 17)

Clients living with HIV require help in planning for hospitalizations and debilitating illnesses. AIDS-related illnesses can have an astonishingly sudden onset. Often clients and their families or support networks are ill-prepared to cope with decisions that could have been discussed in depth prior to the onset of a medical emergency. It is best to raise the difficult and painful issues discussed in the next section long before there is any apparent need for them. When the client is well, he or she is more likely to have the necessary energy for planning these difficult realities. The worker needs to question clients' unwillingness to discuss concrete plans or desires for a living will or treatment options long before there is an acute medical emergency. Emphasize to the clients that by addressing these issues now they can ensure that they will have a measure of control over what happens to them.

Social workers must overcome their own discomfort about discussing preparing for the end of life in order to help clients and their families and loved ones prepare for this eventuality. It is useful to raise with all clients, but especially those with a life-threatening illness, the issues of having prepared a will, a medical proxy, and a living will. The worker can introduce these issues by stating that although it is clearly much too early to start thinking about some of the difficult realities that accompany a serious illness, the worker feels that it is in the best interests of the client that these sensitive issues begin to be addressed now. This is certainly true if the client is a single parent and has not made any provisions for who will care for his or her children, if he or she becomes too ill to actively parent or for who will have custody of the children following his or her death.

Crucial Points

- The client needs to know which hospital he or she wants to be taken to in the event of an emergency.
- If the client lives alone or with small children, he or she needs to discuss who will be contacted, even in the middle of the night, to help with transportation to the hospital and/or to care for children or pets during the crisis?
- The client should maintain a current and complete list of all prescribed medications and dosages that can be brought to the hospital during an emergency admission.
- The client must discuss advance medical directives, including how aggressively he or she wishes to be kept alive if no reasonable hope for recovery or for a good quality of life exists. A living will needs to be made. These directives must be written down and given to the physician and brought to the hospital to be placed in the chart at the start of each hospitalization.
- The client must designate a health care proxy (a family member or close friend) and ask this person if he or she feels able to ensure that the client's wishes will be followed—*even if those wishes are contrary to what the proxy feels is best.*
- The client needs to be asked "What do you want done in the eventuality that your heart stops beating?" If a client does not wish to be resuscitated, then a "do not resuscitate" (DNR) order should be written and placed in his or her chart.
- The client needs to be reminded that these instructions can be revised if any of his or her feelings change over the course of the illness.

One of the most important functions of the social worker will be as liaison between the client and his or her family, between the client and physician or other health care providers or home care agency, and between the client and social service agencies. Families and other loved ones are often in greater denial than the client and may benefit greatly from speaking with a social worker.

End-of-Life Issues

> Few people who are not profoundly depressed speak about being ready to die or welcoming it, except if they are in the advanced stage of a terminal illness. People with AIDS who have become extremely debilitated after going through extensive treatments often speak of being ready to die since they no longer have a meaningful quality of life. (Rabkin, Remien, and Wilson, 1994, p. 143)

It is imperative for the worker not to judge these feelings and to elicit how the client feels about approaching the end of his or her life. While directly discussing these issues initially makes clients uncomfortable, it is my experience that clients welcome the worker's raising questions about death, dying, and end-of-life practicalities. One useful way to introduce the topic is by asking what the client believes happens after death, and if those beliefs are comforting? Also, exploring a client's feelings or thoughts about the religion in which they were born and raised can be useful in helping discover sources of strengths or of old wounds that might need to have opportunity to heal. I have found that clients are almost always grateful to have the opportunity to speak to a sympathetic clergyperson who will not be judgmental about their having AIDS or how they may have contracted it. A list of such clergy is an important and useful resource for all workers to cultivate, so that one can be called upon to visit with a client who is dying and who feels the need for religious reconciliation.

Funerals and Memorial Services

One way of empowering dying clients is by urging them to discuss what they wish done with their bodies after they have died. Do they want to be cremated or buried? Have they documented their wishes? It can be one very comforting option for some people to plan their funeral or memorial service, specifying who they wish to speak, what music or prayers should be recited, and where the service should take place. On the other hand, confronting these details may be too stressful for some individuals who cannot face what making those plans means regarding the acceptance of their health status. But if the client has been able to discuss these issues during counseling, the next step is to urge him or her to discuss these details with family and loved ones. If the family or loved ones refuse to discuss these issues with the client, the worker should urge the significant others to come in for some sessions to help them work through their feelings of denial, sadness, and discomfort.

These family sessions can help significant others see that once they are clear about the wishes of their loved one, carrying out his or her wishes after he or she has passed away will be much easier. It is a useful intervention to restructure the reality from one of morbid preoccupation with the unpleasant inevitability to allowing the person who is ill to take control over the few areas of his or her life that are still controllable. Another useful intervention is to explain to the loved ones that it is an expression of how much the ill person loves them that he or she does not want them to have to guess what should be done during the extremely stressful period following death. Establishing postdeath details is one way the person who is dying is still able to take care of his or her loved ones.

Pain Management

Rabkin, Remien, and Wilson (1994) note that most people fear they will be in excruciating pain as they near death from a terminal illness. Clients need to be assured that they will not suffer. Most major hospitals have physicians who are pain management specialists who can consult with the patient about helping him or her remain comfortable during this phase of the illness. "Some people prefer to be unconscious, others wish to be alert, but sedated and pain free" (Rabkin, Remien, and Wilson, 1994). People need to be taught how to explicitly describe how much pain they are experiencing in order to effectively communicate this to the physician. Pain can be effectively controlled even if the client decides to die at home. In addition, social workers can help clients who experience pain by teaching them the techniques of self-hypnosis and visualization.

Weiss (1995) states the following:

> [A]ctively chemically dependent patients with AIDS usually require generous amounts of medication while in the hospital. Medical and nursing staff often withhold the very medication these patients need, making them even more irritable and difficult to manage. Making patients comfortable with adequate opiates or sedatives helps them feel they are being heard, enhances their trust, and improves the working relationship between the chemically dependent patient and staff members. (p. 46)

Hospital social workers need to be alert to the above-mentioned dynamic and be prepared to advocate for chemically dependent patients who are not being adequately medicated. Conversely, some patients who are in recovery have unrealistic expectations regarding using any drug that they once may have taken illicitly. Social workers need to remind people that they did not get sober to suffer and that taking prescribed medication to alleviate pain is not the same as abusing drugs.

Choices in Dying

One major issue for dying people is that they are at a point where their ability to control what happens to them has been greatly diminished. Clients at the end of their lives can be empowered by social workers engaging them in a discussion about where they want to die. Many clients may not realize that whether to die at home, in the hospital, or in a hospice is a decision that they and their loved ones can and should consciously make together in consultation with their physician. Explaining hospice care can be enormously helpful. Suggesting that an intake worker from hospice visit the client to describe the program in detail is one useful intervention. These discussions are best held in at least two different sessions. The first is with the client alone to explore all of his or her feelings about this emotionally laden issue. Next, the discussion needs to be continued with the people, if there are any, who will help care for the client in order to explore all the emotional as well as logistical and practical considerations.

As Rabkin, Remien, and Wilson (1994) note, "It can often be difficult for all concerned to acknowledge that 'enough is enough.'" It is the role of the social worker to explore with the client his or her feelings about whether or not to cease treatments or to continue fighting for extra time. It is not the worker's role to give permission for one choice or another, though the client may be asking the worker either directly or obliquely for his or her opinion about what course of action seems best. Dying can be a quality time both for the terminally ill person as well as those who love him or her. As Hines and Peura (1995) explain,

> . . . at a certain point, we must all let go of living well and begin to consider what it means to be dying well. This can become a very attractive concept for the client, the significant others, and the worker. Many of us associate the dying process with all the worst things, from pain to mental deterioration, But through counseling, a skilled worker can help the client explore what it would mean for him or her to die well, and what steps need to be taken in order to promote this outcome. (p. 1)

One way to help ensure this is for the social worker to ask the client questions that will offer him or her options and some control over the process. Rabkin, Remien, and Wilson (1994) correctly note that it is far easier to believe in the right to choose the timing of one's death when the person is actively dying and when his or her remaining time is likely to be hours or days. The strength of this conviction is tested when the person is not acutely and severely ill but untreatable, and may have weeks or months to go before an inevitable death. Such a person may be able to survive physically but with such chronic discomfort and diminished hope for any good quality of life that he or she sees no reason to remain alive. Is this person entitled to say "Enough is enough?" Many health care providers who work with terminally ill people believe so. Once the client has decided to discontinue medical procedures or drugs, often IV morphine is started with the double purpose of alleviating pain and accelerating the timing of death. After its initiation, a period of alertness for several days, or even weeks, may ensue before death occurs, but often a person becomes unable to communicate once the morphine drip has begun. Therefore, prior to beginning a morphine drip, the counselor or nurse should look for opportunities to facilitate conversations between the dying person and his or her loved ones and family members.

Some key questions to ask are as follows:

- Do you feel that you are going to die soon?
- If so, how do you feel about this?
- How will you know you no longer wish to continue medicines, treatments, or supplemental feedings? (It is important to reflect to the client that what he or she feels is intolerable may in fact change. Most people with AIDS surveyed felt that blindness, dementia, and incontinence were hallmarks of life not being worth continuing.)
- Do you prefer to die at home, in a hospice, or in a hospital?
- Whom do you wish to be with you?
- Would you like to have a clergyperson make a final visit?
- Is there anything you still need to say to your loved ones?
- Is there anything else you need to do or complete?
- Have you thought about letting go since it seems to me that you are suffering a great deal?

Some salient points for significant others to consider in conversations with a person who is dying are as follows:

- Is there something you still need to say?
- Have you told the person that it is okay for him or her to go now?

- Discuss what specific things or events will always make you think of him or her.
- Remind him or her of a special moment you two shared that will be with you forever.
- Say that you love him or her, and thank him or her for the relationship you had.
- Say "good-bye" and relate how much he or she will be missed.
- Give assurance that though you will miss him or her, you will eventually be alright.

POTENTIAL BARRIERS TO SUCCESSFUL INTERVENTION

The major obstacles to beginning work with people with HIV or AIDS is the social worker's own degree of discomfort with a variety of issues. First, the worker may be uncomfortable with members of sexual minorities, specifically gay men, or with racial minorities or people who have used illicit drugs. These prejudices all must be acknowledged in order to be addressed. Second, as social workers, like most people, we have internalized an illusion of our own immortality. Working with young people who are dying forces us to confront our own mortality, which is a formidable task for any human being. Third, working closely with someone who is becoming progressively sicker and deteriorating physically is extremely painful. Yet it is precisely by facing these challenges directly that each social worker has the opportunity to grow enormously professionally, personally, and spiritually.

RECOMMENDED READINGS

Face to face: A guide to AIDS counseling, J. Dilley, C. Pies, and M. Helquist (Eds.), 1989, Berkeley, CA: Celestial Arts Press.
Good doctors, good patients: Partners in HIV treatment, J. Rabkin, R. Remien, and C. Wilson (Eds.), 1994, New York: NCN Publishers.
The second decade of AIDS: A mental health practice handbook, W. Odets and M. Shernoff (Eds.), 1995, New York: Hatherleigh Press.
AIDS health and mental health: A primary sourcebook. J. Landau-Stanton, C.D. Clements and Associates, 1993, New York: Brunner/Mazel.

REFERENCES

Cargill, V. (1995). African-Americans and AIDS. *HIV Newsline*: 39-41.
Gaies, J., and Knox, M. (1991). The therapist and the dying client. *FOCUS: A Guide to AIDS Research and Counseling* 6(6), 1-2.

Hines, B., and Peura, S. (1995). Hospice: A place for dying well. *FOCUS: A Guide to AIDS Research and Counseling 10*(8): 1-4.

Hunt, M. (1974). *Sexual behavior in the 1970s*. Chicago: Playboy Press.

Hyde, S. (1982). *Understanding human sexuality*. New York: McGraw-Hill.

Kinsey, A., Pomeroy, W., and Martin, C. (1948). *Sexual behavior in the human male*. Philadelphia: W.B. Saunders and Co.

Kolata, G. (1987, October 19) "AIDS is killing women faster, researchers say." *The New York Times*: A1.

Marks, R., and Goldblum, P. (1989). The decision to test: A personal choice. In J. Dilley, C. Pies, and M. Helquist (Eds.), *Face to face: A guide to AIDS counseling*. San Francisco: University of California AIDS Health Project, pp. 49-58.

Newmeyer, J. (1989). The epidemiology of HIV among intravenous drug users. In J. Dilley, C. Pies, and M. Helquist (Eds.), *Face to face: A guide to AIDS counseling*. San Francisco: University of California AIDS Health Project, pp. 108-117.

Ostrow, D. G., and Wren, P. A. (1991). Comprehensive HIV/AIDS Mental Health Education Program: Volume 1: Mental health aspects of HIV/AIDS: Curriculum modules, unpublished text, University of Michigan Comprehensive HIV/AIDS Mental Health Education Program.

Rabkin, J., Remien, R., and Wilson, C. (Eds.). (1994). *Good doctors, good patients: Partners in HIV treatment*. New York: NCN Publishers.

Springer, E. (1991). Effective AIDS prevention with active drug users: The harm reduction model. In M. Shernoff (Ed.), *Counseling chemically dependent people with HIV illness*. Binghamton, NY: The Haworth Press, pp. 141-158.

Verghese, A. (1994). My own country: A doctor's story of a town and its people in the age of AIDS. New York: Simon and Schuster.

Walker, G. (1995). Family therapy interventions with inner-city families affected by AIDS. In W. Odets and M. Shernoff (Eds.), *The second decade of AIDS: A mental health practice handbook*. New York: Hatherleigh Press, pp. 85-114.

Weiss, C. (1991). Working with chemically dependent HIV-infected patients on an inpatient medical unit. In M. Shernoff (Ed.), *Counseling chemically dependent people with HIV illness*. Binghamton, NY: The Haworth Press, pp. 45-53.

Multicultural Competence

Lana S. Ka'opua

WHY DO THIS?
STATEMENT OF THE PROBLEM AND ISSUES

Three competencies or proficiencies have been identified for use in the HIV-related intervention with the client who is culturally different from the practitioner. These cultural competencies include observation of entry etiquette, elicitation of cultural information and negotiation of understanding (Berlin and Fowkes, 1983; Gallego, 1989; Sue, Arredondo, and McDavis, 1992). Working with a client who is culturally different can raise some anxiety for the social worker and it is natural for the practitioner to want some knowledge, perhaps a list of pertinent cultural values and practices, or a few salient pointers for working with members of a particular group. However, the "cookbook" approach to working with the culturally different client can run dangerously close to stereotyping the client, and while helpful for general understanding of cultural group, such an approach must be used with caution in assessing the individual client. While there is no recipe for effective intervention, the three essential competencies identified here can guide the frontline social worker in minimizing conflict, in making a more accurate assessment of cultural influences, and in working with a culturally different client to develop meaningful intervention. The social worker who is armed with these proficiencies can collaborate with the client to determine what constitutes culturally compatible intervention.

Culturally competent service assumes client involvement and ideally resides in a system with culturally competent policies and programs. The literature identifies numerous competencies that address systems issues (Cross et al., 1989; Chau, 1991; Sue, Arrendondo, and McDavis, 1992). However, this chapter discusses those competencies most relevant for direct practice in the HIV-related social work intervention.

The HIV pandemic has been viewed as a series of many diverse epidemics (Daniels, 1995). Hence, the needs and practices of the homeless in

51

a major city may be strikingly different from that of ethnic women living in a rural community or from that of *mahu** working in the sex industry of a tourist mecca. Cultural groups are distinguished by their unique socialization process (McDermott, Tseng, and Maretzki, 1980). Members of a cultural group may share a sense of history that includes a history of stigmatization or being viewed as deficient on the basis of difference from mainstream society. In health/mental health care services, culturally different clients have often been misunderstood by professionals, which has resulted in misdiagnosis and inappropriate treatment (Hines and Boyd-Franklin, 1982; Jones, Gray, and Parson, 1983; Sata, 1990).

In the cross-cultural encounter, the frontline social worker is faced with a potentially difficult task: delivering the best possible services in a culturally sensitive manner to clients who may not always understand, recognize, or trust the value of social services. When the client and social worker are culturally different, misunderstanding and conflict can result in premature termination of services and the client's seeming reluctance to follow through with service plans. Communication between the social worker and client in a HIV-related situation may be further complicated by the need to address highly value-laden issues such as illness, healing, sexuality, and death and dying. For the frontline social worker, the fundamental challenge remains understanding the person-in-environment and the implications this may have for practice.

CULTURAL COMPETENCY CONSIDERATIONS

While general knowledge of a cultural group is important, this knowledge in and of itself may be insufficient to obtain successful outcomes (Proctor and Davis, 1983; Chau, 1991; Nakanishi and Rittner, 1992). The balance lies in understanding the uniqueness of each group, as well as the diversity within each group (Brislin, 1993). Great variation exists among members of the same cultural group. Therefore, a cultural assessment of each client is necessary to avoid stereotypic understanding and inappropriate treatment.

Cultural matching of social worker and client is only useful in certain situations. That is, a social worker may belong to the same ethnic, racial, or cultural group as the client, but this shared membership does not naturally endow the social worker with competencies necessary to effect inter-

---

* *Mahu* is a term used in Polynesia to describe a person born with male genitalia and taking on male and female roles.

vention. A more relevant process outcome is the development of cultural compatibility in assessment and intervention (Sue, 1981). The following discussion identifies value, knowledge, and skill competencies that may be useful in developing cultural compatibility between social workers and clients. Case illustrations have been excerpted from actual cases.

Observation of Entry Etiquette

Entry etiquette refers to the way in which the social worker makes initial contact with the client and the client's significant others. In many ethnic cultures, demonstration of certain behaviors signifies respect and knowledge of what is polite and respectful (J. Gallego, 1994; Higginbotham, 1987). For example to meet Hawaiian expectations, the provider may need to engage the client at the personal rather than the professional level (Higginbotham, 1987; Mokuau, 1987).

Case Study

Upon arrival for an initial home visit to a Pacific Islander family, the social worker is greeted pleasantly and asked if he would like something to drink. Over refreshments, the family asks the social worker to share something about himself. As the social worker begins to discuss what he does in the agency, the eldest family member interrupts and asks: "No, who are you?"

Process questions: How might the social worker assess what is meant by the question? What function does this question have in the building of the therapeutic relationship? How might the social worker answer?

The client's perceptions of the social worker as a credible and competent helper may be influenced by the social worker's attention to culturally appropriate protocol at the initial meeting. The style of communication and the pace of communication are important here. "Cutting to the chase" and "getting down to business," if advanced prematurely, may be unproductive in building a therapeutic relationship with the culturally different client and his or her family.

The offering of refreshments may be a cue that different cultural rules of etiquette are in operation. Seemingly innocuous communication may actually provide opportunities for the social worker to demonstrate credibility as a helper. By accepting refreshments, the social worker begins a process of joining with the client and the client's significant others. The family's desire to know more about the social worker represents a marker in the purposeful movement toward discussion of sensitive subjects.

The key issue at hand for the culturally different client and family may be that of the social worker's credibility, or that constellation of characteristics that make certain individuals appear trustworthy and capable. The client is more likely to engage in productive relations with a helper who is seen as credible (Sue, 1981). Hence, when the client family member asks the social worker to share something about himself, the issues raised might include the following: Who is this person who comes before us? Can this person provide the kind of help we need? Has this person ever lost someone to HIV/AIDS? Is there something in this helper's background that indicates a capacity to understand the family situation and its cultural orientation?

For families that have experienced discrimination on the basis of ethnicity, race, or culture, additional issues may exist, including the following: Will this person attempt to impose other values and practices? Will there be negative consequences if the family works with this helper? How confidential are these services?

The competence of the worker in responding to the family's request for personal information may enhance the perception of worker credibility and thus facilitate the family's willingness for deeper disclosure during the course of the therapeutic relationship.

Professional credentials or expert status may only be a part of what is being asked by the family. For example, in traditional Hawaiian families, the process of finding mutual relationships, friends, or similar experiences facilitates the perception of worker credibility (Rocha, 1985). The process of building common ties between helper and client is a process of discovering commonalities and involves considerable self-disclosure from all involved parties.

The social worker who is unfamiliar with such a tradition may experience discomfort and may even question if the client and family are trying to reduce the professional relationship to one of friendship. However, in some cultures, the boundaries between helping relationships and personal relationships are more fluid than in Western culture. When disclosure of self and personal networks is a cultural norm, the social worker may need to adjust. In building a therapeutic alliance with the culturally different client and family, the social worker must seek to balance personal comfort with purposeful self-disclosure.

One persistent myth is that culturally different clients avoid discussion of sensitive subjects such as sexuality and death and dying. In fact the therapeutic issue may be more one of establishing the social worker's credibility in the therapeutic relationship. During the initial stages of a relationship, the frontline social worker may find it productive to observe appropriate entry etiquette and to respect cultural differences in the pacing and approach of sensitive discussions.

To ensure competence in entry etiquette, the social worker can do the following:

1. Consult a cultural resource to become familiar with values and practices specific to entry etiquette, help-seeking, and caregiving. Seek to find out if any specific customs should be observed in an initial meeting; as well as what the preferred style of communication is. Also seek information on how the client may perceive social work services. Are there stereotypes of service that might be anticipated and addressed by the social worker in the initial meeting?
2. Address issues of confidentiality. Clarify with the client what he or she wishes others to know. Be specific about the kind of confidentiality that can be ensured.
3. Take time in the initial interview to observe how a client communicates. Is the pace different from yours? Is the client's style of communication relatively formal or informal? Is the client generally direct or indirect in communication? Consider mirroring the client's pace and style of communication.
4. How are sensitive subjects framed by the client? It may be necessary to use metaphors and stories from the client's culture to discuss sensitive topics such as sexual practices, help-seeking, illness, death and dying. As much as possible, use the client's terms.
5. Know personal biases and preferences regarding entry etiquette. Be flexible and suspend judgment about client behaviors that seem unfamiliar.
6. Acknowledge that there may be differences and explore what those differences might be with the client. This is an important step in the development of the therapeutic relationship. The social worker might begin by saying:

   I know that families have their own ways of staying healthy, of healing, and of caring for their loved ones. So it's important for me to understand your ways. As we get to know each other better, I invite you to tell me what is important to you, what you need, and how I can best be of help to you.

7. Apologize in advance for any inadvertent cultural mistakes. In some cultures, this is preparatory for the discussion of sensitive subjects. Be clear with the clients about the importance of such discussion.

This might be followed by more specific questions about beliefs and practices.

Elicitation of Cultural Information

The elicitation competency requires listening for and seeking information about cultural values, beliefs, and practices (Berlin and Fowkes, 1983; Katon and Kleinman, 1981).

Case Study

The caregiver continues to feed her sister, despite professional recommendations that the feeding stop. The social worker has tried on several occasions to counsel the caregiver. The social worker has provided information about how the body systems shut down in the final stages of AIDS and how eating may cause the patient discomfort. The caregiver is feeling frustrated and resentful of the social worker's repeated instructions. The caregiver has stated that the social worker's explanations "don't make sense" and that she cannot stop feeding her sister. The social worker is concerned about the comfort of the identified client, the dying woman. She is angry and is sure that when she leaves, the feeding will continue.

Process questions: What are the social worker's biases in this situation? How does this influence her behavior toward the sister? What does the social worker need to learn about culture and caregiving in order to understand and make appropriate intervention?

The elicitation competency is grounded in the social worker's awareness and acceptance of difference in worldviews. Elicitation is the intentional process of drawing out essential cultural information. It involves obtaining the client's statement of the problem, as well as obtaining the meaning assigned to the problem.

In the case illustration, the caregiver indicates that the social worker's explanation "does not make sense." This is a cue that a difference of worldviews probably exists and suggests the need for further exploration on the part of the social worker. Reiteration of the biomedical explanation for cessation of eating and feeding assumes that the social worker and client share the same understanding of the symptoms of the disease, the cause of the disease, how the disease will progresses, and how to heal the disease and its symptoms.

The social worker's explanation reflects the view that the disease is based in human biology. She does not consider that the caregiver's view of the symptoms may not based in the same framework. Hence, she continues to offer variations of the same explanation. These explanations are unsatisfactory to the caregiver, who is a product of both Western and traditional Hawaiian socialization.

In contrast to the Western biomedical view of illness and disease, many non-Western cultures conceptualize disease and illness from a more holistic perspective, which may include spiritual, emotional, and social aspects. For example, in the traditional Hawaiian view, health involves a balance of relationships between person, social system, physical environment, and the spiritual world (Blaisdell, 1983). Being ill was not just a physical discomfort, but moreover an imbalance of a spiritual or psychological well-being (Chun, 1986). Diagnosis involved discovering the cause for the loss in balance in one or more of the key relationships and in healing that relationship.

In the case example, the social worker needs to elicit how the caregiver understands her sister's illness, the cultural prescriptions for healing, and the role expectations of caregiver and sick person in the healing process. Hence, the social worker might inquire about the client's health paradigm with questions like: What do you believe is happening to your sister? What do you believe has caused this problem? Have you or any member of your family ever been in a similar situation? What did you do in that situation that might be appropriate for you to do in this situation?

In eliciting specific information about the meaning of eating and feeding, the social worker might ask the following questions: Besides yourself, who in your family is responsible for deciding how to care for your sister? Does eating and feeding have a special meaning in your family? Are there special family/cultural rituals that involve the offering of food? What do you/your family believe happens when someone is dying? Dies? What are the family responsibilities at these times? What does your family expect you to do?

The social worker ensures accurate assessment by periodically checking understanding of the client's beliefs, values, and practices. This understanding might then be summarized and integrated into recommendations of how to proceed.

To ensure competence in elicitation of cultural information, the social worker can do the following:

1. Monitor personal biases. Refrain from stereotyping the client's behavior and seeing it as a cultural deficiency.
2. Remember views about health can be culture-bound.

3. Assess the presence/absence of shared views with the client and the client's caregivers. Expect different views concerning family structure, roles of caregivers, roles of the sick person, illness, disease progression, healing strategies, coping strategies, spirituality, and death and dying. Healing and problem resolution occur within the *client's* cultural frame of reference.
4. Listen for information about educational background, familiarity with medical terminology, socioeconomic level, and degree of Westernization/degree of adherence to traditional belief systems.
5. Ask open-ended questions to elicit differences in worldview.
6. Stop periodically to check your understanding of the client's worldview.
7. Seek information from the client and caregivers regarding how decisions are made about health, illness, and caregiving.

Negotiation of Understanding

The negotiation of a shared understanding of the illness and its symptoms is regarded as the most critical of the essential competencies in the cross-cultural helping encounter. Negotiation builds on the previous competencies and involves reaching agreement through discussion.

Case Study

The client is a twenty-four-year-old Asian American who lives in a residence for people living with HIV/AIDS. He has an advanced case of Kaposi's sarcoma (KS). As part of the residential program, he has been assigned a social worker whose primary responsibility is to provide mental health counseling.

In the initial meeting the social worker elicits relevant cultural information. The client was born in a Southeast Asian country but has been living in the United States for ten years. The client considers himself bilingual with English as his second language. The client states that he was once regarded as extremely desirable and attractive, but now feels abandoned by his friends and former lovers. He has minimal contact with his family.

The client complains of "depression." Because of his KS lesions, he feels disfigured and can no longer wear fashionable outfits. He experiences this as a great loss. In the initial meeting, the client cries as he relates this information, and the social worker responds with active listening and reflection of the client's feelings. Although the relationship appears off to a good start, the social worker feels that subsequent meetings amount to little more than a social hour with the client talking at length about his once fashionable past.

Process questions: What are some of the barriers that this client might have to the utilization of mental health services? Why was the client unwilling to explore his feelings in subsequent meetings with the social worker? What are the areas that may need to be negotiated by the social worker?

In the social work intervention, negotiation specifically involves an assessment and acknowledgment of differences in values and practices, the development of common aims, the shared understanding of options, recommendations of how to proceed, and discussion to a point of agreement. The goal of negotiation is to reduce conflict in a way that strengthens the therapeutic alliance and encourages cooperation. Negotiation might be conceived as the key to "customizing" intervention to the client.

While negotiation is central to effective cross-cultural relations, an important caveat exists: In certain cultures and among particular ethnic groups, the helping professional is expected to be the authority and to give active direction about what is done (Markoff and Bond, 1980; Ponce, 1995). In such cases, a negotiation model may represent an inappropriate imposition of values and it may be inappropriate to alter the relationship along such lines. However, the decision to dispense with negotiation must be carefully assessed by the social worker. In the HIV-related counseling situation, there are many barriers to the client's utilization of services. As in the case illustration, an assessment of mental illness such as depression warrants psychiatric evaluation. There are many complex ways in which biological, psychological, and social factors intersect to cause the depressive symptomatology of a person with HIV/AIDS. Obtaining a psychiatric consultation allows the social worker to rule out depression resulting from drug side effects or effects of HIV-related opportunistic infections on the brain.

Following the ruling out of organicity or drug complications, the social worker may proceed to assess other potential barriers to service utilization, including the cultural unacceptability of mainstream services. Three areas are important to assess and negotiate:

1. *Use of language,* including the use of English as the primary language in counseling or the use of terms and metaphors that are culturally dystonic for the client.

2. *Counseling goals and outcomes,* including those that are based only on mainstream values and that conflict with the client's cultural paradigm.
3. *Models of practice,* including the therapeutic orientation of the provider and the use of strategies and techniques that are incompatible with the client's worldview and style of communication.

Use of Language

In the initial interview the client has indicated that he is bilingual with English as his second language. This is a cue that some discomfort may exist in using the English language. While the client may have no apparent difficulty in understanding English, he may feel more comfortable discussing certain issues in his native tongue. Some cultural terms are idiomatic and do not readily translate into English, yet may have powerful meaning to the client. When there is great language dissimilarity, the social worker might propose referral to a bilingual/bicultural counselor. Even when both the client and social worker are comfortable using English, the social worker will need to give ongoing attention to conceptual differences of terms used; a cultural consultant may be helpful in this situation. For example in traditional Japanese culture, *amae,* or "dependency," has a positive connotation and reflects the value priority of interdependence between people. Individuality threatens the collective identity of Japanese culture and, in some instances, can even be perceived as a danger to the self. Thus, Western connotations of dependency may lead to erroneous conclusions about the client who subscribes to more traditional Japanese values.

Nonethnic cultures, such as gay culture or professional culture may also influence the client's worldview. In the case illustration, the client suggests multiple cultural identifications: gay culture, Western culture, traditional ethnic culture, and possibly a religious culture outside of the Judeo-Christian tradition. The presence of multiple cultural identifications may require the client and social worker to blend primary, secondary, and perhaps even tertiary worldviews in order to adequately interpret the client's experience of HIV illness. The Asian-American man in the case illustration may be depressed about his early death and may need a view of mortality that incorporates the traditions of his ethnocultural background with the Western values and practices of his adult life. Again, a cultural consultant may be useful in helping the social worker to identify language, stories, and metaphors that will make sense for this client.

Counseling Goals and Outcomes

Experts in cross-cultural counseling have raised concerns about values implicit in Western mental health services, including the high premium placed on verbal, emotional, and behavioral expressiveness and the value of insight as a process goal to positive change (Sue, 1981). According to the experts, values implicit in counseling may be in direct conflict with cultural groups who value emotional restraint, indirect communication, and the use of natural helpers. The culturally different client may find it either unfamiliar or undesirable to discuss intense feelings with someone he or she has just met. These differences can truly challenge the social worker to suspend judgment and to assess a client from the appropriate cultural context.

In the case illustration, the client operates from traditional ethnocultural norms that value restraint of emotion. From this client's experience, intimate details are generally shared in close friendships that have been forged over prolonged periods of contact. Because the client expressed considerable emotion in the initial interview, the social worker erroneously assumed that such expression was normative for this client. In fact, the client was unfamiliar with the experience of verbalizing intense feelings, and after the initial meeting, he had experienced emotional flooding. As a result, he chose to exercise more caution in subsequent meetings with the social worker. The client's caution in the therapeutic relationship was exacerbated by his perceptions that he had been abandoned by his friends.

Models of Practice

In the case illustration, the social worker assessed the need to adapt his style of counseling. In negotiating a different style of work, he proposed a psychoeducational approach that would focus on reduction of symptomatology. The social worker and client collaborated on the development of short-term goals and agreed to evaluate progress at specified points in time. Immediately following the renegotiation of the relationship, the social worker offered the client a "gift" or a gesture of caring. The social worker could not simply raise the expectations of the client about outcomes. He realized that the client needed to experience a direct benefit or gift from the new arrangement. Thus, he offered the client a means of understanding the confusion and emotional chaos that can accompany the experience of HIV illness. Through psychoeducational techniques, the therapist helped the client to "normalize" reactions to illness. Since the client did not ordinarily talk to others, he was greatly relieved to discover that others suffered from similar difficulties.

To ensure competence in negotiation, the social worker can do the following:

1. Check to see if negotiation is appropriate from the client's frame of reference.
2. Check for potential conflict in models of intervention, therapeutic style, culturally biased assumptions about the client, and linguistic and cultural differences. As necessary, recommend changes and confer with the client to a point of agreement.
3. Consider referral to a bilingual/bicultural counselor or consider using a cultural consultant.
4. Exercise patience in the development of the therapeutic relationship.
5. Increase credibility by "gift giving." Culturally different clients may wonder how disclosure of personal problems can result in the alleviation of emotional and behavioral distress. In gift giving, the therapist offers direct benefits that can be experienced by the client early in the treatment process.

CONCLUSION

The underutilization of HIV services by ethnically and culturally diverse peoples is often a function of the cultural unacceptability of services rendered. In the cross-cultural intervention, the key to successful outcomes lies in the "goodness of fit" between services and the cultural reality of diverse clients. The frontline social worker can maximize goodness of fit in services by becoming proficient in observance of entry etiquette, elicitation of relevant cultural information, and negotiation of understanding and intervention. These competencies are essential when addressing the many sensitive issues raised by HIV disease and illness.

RECOMMENDED READINGS

Berlin, E. A., and Fowkes, W. Jr. (1983). A teaching framework for cross-cultural health care. *Western Journal of Medicine 139:* 934-938.

Brislin, R. (1993). *Understanding culture's influence on behavior.* Fort Worth, TX: Harcourt Brace College Publishers.

Ka'opua, L. S. (1992). *Training for cultural competence in the HIV epidemic.* Honolulu: Hawaii Area AIDS Education and Training Center.

Ka'opua, L. S. (1994). Cultural competency in the HIV epidemic. In *1994 National HIV frontline forum.* New York: NCM Publishers, Inc.

Leukefeld, C. G., and Fimbres, M. (Eds.) (1987). *Responding to AIDS—Psychosocial initiatives.* Silver Spring, MD: National Association of Social Workers, Inc.

Morales, J., and Bok, M. (Eds.) (1992). *Multicultural human services for AIDS treatment and prevention: Policy, perspectives, and planning.* Binghamton, NY: Harrington Park Press.

Sue, D. W. (1981). *Counseling the culturally different.* New York: John Wiley and Sons.

Sue, S. (1994). Mental Health. In N. Zane, D. Takeuchi, and K. Young (Eds.), *Confronting critical health issues of Asian and Pacific Islander Americans.* Thousand Oaks, CA: Sage Publications, pp. 266-288.

REFERENCES

Berlin, E. A., and Fowkes, W., Jr. (1983). A teaching framework for cross-cultural health care. *Western Journal of Medicine 139:* 934-938.

Blaisdell, R. K. (1983). Health section of Native Hawaiian study commission report. *Native Hawaiian Study Commission Report.* Honolulu: E Ola Mau.

Brislin, R. (1993). *Understanding culture's influence on behavior.* Fort Worth, TX: Harcourt Brace College Publishers.

Chau, K. (1991). Social work with ethnic minorities: Practice issues and potentials. *Journal of Multicultural Social Work 1*(1): 23-39.

Chun, M. N. (Trans.) (1986). *Hawaiian medicine book: He buke laau lapaau.* Honolulu: The Best Press.

Cross, T., Bazron, B., Dennis, K., and Isaacs, M. (1989). Toward a culturally competent system of care: A monograph on effective services for minority children who are severely emotionally disturbed. Washington, DC: Georgetown University.

Daniels, E. (1995). Address to Ryan White grantees and representatives from the National Area AIDS Education and Training Centers, National ETC teleconference, March 16, 1995.

Gallego, J. (1994). The ethnic competence model for social work education. In B. White (Ed.), *Color in white society.* Silver Spring, MD: National Association of Social Workers, pp. 1-9.

Gallego, S. (1994). Women and HIV. In *1994 national HIV frontline forum.* New York: NCM Publishers, pp. 24-29.

Higginbotham, N. (1987). The culture accomodation of mental health services for Native Hawaiians. In A. Robillard and A.J. Marsella (Eds.), *Contemporary issues in mental health research in the Pacific Islands.* Honolulu: Social Science Research Institute, pp. 94-126.

Hines, P. M., and Boyd-Franklin, N. (1982). Black families. In M. McGoldrick, J. Pearce, and J. Giordano (Eds.), *Ethnicity and family therapy.* New York: Guilford Press.

Jones, B., B. Gray, and Parson, E. (1983). Manic-depressive illness among poor urban Hispanics. *American Journal of Psychiatry 140:* 1208-1210.

Katon, W., and Kleinman, A. (1981). Doctor-patient negotiation and other social science strategies in patient care. In L. Eisenberg and A. Kleinman (Eds.), *The relevance of social science for medicine*. Dordrecht, Holland: D. Reidel Publishing Co., pp. 253-279.

Markoff, R. A., and Bond, J. R. (1980). The Samoans. In J. F. McDermott Jr., W. Tseng, and T. Maretzki (Eds.), *People and cultures of Hawaii*. Honolulu: University of Hawaii Press.

McDermott, J., Tseng, W., and Maretzki, T. (Eds.) (1980). *People and cultures of Hawaii*. Honolulu: University of Hawaii Press.

Mokuau, N. (1987). Counseling Pacific Islander Americans. In P. Pedersen (Ed.). *Handbook of cross-cultural counseling and therapy*. New York: Praeger, pp. 147-155.

Nakanishi, M., and Ritter, B. (1992). The inclusionary cultural model. *Journal of Social Work Education 28*(1): 27-35.

Ponce, D. (1995). Consultation on working with Filipino-Americans in the HIV-related mental health encounter. Interview conducted by faculty of the AIDS Education Project, University of Hawaii, Department of Psychiatry.

Proctor, E. K., and Davis, L. E. (1983). Minority content in social work education: A question of objectives. *Journal of Education for Social Work 19*(2): 85-93.

Rocha, B. A. (1985). "Toward an understanding of Hawaiian thinking about mental health." Interview recorded by N. Higginbotham and K. Wight, University of Hawaii, Department of Psychology.

Sata, L. (1990). "Working with persons from Asian backgrounds." Paper presented at the Cross-Cultural Psychotherapy Conference, Hahnemann University, Philadelphia.

Sue, D. W., Arredondo, P., and McDavis, R. J. (1992). Multicultural counseling competencies and standards: A call to the profession. *Journal of Counseling and Development 70:* 477-485.

Sue, D. W. (1981). *Counseling the culturally different*. New York: John Wiley and Sons.

Sue, S. (1994). Mental Health. In N. Zane, D. Takeuchi, and K. Young (Eds.), *Confronting critical health issues of Asian and Pacific Islander Americans*. Thousand Oaks, CA: Sage Publications, pp. 266-288.

Back to the Future:
Survival, Uncertainty, and Hope

Avi Rose

THE ROLLER COASTER OF HOPE

In the June 1997 issue of FOCUS, Michael Shernoff accurately referred to the history of HIV treatment as a roller coaster. Since the beginning, there have been frequent flurries of excitement based on rumors, anecdotal stories, clinical trials, and our deep longing for hopeful news to sustain us. Treatment alternatives have developed, and we have progressed, with many people with HIV living longer and healthier lives. But there have also been many promising developments that ended in disappointment, or at least fell short of initial expectations. Riding this roller coaster has always been part of the picture for people living with HIV as well as all those who provide care for them.

In 1996, with the advent of protease inhibitors and triple-combination antiretroviral therapy, hopes rose to new heights. Among those who have had access to these powerful drugs, many have responded very well, with viral loads plummeting to undetectable levels, immune system measurements rebounding, dramatic reductions of opportunistic infections and symptomatic problems, and miraculous surges of energy. As this chapter is being written in fall 1997, this trend continues for some, though both studies and anecdotal evidence reveal that many are not necessarily staying well on the new medications. The roller coaster continues.

Those who are doing well are finding that living with HIV as a chronic manageable condition is not necessarily as simple as "the epidemic is over for me and I'm getting on with my life." People face a complex set of issues in going about the profound task of reconstructing the future. This chapter will briefly address some of these psychosocial issues, primarily issues of hope, uncertainty, and survival.

This chapter is adapted by the author from his article of the same title published in the June 1997 edition of *FOCUS: A Guide to AIDS Research and Counseling,* a publication of the University of California San Francisco AIDS Health Project.

First, an important caveat, already implied. Especially when viewed globally, it is clear that most people living with HIV do not have access to quality health care and expensive medications; many have no access to simple antibiotics. In the United States, current statistics that show declining death rates and drops in the incidence of opportunistic infections reveal disparities closer to home—that women and people of color, particularly African Americans, are less likely to have adequate access to care and medications. As social workers, we always have a mandate to advocate in the face of such inequities while continuing to provide care to individuals. In this case, our clients' lives may depend on it.

POSITIVE TRENDS

For those who do have access to care and are currently doing well with combination therapy, many positive trends may be acknowledged and celebrated (something we and our clients often do not take the time to do). Many people are feeling strength and vitality that they have not felt in years. Some are returning to work or to school or are thinking about life in ways that they never thought they would again. Others are building new relationships, while some are mustering the courage to leave unhealthy relationships. Some people are feeling new energy and joy in their sexuality. Still others are feeling more motivated to deal with their addictions to alcohol, tobacco, and other drugs, and some are getting back to the gym or other kinds of physical activity. Overall, many individuals feel that now they have a real chance to have a future again. a profoundly hopeful shift away from the despair many have felt in the past.

Certainly, some HIV-positive people have always believed that they would survive for a long time and have lived accordingly, or at least that "you might as well live as though you're going to live." For some of these people, the new surges of hope have not necessarily changed their positive course. But it seems that for everyone touched by the epidemic, no matter how optimistic or pessimistic one was before triple-combination therapy, all have been affected in some way just by having more hope in the air. It affects us to breathe it in.

LIVING WITH UNCERTAINTY

The relative success of triple-combination therapy has been exhilarating. But while exhilaration is hopeful and exciting, it can also leave one feeling dizzy and disoriented. There is still a strong underlying current of uncertainty. Inevitably one wonders how long the new treatments are going to remain effective, whether particular strains of the virus are going to become resistant, what side effects might develop, and whether the next wave of treatment alternatives will come along in time. Some are fearful that they will make major changes in their lives, get sick again, and then be more vulnerable than ever. The risks are not only emotional, but are also directly related to one's finances and the ability to access health care.

Uncertainty is a fact of life. That can be difficult for anyone to accept, let alone those who are living with HIV and whose lives are directly at stake. All of us are challenged by the life task of learning to tolerate uncertainty, let alone to embrace it.

As difficult as that task may be, I have seen individuals find much relief and comfort in constructing ways to face uncertainty head on and live with it, instead of trying to get around it or simply pretending it isn't there. I have seen people find ways to affirm life and keep moving forward and doing what needs to be done, while knowing that anything could happen, and it could happen tomorrow. I am thinking, for example, of a man with AIDS who performed stand-up comedy in between bouts of pneumonia, doing what he felt passionate about and unfusing his humor with the honesty and depth that many experience when confronting their own mortality.

For social workers and other care providers, it is important to help people figure out how to hold different possibilities at the same time and to not get caught just on one end of the spectrum. For example, some deal with uncertainty by expecting only the worst things to happen, which may prepare that person for downturns or disasters, but she or he then runs the risk of not noticing that life is going on in the meantime. On the other hand, some deal with uncertainty by expecting only the best things to happen, but in a way that they pretend that symptoms or limitations simply do not exist, which can actually be dangerous and lead to worse problems. It is important to note that facing uncertainty head-on does not mean the one needs to like it, but it does mean learning to live with it.

Related to this issue of uncertainty is the fact that some persons have a difficult time adjusting to new treatments and attendant hopes simply because they represent change, which requires that once again, a person's sense of certainty needs to shift. Many of those infected with HIV have lived with the expectation that over the next several years, they would gradually get sicker and then die. People have planned their lives according to that scenario, and now they need help to reformulate those plans in order to face a future with new possibilities.

In working with issues of uncertainty, social workers and other care providers need to be scrupulously honest about what we do not know. For some of us, that means dealing with our own discomfort about uncertainty, our own feelings of omnipotence, or our own feelings of responsibility to fix things that are far beyond our control. If we do not pretend to have answers to unanswerable questions, we need to be prepared to deal with—and to honor—clients' anger about that. We need to acknowledge and empathize with the fear, skepticism, weariness, and other feelings behind those questions, and not to fend them off out of our own discomfort. We need to understand how frightening it can be not to have answers. While people of course desire "answers," I am convinced that ultimately people are more deeply reassured by honesty than by pretense, and that maintains the integrity of care providers as well.

In dealing with uncertainty, it is inevitable that we deal with issues of faith and spirituality. I have found it very important to support people's faith and to actively encourage them to explore and strengthen it. For some, it is important to hear that sustaining one's spirit by believing that good things are possible is completely different from pretending that bad things could not possibly happen. And for some, it is also important to hear that it is, in fact, possible to have faith and also be skeptical, which sounds contradictory but nevertheless seems to be true for the majority of HIV-positive people I have encountered. It is also resonant in the experience of many with HIV that their personal relationship with faith and spirituality may have little to do with traditional religious institutions, though an increasing number of those institutions have opened their doors and their hearts to those living with HIV.

PAST, PRESENT, AND FUTURE

Recreating a sense of having a future is an awesome, complex task. Much of it is joyful, but that depends in part on what the future looked like before someone's life was transformed by becoming infected with HIV. No adult came to HIV as a blank state; each already had his or her own history, circumstances, and character. For those who were fortunate to have a sense of purpose and direction in life, felt good about themselves, did meaningful work, had positive and fulfilling relationships with friends and family, and felt connected to a community, going back to the future is likely to be joyful. But for the growing numbers of HIV-positive individuals who had limited job skills and opportunities or were doing work they did not like; felt isolated, anxious, stressed, or depressed; struggled with major addictions; or were barely able to make ends meet, going back to the future may be more fearful. On the one hand, anything is possible; on the other, obstacles, especially those whose prominence were eclipsed by HIV infection, are daunting. And for an increasing number of HIV-positive individuals, dealing with the loss of government benefits or the impact of punitive immigration policies may make it difficult to feel hopeful about the future, no matter how promising new treatments may be. Again our role as advocates comes to the fore, and applies far beyond narrowly defined parameters of "HIV issues."

Facing the future is sometimes complicated by those who feel they were left behind by their uninfected friends in the past. Understandably, people living with HIV measure themselves against their uninfected peers. For those with middle-class opportunities and expectations, this means looking at those who may have settled down to careers, families, financial security, and retirement planning. This is especially difficult for the large number of people whose lives were interrupted by HIV during a stage of life when they ordinarily would have been building the foundation for a seemingly secure future. It is important, though sometimes very difficult, to face feelings of envy, anger, and resentment toward those who are not infected. It is important as well to mourn the lost opportunities of the past in order to move forward in the present and future.

Feelings of abandonment are understandably evident among people for whom new medications are not working well. There have always been disparities in treatment success among people with HIV disease, but the differences now have wieghtier implications attached. Successful treatment is likely to bring exhilaration; treatment failure may lead to feelings of inadequacy, shame, and isolation. This is particularly true in communities hardest hit by the epidemic, where the celebratory atmosphere is inescapable. Shared adversity often fosters camaraderie, and for those who have not yet been doing well with new treatments, the treatment success of others can engender a feeling of being left behind by their treasured comrades. For those who are doing well, it can be difficult to not succumb to survivor guilt, even if survival still feels precarious.

As social workers and other care providers, it is especially important for us to ensure that community and emotional support embrace everyone. We must also be careful not to abandon those who might make us feel impotent and uncomfortable when they do not do as well as they are "supposed to." We need to ensure that there is ample room for the despair of some of our clients, the excitement of others, and the community and solidarity which is still crucial to everyone.

A HISTORY OF SURVIVAL

For years now, there have been those who have identified as long-term survivors of the epidemic. With the advent of combination therapy, growing numbers of HIV-positive people are thinking of themselves as survivors, able to contemplate living a normal life span. Even though the epidemic is not yet over, it is important to think about survival and its implications and also to think about posttraumatic stress. This epidemic will end at some point, and it is not too early to face the challenge of envisioning a future beyond AIDS.

As the AIDS epidemic has taken a more hopeful turn, some social workers and others have begun to reflect on past work with other groups of people who have survived ongoing life-threatening trauma, including survivors of the Holocaust. In reflecting on the experience of previous survivors, we are reminded that there is a long, rich, complex history of human survival. We are not the only people in history who have survived or witnessed massive trauma; it is not only people living with HIV who have returned from the edge of death to another chance to build their lives.

The primary lesson we learn from the past experience of survivors is that "back to the future" is not the same as "back to normal." There are other lessons as well: that it is hard to reconstitute life when so many from the past have not survived; that some individuals numb themselves to get through a traumatic experience and do not know how to reopen themselves to the whole spectrum of human emotions afterward; that for some, the trauma becomes so enveloping that it is hard to figure out how to live without it. We learn from past survivors that those who resisted and stood up (or "acted up") for themselves and for others, even in small ways, often do better afterward. We learn that it helps people to stay connected to the community of others who have gone through the traumatic experience, although it is from these connections that some individuals most want to flee.

We learn from past survivors that it is essential to remember, but not to live only in the past; that it is important for people to tell their stories; and that they remember for their lifetimes who stood with them and who did not. We learn that we all need to remember and honor those who died, participating in individual and communal ritual and acts of affirmation and renewal. We learn that traumatic wounds are deep, and they do not necessarily heal easily or at all. But we also learn from experience that some survivors do go on to create lives that are powerful, beautiful, and inspiring.

The work of survival is both deeply psychological and profoundly mundane. Social workers are particularly well suited to assist people not only with the complex psychological tasks of reconstructing their lives, but also with the concrete tasks of setting goals, choosing priorities, and accessing resources. Even if we continue to ride the roller coaster for a long time to come, there will always be some people engaged in these tasks of reconstruction, and many will need our assistance.

THE WELL OF GRIEF

Grieving in the face of AIDS has become intimidating. There is simply too much of it, and it has become easy to feel that so much has accumulated that people will never be able to catch up with themselves. It is necessary to grieve not only for those who have died, but also for shattered dreams, missed opportunities, and lost hopes. It is easy to understand why some want to run in the other direction from all that grief. But for some, going into that well of grief is the only thing that will make it possible to recover resilience, faith, and a full-hearted commitment to life.

Some of this grief is hard to get at individually and is more easily accessible in the context of community rituals. We—HIV-positive people together with care providers—need opportunities to remember those we have known and loved, recalling them as they really were, not limiting ourselves to a saintly romanticized version. We need to celebrate the lives of those who have died, but not in a way that does not allow us to feel our sorrow.

While listening to and assisting people spill out their pain, social workers need to be clinically vigilant about each person's psychic limitations in coping with trauma. In the face of chronic overwhelming loss, the role of the social worker may be to help people contain their grief as well express it. Those who feel as if they are drowning in sadness, especially those who experience little or no respite from intrusive thoughts and images of death, may need help to define boundaries of grieving, while understanding that such boundaries can change over time.

For social workers and other care providers working with survivors, our simple yet formidable challenge is to be deeply present, respectful, and compassionate with those we serve. This work is formidable primarily because many providers carry our own HIV-related numbness and despair. In the face of overwhelming loss, trauma becomes normalized, and we tend to minimize losses, including (or especially) our own. This is work that absolutely must include collegial support, supervision, and consultation—no one can or should do this work in isolation.

CONCLUDING THOUGHTS

Most people who do HIV work feel passionate about it. That passion has been evidenced by deep commitment and stunning creativity. However, I have seen care providers unwittingly become passionately attached to being needed by their clients. As people live longer and healthier with HIV, some needs do in fact diminish, and some want to pull away from their providers, at least to some degree. Providers may be helpful and supportive, but we also represent AIDS to people who are trying to build new lives that do not revolve around the epidemic. This is not only understandable, it is cause for celebration.

As care providers, we need to be careful not to foster dependence that is unnecessary and unhealthy. To some clients, we may need to directly express our concerns that they may be pulling away too quickly or in ways that may actually endanger their health and well-being. But in most cases, we simply need to be willing to let go and let clients be as independent as they desire, while making sure they know that they can come back to use whenever necessary.

We need to make sure that what we offer clients matches what they currently need, not what they used to need. We need to adapt, helping people figure out what they want to do with their lives now and supporting them as they move forward, not only in terms of work or school, but also in other aspects of life—dating, quitting smoking, cleaning up a police record, dealing with bad credit history, or beginning to job again.

The future is filled with possibilities. We need to hold out that hope for those we care for and for ourselves, without denigrating it or invalidating it as "false hope." Hope is never false. Our proper role as social workers and as human beings, no matter where the roller coaster takes us, is to be the nurturers of people's hopes.

SECTION II:
PRACTICE SETTINGS

Case Management
in AIDS Service Settings

Bruce J. Thompson

WHY DO THIS?
STATEMENT OF THE PROBLEM AND ISSUES

Although case management may be a component of social work services in all practice settings, it is also frequently seen as practice modality unto itself in many AIDS service settings. In this section, the process of AIDS case management and suggestions for increasing the social worker's competence and intervention skills will be presented.[1]

Social workers have long been familiar with case management as a method for minimizing problems in the provision of services to complex client populations such as the deinstitutionalized mentally ill, the frail elderly, and individuals with chemical dependencies. The concept developed from an approach to care that embodied two goals: (1) advocacy and coordination for clients who were dealing with multiple and complex service systems, and (2) efficiency and cost-containment in services allocation. With the increasing emphasis on managed health care in the past decade, case management has become a primary method for monitoring the utilization of health and mental health care services. As case management has evolved in more and more sectors—from the private insurance industry to community-based organizations—its goals and outcomes have not been entirely clear. Studies related to its effectiveness in the provision of service and its efficiency in the containment of costs have been equivocal, particularly so in looking at more vulnerable populations. However, in most parts of the United States, case management is an integral part of services for people with AIDS, and social workers frequently either provide case management or interact with case management when providing services.

Most of this material is derived from the results of the evaluation of the Robert Wood Johnson Foundation AIDS Health Services Program found in Mor, V., Fleischman, J.A., Allen, S.M., and Piette, J.D. (1994), Networking AIDS Services, Ann Arbor, MI: Health Administration Press.

THE PROCESS OF CASE MANAGEMENT

Case management can be subdivided into five basic functions, which are all familiar to social workers: assessment, care plan, linking clients with services, monitoring, and advocacy.

Assessment

The case manager meets with the client and collects information about the person's physical and psychological functioning and about the social environment in which the person lives. Assessment can be done when the client enters the case management system to determine if case management is necessary; this is called triage. Once it has been determined that case management is needed, further assessment may be done so that the client might be assigned to the case manager whose skills (and/or caseload) may best match his or her needs. After assignment, the case manager, working with the individual and his or her significant others, can complete a more thorough assessment for the purpose of developing a care plan. It is important to note that if some triage component is not included in assessment, all clients with HIV may be admitted to the case management system of the agency; this can create an overwhelming caseload for the case managers, create a crisis mode of intervention, and leave no opportunity for the case manager to triage clients out of the active caseload if needs for service lessen. There are a number of standardized case management assessment instruments, some specifically for AIDS service organizations (see Appendix).

Care Plan

Based on information obtained through the assessment, the case manager develops a care plan that identifies the resources which will best meet the client's needs. The care plan frequently is complex and involves many agencies and providers as well as the client. Depending on the setting, the care plan can be developed by an interdisciplinary team or by the case manager with less formal input from the client's providers and significant others. The care plan should be documented in the client's medical record for purposes of accountability, ease of transfer if the case manager changes, and accurate monitoring services and changing needs over time.

Linking Clients with Services

Based on the care plan, the case manager links the client with financial, medical, and social services both inside and outside the agency. This core function of case management is frequently very time-consuming and requires smooth working relationships between the case manager and the rest of the client's medical and social services systems. The case manager obviously should include the client and significant others in the scheduling of appointments and may need to help them create a plan for keeping appointments (e.g., obtaining child care services). Depending on the setting, the case manager may accompany the client to appointments. Linking activities should always be documented in the client's record.

Monitoring

To ensure that the care plan and linking activities are in effect, the case manager will need to monitor the clients in his or her caseload over time. This is particularly important with clients with HIV since their needs may change with crises and plateaus in the course of disease progression. Some needs may be continual such as the need for emotional support; other needs may be intermittent such as the need for home health care after an acute episode. Monitoring can be done through regular appointments with the client at the agency, through home visits, or through telephone contact. Monitoring sometimes works best when the case manager meets for case conferences with others involved in the client's care, even including volunteers. In addition, monitoring functions can be facilitated by software programs that track clients over time. Monitoring activities should be documented in the client's record, and the care plan should be revised as needs change.

Advocacy

Case managers frequently advocate to eliminate barriers to services or to generate needed services for their individual clients. In addition to this client-specific advocacy, they also may become involved in advocacy for systemic changes that may benefit large numbers of clients (Piette et al., 1993). Depending on the setting, the advocacy function of case managers will have more or less prominence and support from agency administration.

ACTION STEPS FOR SUCCESSFUL INTERVENTION

Although the individual social worker will bring his or her practice wisdom and intuitive sense to the functions of case management with people with HIV, the following suggestions may help in each of the five areas outlined.

Assessment

- If a triage system is not in place in your agency, discuss the importance of this with your administration. Meanwhile, design a system of triage within your own caseload, prioritizing clients in terms of acuity of need.
- Ask each client to invite significant other(s) to intake session. Do not assume that your client wants others present without asking before the meeting by phone. Make sure that the meeting place is private and is appropriate for the number of people attending. Allow enough time for establishing a relationship and for completing an adequate assessment.
- Acknowledge that it is frequently difficult for people to ask for help, and be clear about your role as a case manager whose job it is to help the client negotiate the complex system of services he or she may need. If part of your assessment is going to be whether the client currently needs case management (triage), be clear about this at the outset.
- Find out if there are other case managers (from hospital or community settings) involved with your client. Be clear with your client if you intend to confer with them, and make sure that there is a signed "release of information" form that covers all of your potential interactions with people involved in the client's care.
- Use a standardized form (such as the exemplary assessment form of the Institute de Salud Latina/Latino Health Institute, Boston, Massachusetts—in appendix) to gather service need information; such a form will help you to determine the acuity of need. If the form is unclear, not specific enough, or lacking in cultural sensitivity, "translate" it for the client. Ask for elaboration on answers and for input from significant other(s) as appropriate.
- Although you may be using a standardized form, let it "guide" the interview in a manner that allows you to be empathic, nonjudgmental, comfortable with your competence, and kind. Remember that this interview may be the first time that this client has asked for help.
- If needs are identified that clearly cannot be met by the AIDS service system in your community as it exists, let the client know this while taking the need seriously. Do not make promises you cannot keep.
- At the end of the interview, be clear with the client about how, when, and with whom the care plan will be developed and how he or she will be involved in its development.
- Explain the idea of monitoring the care plan and the need for ongoing contact either in person or by telephone. If your policy is that the client

needs to make an appointment to see you, explain this at this meeting. Set up the next contact before ending the assessment session.

Care Plan

- Involve the client and significant other(s) (if desired by the client) in the development of the care plan if you want the plan to be successfully implemented. Start at an appropriate level for the client; do not impose an elaborate "state of the art" care plan on a client who is not ready to use it.
- Whenever possible, use an interdisciplinary team to develop the care plan. The plan will be more successfully implemented if caregivers do not feel that it is being imposed on them. At the very least, obtain informal input from the client's service providers; do not be afraid to call the client's physician or clinic.
- If care of the client is going to affect other family members (e.g., children or elderly parents), include their needs in the care plan. You may need to plan for child care for your client to attend a support group, or you may need to get temporary help from another family member in caring for an elderly parent if your client needs to be hospitalized.
- Be clear with your client that the care plan may change over time as his or her needs change. It may be appropriate to be honest with the client that the care plan may need to be changed because of future changes in program funding.
- Document the entire care plan in the client's chart. Include copies of written correspondence and application forms for entitlement programs, experimental drug protocols, participation in compassionate use pharmaceutical programs, etc.
- Give the client an outline of the care plan with names, telephone numbers, addresses, appointment times, and any other relevant information. Leave plenty of time for questions and reassurances. If your client does not have an appointment book, suggest that he or she get one and use it.

Linking Clients with Services

- Whenever possible, "clear the road" for the client who is going to meet with providers, particularly for the first time. For example, let the support group leader know that the client is coming to the group for the first time.
- Learn who to call in which agency or health care facility to help the client negotiate that particular system; it may very well be your social work

colleague in that agency. This may also apply to entitlement agencies, such as Medicaid, Medicare, or SSI, some of which have particular workers assigned to help people with HIV.

- If your client is being admitted to the hospital and you are a community-based case manager, contact the social work or discharge planning office so that you can be a part of the discharge care plan. If you are a hospital case manager, contact the community-based case manager and invite him or her into the discharge planning process.

- Be as familiar as you can with eligibility criteria, application procedures, etc., for programs that your clients may need, and explain these criteria and procedures to clients. This will include being familiar with anti-HIV therapies, access to and insurance coverage for these therapies, and programs designed to facilitate access (e.g., compassionate use programs, state-funded programs for medication assistance, buyers' clubs, etc.).

- Learn from co-workers how to best negotiate systems of care. If your agency does not have protocols for linking clients with services, you may want to help develop them so that each new worker does not have to "reinvent the wheel."

Monitoring

- When possible, use on-line systems to monitor your clients. This will help to remind you of follow-up times, scheduling, etc., particularly if your caseload is large and complex. It will also help the agency develop a database if it does not already have one.

- For clients with time-limited concerns such as the process of entitlements, monitoring may mean telephoning the client to see if the service has been provided. For clients with intermittent or continuous concerns such as home health care or psychological support, monitoring may mean regularly scheduled meetings at the agency or at home. At the least such clients will require scheduled" phone time.

- Be prepared for changes in the client's functioning—and consequent changes in the care plan. If the client's functioning worsens, it may be time to add new services to the care plan. Similarly, if a client's functioning improves, some services may be no longer necessary. Reassuring the client that services will be resumed if necessary may be helpful, but do not make promises you cannot keep.

- When possible and appropriate, use a case conference approach to monitoring. Meeting with representatives of other agencies involved in the care of your client can be very helpful as long as releases have been obtained and confidentiality issues do not supersede the sharing of information. It may be helpful to include volunteers involved with your client in the case conferences or to confer with them individually.

* Document all monitoring activities in the client's chart, including changes in the care plan. Be prepared to close the case if your client is functioning so well that he or she no longer needs case management services or upon your client's death.

Advocacy

* You may find it useful to distinguish between "client-specific advocacy" and "systems advocacy" and to be clear what your role is as a case manager in your setting. You may be in a unique position to help your client overcome barriers to service, to identify gaps in services, and to suggest creative new ways for health care and social service systems to provide services to clients. Or you may need to "pick your battles" based on your agency's purpose and support or your caseload.
* It is easy to get caught up in the battles and to neglect the service components of case management. Your agency may need to clearly assign systems advocacy and to help you maintain your boundaries in the role of client-specific advocacy. However, no hard and fast rules exist for this issue.
* Finally, you may want to advocate for yourself for the following reasons: (1) so your caseload does not become so large that you cannot perform the functions of case management and become strictly crisis-driven; (2) so you can absorb the trauma of this work and not become overwhelmed and burned out from it; and (3) so you can provide your clients with the compassion, competence, and kindness they need.

RECOMMENDED READINGS

Piette, J., Fleishman, J.A., Mor, V., and Thompson, B. (1992). The structure and process of AIDS case management. *Health and Social Work, 17*(1), 47-56.

Piette, J.D., Thompson, B.J., Fleishman, J.A., and Mor, V. (1993). The organization and delivery of AIDS case management. In V.J. Lynch, G.A. Lloyd, and M.F. Fimbres (Eds.), *The changing face of AIDS: Implications for social work practice* (pp. 39-62). Westport, CT: Auburn House.

National Association of Social Workers. (1991). *NASW standards for social work case management.* Silver Spring, MD: NASW Press.

Appendix

LATINO HEALTH INSTITUTE
SCREENING/INITIAL REQUEST FOR SERVICES

Has the eligibility criteria for the services/program been explained to the caller? ☐ yes, ☐ no.

Is the caller clear that many of the programs are only for persons living with HIV/AIDS? ☐ yes, ☐ no.

Does the consumer meet the basic eligibility requirements for the service of interest? ☐ yes, ☐ no.

If you answered yes to all three questions then continue. If you did not then the referral may not be appropriate.

If the caller would like to continue, let them know that you will be asking a few questions that will help you both determine if LHI is the best place for them to be receiving services.

Name of caller_____ phone_____

Agency and address_____

What is the caller's relationship to the consumer?_____

What is the reason for the referral?_____

_____

_____

_____

_____

Consumer's name:_____phone_____

Current address_____ zip code_____

May we leave a message?_____   Primary language_____

	yes	no		yes	no
Does he/she have a history of substance abuse?	☐	☐	History of mental illness?	☐	☐
Is he/she actively using?	☐	☐	Psychiatric hospitalizations?	☐	☐
How long has he/she been clean?	☐	☐	Previous suicide attempts?	☐	☐
Is individual homeless?	☐	☐	Is he/she under psychiatric care?	☐	☐
			Is he/she prone to violence?	☐	☐
			Is he/she actively suicidal?	☐	☐
			Is he/she actively psychotic?	☐	☐

*If you answered yes to any of the bolded questions, and the caller **is not** under psychiatric care, you should inform the caller that LHI is currently not staffed to offer the type of intervention this person needs. The exception is if they are interested in the SSI program.*

Check the type of services that are being requested

Housing   **Inter/Advocacy**   **HIV case management**   **Benefits**   **Breast cancer**
perm ____   —   info/referral ____   SSI ____   screening ____
trans ____   long term ____   follow-up ____

Developmental Disability   **Comadres**
child ____   pregnant ____
adult ____   baby under one year ____

HIV SERVICES
CONSUMER INFORMATION AND NEEDS ASSESSMENT

Identifying Information

Client Code # _____ D.O.B._____ Age _____ Gender_____

Name_____

Address: _____ Telephone # _____

Primary language _____ Ethnicity _____

Who may we call in case of an emergency? _____

Telephone # _____ Does this person know your HIV status?   yes   no

Employment (current) _____ Telephone # _____

May we leave messages at your work?   yes   no   May we leave a message at home?   yes   no

Does your employer know your HIV status?   yes   no

Referred by: _____ Agency: _____

What other agencies or people are helping you?

_____ contact_____ #_____

_____ contact_____ #_____

_____ contact_____ #_____

_____ contact_____ #_____

Transportation

How do you get to the doctor, shopping, errands, etc.? _____

Is transportation a problem for you?   yes   no   sometimes

If answered sometimes, ask him/her:

In what situations is transportation a problem? _____

Do you have: MBTA pass _____   taxi vouchers available to you _____   Medicaid transportation _____

DOES CLIENT NEED TRANSPORTATION ASSISTANCE? _____

Financial

Are you employed?   yes   no

Have you ever applied for benefits?   yes   no   If yes, When? _____

Are you receiving benefits?   yes   no   **IF YES, CIRCLE ALL THAT APPLY**

AFDC   SSI   SSDI   GR   Unemployment   Food Stamps   WIC   Sect. 8   other _____

What is your monthly income? $_____

Are you able to support yourself and your family on this amount of money?   yes   no

DOES CLIENT NEED HELP WITH BENEFITS OR MONEY MANAGEMENT? _____

Legal

Have you ever been
   convicted of a crime?   yes   no   Name of parole/probation officer_____

Are you on probation or parole?   yes   no   Telephone # _____

Does your probation/parole officer
   know your HIV status?   yes   no

Do you have any open court cases?   yes   no

Do you have any outstanding warrants?   yes   no

Do you have any of the following?

Power of Attorney _____ (If you were unable to care for yourself for any reason, a power of attorney allows you to name someone whom you trust to take care of your personal business, such as writing and depositing your checks, dealing with your landlord, etc.)

Living Will _____ (This is a legal document that allows you to give instructions on how you would like your affairs dealt with if you should die. People include things like who will raise their children, burial wishes, desires not to have their lives prolonged by machines.)

Health Care Proxy _____ (This is someone whom you have legally chosen to make all of your health care decisions for you if you are too sick to do so yourself.)

Affidavit of Guardianship _____ (If you have children, this is where you name someone whom you want to continue to raise your children. If you have someone in mind, but have not filed an affidavit, the arrangement is not legal and could be challenged by other family members.)

Would you like information on how to make any of the arrangements just mentioned?

     yes   no   maybe in the future

DOES CLIENT NEED HELP WITH ANY LEGAL ISSUES?_____

Medical

Physician: _____ Telephone # _____

Address: _____

When were you diagnosed with HIV? _____

Do you have any ideas about how you got the virus?   yes   no

How? _____

Are you seeing any other doctors or specialists?   yes   no   If **yes**, for what condition?_____

_____

Please describe how your health has been within the last six months.

_____

_____

What is your T-cell count? _____

What medications are you taking?

_____   _____   _____

_____   _____   _____

How often do you see the doctor? _____

Do you feel that you understand everything your doctor tells you about your health? _____

_____

Do you need someone to translate for you during your medical appointments?   yes   no

DOES CLIENT NEED INTERPRETATION/ADVOCACY SERVICES? _____

DOES CLIENT NEED MEDICAL INFORMATION? _____

Social and Family

Marital status:

_____single _____married _____divorced _____separated _____ living with partner _____widowed

Is your family there for you when you need them? yes no sometimes

Do they know your HIV status? yes no Who in your family *does not* know? _____

Who do you turn to when you need help? _____

In what ways are they helpful to you? _____

Do you have any children? yes no (Gather the appropriate information listed in boxes.)

CHILDREN

name	sex	birthday	custody*	whereabouts	health problems

*specify voluntary or involuntary, and with whom children are currently living

Do you have anyone who helps you take care of your children? yes no

Have you ever been involved with the Department of Social Services?

When? _____ Reason _____

What happened? _____

Is there any information about your family that is important for me to know? (Secondary client information)

_____
_____
_____
_____
_____

DOES CLIENT NEED SUPPORT/REFERRAL WITH CHILDCARE? _____

COULD CLIENT BENEFIT FROM ADDITIONAL SUPPORT? _____

Housing

Where have you been living?

___ street   ___ shelter   ___ transitional housing   ___ substance abuse treatment facility
___ psychiatric facility   ___ hospital   ___ jail/prison   ___ living with family friend
___ other—specify _____   ___ living in own home

Are you:

___ paying more than 50 percent of your income for rent?

___ living in physically substandard conditions?

___ facing an eviction within 1 to 3 months?

DOES CLIENT NEED HELP WITH HOUSING ISSUES? _____

Substance Abuse History

Have you ever been in a detox program or residential treatment program? If so, include dates and the name of center._____

Are you currently using drugs?   yes   no   If yes, what do you use? _____

How much? _____   How often? _____   When did you last use? _____

IS CLIENT IN NEED OF A DETOX OR TREATMENT PROGRAM? _____

If **not** using drugs, How long have you been drug free? _____

How many times before this time have you tried to become drug free? _____

Please tell me what you are doing to stay away from drugs _____
_____

IS CLIENT IN NEED OF A REFERRAL TO AA, OUTPATIENT PROGRAM TO SUPPORT HIS/HER SOBRIETY? _____

Mental Health

Do you experience any of the following?

___ no energy   ___ nervousness   ___ depression   ___ hear voices

___ falling/staying asleep   ___ angry outbursts   ___ poor appetite   ___ excessive worry

___ poor memory   ___ sadness   ___ anxiety   ___ very happy and then very sad

Have you ever tried to kill yourself?   yes   no   If yes, when and how? _____
_____

Have you ever spoken to a psychiatrist before?   yes   no   If yes, what was the problem; when did it happen, and where were you treated?

Problem   When   Where treated

_____
_____

Are you seeing a psychiatrist now?   yes   no

Name _____ Telephone # _____

Did they give you any medication?   yes   no

Do they know your HIV status?   yes   no

Do you have a counselor or therapist? yes   no

    If yes, how long have you been seeing them?

Name _____ Telephone # _____

DOES CLIENT NEED A MENTAL HEALTH REFERRAL? ____

Questions to Staff Person

(Assessment of need) What does this person need help with?

_____

_____

_____

_____

_____

_____

Immediate intervention and Service Plan (What are you ACTUALLY going to do?)

_____

_____

_____

_____

_____

Documentation

Has client signed all of the appropriate releases   yes   no

    (doctor, service providers, etc.)?

Has HIV status been verified?   yes   no

    Type of documentation? _____

Has income been verified?   yes   no

    Type of documentation? _____

_____   _____

Your Signature   Date

PART A:
SERVICES IN HEALTH SETTINGS

Discharge Planning in Acute Care

Judith Hanson Babcock

To know AIDS is to know social work.

—Harvey Gochros

WHY DO THIS?
STATEMENT OF THE PROBLEM AND ISSUES

All of us are affected by the stigma associated with HIV/AIDS. We have grown up in a society in which homosexuality and IV drug use are taboo. Many people in this country, in our own communities, in our own workplaces, perhaps even in and among our own families and friends believe that "people who get AIDS deserve it!" No person you meet who is living with HIV or who cares about someone who has HIV/AIDS will be unaffected by this societal context. Nor will the health care professionals with whom you work. Nor will you be unaffected. People will ask you, "Why are you working with people with HIV/AIDS? Why do you care?" Initially, the answer may be, "Because it's my job. I'm responsible for discharge planning for all patients who come to my unit."

Although hospital social workers are more likely to encounter people with HIV if they live in areas where there are populations who are at greater risk, it is essential that we consider the possibility that anyone we meet may have contracted HIV, regardless of age, sex, sexual orientation, or other sociocultural factors. Many people have gone undiagnosed because they did not fit some stereotype of people considered by the health care provider(s) to be "at risk." (In my experience this has been particularly true of women, who may be less aware of the possibility of infection; however, many men who have had sex with other men, and many men and women who have shared needles in the past are reluctant to share such "taboo" information with a doctor or nurse.)

A social worker who is comfortable taking a history that includes asking about possibly risky behaviors in a matter-of-fact, nonjudgmental way may actually help to determine an otherwise "missed diagnosis." (He or she may also help prevent HIV infection by providing education about behaviors that put people at risk.)

EXAMPLES OF HOW THE ISSUE MAY PRESENT

In any community in the country, a person with AIDS may be returning to the home of his or her family for care. This person may be the first—or one of a few—cases of HIV to present to the local hospital. Even if the staff members have been taught "the facts" about HIV/AIDS, their lack of experience and/or their fears and prejudices may interfere with sensitive care of the patient and the patient's caregivers. Staff members may think the patient should be transferred to a larger medical center where there's more expertise with AIDS; and the advantages and disadvantages of this option need to be weighed with the patient and caregivers, just as it is with other serious illnesses. (Sometimes care can be provided locally with consultation from the larger medical center, as is often done with cancer patients.)

If the patient needs home care or placement in another facility, again the providers may have no experience with the medical or psychosocial needs of the patient and his or her family. Nursing homes have often been reluctant to take people with AIDS, ostensibly because of their labor-intensive needs. (People in need of nursing home care are often those whose dementia or severe debilitation from chronic diarrhea; thus, they require frequent attention from the staff). However, with levels of care being continually redefined by the "health care reform process," a patient may need a place to go between a skilled nursing facility or chronic care hospital (which may keep him or her only as long as IV medications are being administered) and home with hospice care. In addition, many people with AIDS choose to remain on active treatment to prevent blindness from CMV (cytomegalovirus) retinitis or to control intractible diarrhea, for example, from MAC (mycobacterium avium complex) or cryptosporidium, which may prevent them from being eligible for in-patient or at-home hospice services, even in the final weeks of their lives.

The hospital social worker can provide a valuable contribution to the care team by helping to clarify the following: (1) what the preferences of the patient and caregivers are; (2) what options exist to fit those preferences; and (3) what care can be covered by the patient's insurance.

FACTS THE SOCIAL WORKER NEEDS TO KNOW BEFORE PROCEEDING

The social worker must know the following basic information about concrete services.

What resources are available in your community for providing AIDS-sensitive support?

Where is the nearest AIDS service organization, and what resources can it provide to someone in your community? Examples of such resources are pro bono legal services to help with discrimination issues and/or making a will, etc., and AIDS education and training to local caregivers, including health care professionals.

What help can your state's Department of Public Health offer? Examples include providing the training necessary for a local home care agency to deal with a patient with AIDS and providing financial assistance for AIDS-related medications?

Does your patient's insurance company have HIV case management services? (Such a case manager can help advocate for coverage for less expensive alternatives to hospitalization, for example, home or hospice care, even if those benefits are not in the patient's policy).

If you are in a community that has not had much, if any, experience with HIV/AIDS, what people or organizations (for example, churches, home care agencies) may be willing to provide assistance with the development of resources that are needed, for example, transportation, meals, respite care, and pastoral care?

The social worker must know the following basic information about the psychosocial issues of those affected by HIV/AIDS.

This is not just another "terminal illness." If this same "too young" person presented with an equally life-threatening diagnosis of leukemia, he or she would probably call family and friends for support. In contrast, people diagnosed with HIV often choose to keep their diagnosis a secret. They may even express the hope that they will die in an accident, or that their elderly parents will die before learning of their diagnosis. Coming into the hospital may expose people with HIV to the critical scrutiny of people who consider their lifestyles taboo. They, and in turn their partners and families, are often forced to "come out." Because families share the stigma, people with HIV often choose to lie about the diagnosis to other family members and friends, which adds to their sense of isolation and shame.

For the patient, each hospitalization is a "predictable crisis" (see appendix). In addition to his or her exposure to the disease (people with HIV are often repeatedly asked, "How did you get this?"), the patient is likely to be experiencing fear that the cause of the current problem may not be found, and/or that a helpful treatment may not exist. In their weakened, exposed state, patients are vulnerable to feeling that "maybe society is right: maybe I deserve this!" One can only imagine the impact of meeting a doctor, nurse, or clergyperson who shares this view!

What social workers need to know in this context is that our basic training and values make a critical difference. "Start where the client is." Respect the worth of each individual. Nonjudgmental acceptance and caring are the strongest antidotes to shame. You do not have to know everything about HIV to be helpful! Our best help is often that of listening to the patient (and caregivers) and then clarifying for the team what is the patient's/family's experience of this particular phase of the illness. The awareness that we do not have all the answers can help us to remain open to the unique way in which each individual responds to the complexities of living with HIV/AIDS.

KEY QUESTIONS TO ASK THE CLIENT

Before you begin asking the client questions, ask yourself, "What do I need to know?" For example, do you need to know how the client got infected? Many people say, "I have HIV or AIDS; what difference does it make how I got it?" (*Note:* People appreciate being given the opportunity to disclose what they are ready to share instead of being asked directly.)

It can be helpful to know the following information, but it is important to check with the patient about his or her comfort level with the questions as you proceed. A good way to begin is to ask the following questions:

1. What do you think I need to know to understand your situation? (How much of your story would you like to share?)
2. How long have you known you were HIV positive?
3. What made you decide to get tested? (This is where the risk factors may be disclosed.)

4. How was it for you to find out?
5. What has changed over the weeks/months/years since diagnosis?
6. What has helped?
7. What has been less than helpful?
8. Who knows about your diagnosis and why you may have been at risk for HIV? (*Note:* If the person shares with you that he or she is gay, asking about whether the family members know and what their response was/is can be an indication of what the patient faces in disclosing his or her HIV diagnosis. In general, I have found that if someone is comfortable being open with his or her family about being gay, he or she finds it less daunting to disclose the diagnosis of HIV.)
9. Is that okay for now, or are there other people who need to be told?
10. Does your family (that is, next of kin) know? If not, have you designated someone as your health care proxy (or durable power of attorney)? If not, are you aware that a doctor has to contact your next of kin (spouse, parent, sibling) if there is an emergency situation (for example, a car accident) in which you cannot tell the doctor what you want him or her to do unless you have legally designated an alternative person (partner, friend, sibling, etc.)? If your family does not know, do you want help telling them? If your family does know, have they been able to tell other people, or do they need support?
11. Do you have enough support? (financial, physical, emotional, spiritual?) Who is there for you? Is (are) that person(s) OK? (*Note:* The person's caregiver(s)—whether partner or parents—may not be capable of providing the support that's needed because of their own illness or substance abuse or fear or many other factors). Would you and/or your caregivers be interested in a support group (if one is available)?

QUESTIONS SPECIFICALLY RELATED TO DISCHARGE PLANNING

First, ask yourself the following questions:

1. What level of care will the patient need, and what options exist to provide that care?
2. Is there any question that the patient's judgment is impaired, either by HIV dementia, or because his or her illness or chronic drug/alcohol abuse?
3. Does the patient's competency to make his or her own decisions need to be determined before a discharge plan can be completed?
4. Does the patient need substance abuse rehabilitation? Inpatient or

outpatient? Is the patient willing to participate? Is there a facility or program available that has experience with people with HIV/AIDS?
5. Does the hospital staff have any concerns about the patient's safety if he or she were to return home alone?

With this information in the background, you may then ask the patient the following questions:

1. What help (if any) do you think you may need when you leave the hospital? Are you strong enough to get to the bathroom, to fix your own meals, to do your own laundry, to go grocery shopping, or to do your cleaning?
2. If there is (are) a care partner(s) available, you may ask whether that person(s) feels comfortable with the patient's plan of care. If serious differences exist about what is needed, a team meeting with patient and caregivers may help to develop a plan everyone can live with. (*Note:* A patient may be able to hear from the hospital team what he or she would not be willing to hear from family or friends about what help may be needed at home. Also, such a meeting can give family and friends a chance to clarify their limitations. They may need permission and/or urging to take care of themselves before the care needs become overwhelming. This can be one of the most important contributions of social work to the discharge planning process, that is, setting up adequate supports for both the patient and the caregivers.)
3. Finally, I ask the patient, "Is there anything you want help with or want to know more about?" For example, depending upon the stage of the illness, "Do you want talk about:
   • telling people at work or where you live; possible consequences of disclosing your diagnosis; laws protecting your confidentiality?
   • other legal issues, for example, your health care proxy, will, or power of attorney?
   • telling your family?
   • telling prospective sexual partners?
   • concerns about changing jobs/insurance?
   • support groups for yourself/partner/friends/family?
   • home care, hospice care, or death and dying?"

The key differences that distinguish the discharge planning process for people with HIV from the discharge process for other patients include the following:

1. The patient with HIV may have more difficulty trusting that the system, including the social workers, can understand and help.

2. The patient may not feel able to ask for help from "traditional" sources of support, for example, family, because of disclosure issues.
3. The patient's family may be unaware of his or her diagnosis, which has legal implications.
4. The patient's judgment may be impaired by HIV-related dementia or substance abuse.
5. There may be a lack of needed resources, especially AIDS-sensitive resources.

CULTURAL COMPETENCY CONSIDERATIONS

We can never fully understand our own sociocultural background, let alone those that differ from our own. But we can try to learn as much as possible about the sociocultural context of our patient population(s). It can be helpful to explore particularly the sociocultural attitudes toward the following:

- Men having sex with other men (In many cultures homosexuality is taboo, but even in our dominant culture, men who have "recreational sex" with other men may not consider themselves or be considered by others to be "gay.")
- IV drug use
- Seeking professional help for health and/or mental health reasons
- The meaning of a "social worker"
- The meaning of "illness"
- Ideas about healing and healers, including alternatives to what *we* consider "traditional" (Western/dominant culture) medicine
- The role of the family and other natural helping systems

Again, we can never assume we understand. You might ask a patient, "Can you help me understand what having HIV means to you and to the family (culture) you come from?"

Regardless of your own cultural background, it is worth exploring what ideas the parents of a gay son have about "how he turned out that way." Heredity? An "overly protective mother"? An "absent father"? Is it "a choice" he made? Can psychiatry or religion change someone's sexual orientation? These beliefs can profoundly affect the attitudes of the parents toward themselves and their son. (*Note:* I often explore with parents the effect of their beliefs on themselves and on their relationship with their son. For example, I might ask, "Is this a preferred way to view yourself and/or your son or would you be interested in exploring other ideas that may fit better with the way you'd like to think and feel about yourselves and your relationship with your son?" This is a narrative therapy technique for introducing the idea that people's "beliefs" are affected by their social context, and that beliefs can be questioned based on the real effects on their lives and relationships. I find this approach enormously helpful in clarifying the basis of the stigma attached to AIDS.)

ACTION STEPS FOR SUCCESSFUL INTERVENTION

1. Start where the client is.
2. Accept the person where he or she is and honor the person's right to make choices with which you do not agree, for example, *not* telling their families, or choosing to have a baby. (Get *excellent* supervision to help you deal with the client's complex responses as well as the ethical dilemmas this work may present for you.)
3. Invite the person(s) to share his or her (their) stories regarding the impact of HIV in the past and present as well as hopes and fears about the future.
4. Look for the strengths the person has drawn on; and expand on that story.
5. Be prepared to advocate for services that are needed and for insurances (including state welfare systems) to pay for those services.
6. Be prepared to educate patients, families, hospital staff, and outside agencies about the psychosocial needs of people affected by AIDS, for example, if an agency is not AIDS-sensitive, call the area AIDS service organization or your state's department of public health to do in-service education and training.
7. Consider starting a support group for anyone in the community who is affected by AIDS.
8. Finally, be prepared to have your life change forever. You will never see things in the same way again. You will become increasingly aware— as you get to know the *people* behind the stereotypes—how many assumptions about various marginalized groups have been part of your own cultural conditioning.

POTENTIAL BARRIERS TO SUCCESSFUL INTERVENTION

1. Our own prejudices and fears—a reflection of our sociocultural background
2. Lack of basic information about AIDS and fear of becoming infected ourselves

3. Lack of information about the medical and psychosocial impact of HIV
4. Lack of information about resources
5. Lack of resources, especially AIDS-sensitive resources
6. Patient's discomfort with the social worker because of differing backgrounds and/or a presumed lack of understanding or acceptance (For example, any member of a minority that is stigmatized or discriminated against, including gay/bisexual men, IV drug users, and people of color, may expect to be treated with the same disrespect or even contempt in the hospital setting that that he or she has experienced in the larger society.)
7. Following our agenda (or the hospital's) instead of the patient's, for example, "She should be telling her family (or spouse or children, etc.) about her diagnosis or prognosis!"
8. Shortened length of stays, which often do not allow enough time to form the kind of relationships needed to deal with such complex issues
9. A lack of understanding within hospital systems of the kind of support social workers need to do this work, including the following:
   • reasonable case loads
   • good supervision
   • time to educate ourselves about complex clinical issues and ever-changing resources
   • time to grieve
   • time to offer (or create) supports of various kinds in the absence of natural support systems, for example, time to do short-term individual, couples, family, bereavement, and group work in the absence of such resources in the community

INFORMATION THE CLIENT SHOULD KNOW BEFORE TAKING ACTION

1. How your hospital system works; patients' rights and responsibilities; and your role as social worker
2. Laws protecting confidentiality of HIV status (Staff in hospital and referral agencies may need to be reminded that it is against the law to disclose someone's HIV status without his or her written consent.)
3. Your limits concerning patient confidentiality, for example, what to do if a patient disclosed that he or she is having unprotected sex with a spouse or partner who has not been informed of his or her diagnosis
4 Benefits he or she is entitled to, for example:
   • state/federal programs through welfare and/or social security
   • availability of case management through Medicaid or private insurance

- specific HIV services available through the area AIDS service organization and/or the department of public health
- options for follow-up health care and support services through the hospital and other agencies

POLICY IMPLICATIONS AND RELATED ACTIONS

Many of the current and proposed changes in the provision and funding for health care, welfare, and housing—for example, handing over power to the states to decide who needs assistance—leaves every stigmatized minority vulnerable to further cutbacks in services. Sometimes people are forced to change health care providers if their workplace changes insurance coverage. For people with life-threatening illnesses who find it difficult to build trusting relationships, this can be devastating. Welfare mothers with HIV who are not quite sick enough to qualify for disability worry that they will be forced to go to work. And with patients' lengths of stay becoming shorter, hospital social workers are lucky if they even get to meet the patients on their floors let alone form relationships with them. This necessitates forming a network with out-of-hospital providers to ensure continuity of care.

Policy

If you have not yet begun—or are just beginning to work with people affected by HIV/AIDS—you may prepare yourself in a number of ways. Reading this book will give you a basic introduction as well as refer you to resources for further information. You may receive training from your local Red Cross or your state's department of public health in basic "AIDS 101." The annual "Social Work and AIDS" conference is a wonderful way to meet people who are presenting basic and innovative approaches to working in a variety of settings.

If you have not yet known anyone with HIV/AIDS, you may want to call your nearest AIDS service organization and volunteer to be a "buddy" or to colead a support group or to provide pro bono supportive counseling for someone in your area who is affected by AIDS.

Wherever you are, you can raise AIDS awareness and provide critical support to people in your area who are affected by someone with HIV/AIDS, even if your hospital has not yet had its first patient with HIV. You can begin by letting the community know you are interested in meeting people who have a loved one with HIV/AIDS and gradually form a "community of care" to provide support and outreach to others.

Appendix

PREDICTABLE CRISES IN THE COURSE OF LIVING WITH AIDS

1. Finding out a present or former sexual partner has tested positive for the virus (HIV).
2. Finding out your own HIV test results. (Don't assume it isn't a crisis if someone finds out he or she is "negative." As one such young man said, "I thought this was something we were going to go through together.")
3. Telling your family of origin (whether it is forced on you by a medical crisis or your own decision that it is time they knew, there's always the fear of rejection and the anxiety about how they will respond).
4. The first progression of the disease (from "asymptomatic" to "symptomatic," even if the symptom is minor; because it is no longer possible to deny that the virus is "alive and well").
5. Starting any drug protocol (even if you are asymptomatic, there's the continual reminder of the presence of the virus).
6. Each new opportunistic infection (again, one's attempt to hold onto the hope that "I'll beat this thing" is chipped away).
7. The first hospitalization for an HIV–related problem (often the first hospitalization since one's birth!).
8. Every subsequent hospitalization. (What's happening now? What more will I have to go through? Is this an infection they can treat?)
9. Having to tell someone at work because of regular absences for medical treatment or for illness.
10. Having to stop work. (How will I survive economically? emotionally? Will I lose my insurance?)
11. Visible signs of the disease (KS lesions, weight loss).
12. Any loss of functioning resulting in the need for help with one's care.
13. The need to change one's living situation, whether for financial or for health reasons.
14. The occurrence of other life crises, e.g., illness or death of friends or family members, that may happen during the course of the illness.

Addendum (1997): With the advent of new drugs that hold the promise that life may be extended, perhaps indefinitely; don't assume that crises may not accompany this new era.

- Many people left work and/or ran up large credit card bills and/or cashed in their life insurances so they could make the most of their "limited" time.
- Many people left work long enough ago that they would not be able to return to the same kind of job (even if they're well enough) without retraining.
- How does one explain an absence from the workforce of one to five years to a potential employer?
- Having a limited time to live "lets one off the hook," for example, it may allow one to make unreasonable demands on others.
- Unhappy relationships are sometimes tolerated because they aren't expected to go on forever or because someone would feel guilty leaving or cutting off contact in spite of impossible demands.
- Having adjusted one's expectations, hopes, dreams, and plans from a seemingly limitless future to a very finite length of time, the readjustment of one's view of his/her own future can be daunting, even overwhelming.
- For those for whom the new drugs are not working or cause intolerable side effects, they are in the painful situation of being left out of "the miracle" they see and hear about happening to others. (Their families may wonder what's wrong with them or their doctors that they *are not* getting better!)

And, for some, life has always been such a struggle (because of severe depression, anxiety, abuse, etc.) that "seeing the dark at the end of the tunnel was a relief!" (to quote one person's comment to me).

So, again, don't make any assumptions about what may constitute a crisis for the people you meet.

Involving Family and Significant Others in Acute Care

Judith Hanson Babcock

WHY DO THIS?
STATEMENT OF THE PROBLEM AND ISSUES

The question of "involving family and significant others" in the hospital care and discharge planning for people with HIV/AIDS reveals complex legal, ethical, and practical issues that we do not usually confront with other patient populations. For example, a cancer patient may not wish to have just any friend, colleague, or family member know his or her diagnosis, but a hospital staff member would not be a risk for a lawsuit if such a diagnosis were thoughtlessly disclosed. Not so with HIV. And for good reason. The cancer patient would not be as likely to risk loss of job, housing, even family connections by disclosure of his or her diagnosis.

Thus, the social worker involved with people with HIV/AIDS needs to be sensitive to a variety of issues—some obvious, some subtle.

- We need to broaden our definition of "family" to include "family of choice," that is, the partner and/or friends that may be the primary support system of many individuals.
- We need to broaden our understanding of, and appreciation for, the reasons why people with HIV/AIDS may not want to disclose their diagnosis to their families of origin. (*Note:* Many people want to wait until they are too sick to keep HIV a secret any longer from their families. Since we are trained to think of the individual in his or her social context, it can be difficult to remain patient and respectful as we think of time running out and the impact on families of having little or no time to absorb and respond to the crisis of disclosure. However, one of the strongest desires expressed by people with HIV is the desire to have as normal a life as possible, not to allow HIV to take over their lives. They know that disclosing their diagnosis to anyone will inevitably change things forever. People often want to postpone this process as long as possible, sometimes to pro-

101

tect others from the inevitable pain of finding out such devastating news, but also to protect their own need for normalcy. We need to be respectful of the patient's sense of timing concerning disclosure.)

- We need to allow the patient to define who, if any, are the "family members" he would want to include in discharge planning. (*Note:* A partner coming into the hospital setting may be facing his or her own coming out issues in terms of lifestyle issues and/or HIV status).
- In spite of the difficulties, including a patient's family can do the following:

    1. Clarify and possibly expand and strengthen the patient's support system and decrease the sense of isolation for both patient and caregivers
    2. Allow the caregivers a chance to express their view(s) about what would be helpful, including increased support to them
    3. Inform caregivers about resources
    4. If the patient chooses to inform his or her partner, family of origin, and/or friends of the diagnosis, we can provide opportunities for them to receive information and support

EXAMPLES OF HOW THE ISSUE MAY PRESENT

1. The family of origin of a gay man with AIDS may, upon learning of his diagnosis and/or hospitalization, arrive on the scene and want to "take over" for the patient and/or his partner or "family of choice." When parents are just learning about the diagnosis when the patient is on his deathbed, their anger and grief can get acted out, for example, against the partner by attempting to override his wishes and even overturn a will, thus disinheriting him.
2. The father (from a heterosexual couple) of young children may not be able to face telling his children that he is going to die, let alone face the questions that may arise from older children about how he became infected. His wife, even if she were aware of his "other life" (bi-sexual or IDU), may be so angry that their cover of respectability has been shattered that she may take out her anger on him by neglecting his care.

FACTS THE SOCIAL WORKER NEEDS
TO KNOW BEFORE PROCEEDING

1. Regardless of the gender, sexual orientation, or means of disease transmission of the patient you are meeting, all are profoundly affected by

the stigma that accompanies HIV. Women who were infected by blood transfusions and men with hemophilia infected by Factor 8 (a clotting factor) may be considered "innocent victims" by some in our society, but they experience many of the same effects of the stigma, including fear of disclosure and rejection.

2. When you are dealing with gay men, the more open they have been about their lifestyle with their families of origin, the easier it may be for them to share their HIV diagnosis. (They are not facing a "double disclosure," and their families are more likely to have some idea that the person is at risk for HIV.)

3. If a gay man experienced rejection because of disclosure of his sexual preference, he is likely to fear rejection now. (*Note:* I choose to be curious about this. There are always other stories we are not hearing. Often the sexuality disclosure accompanied leaving home as a teenager or young adult, a transition that is likely to be "rocky" for anyone, gay or straight. However, the "rejection piece" often gets "frozen in time" and can sometimes be "thawed" if it is revisited and joined with the other stories. For example, I often find that parents—and even siblings—felt as rejected by the gay son as he felt rejected by them when he moved away to some city where he could find a more comfortable niche.

4. There is a higher-than-average incidence of histories of substance abuse in the HIV population. This may be related in various ways to lifestyle issues, including using substances for recreational use and/or to dull the pain of societal abuse, but it may also be the result of childhood family abuse (substance, physical, and sexual abuse).

5. People with histories of IV drug use may have families that are already "burned out" by past difficulties associated with substance abuse. Or they may have families that are already providing care and support for the patient and/or his or her children. (*Note:* People with substance abuse histories may also have had experiences with child protection workers—often referred to as "social workers"—which may affect their reception of our offers to help, especially when we start asking questions about their "families.")

KEY QUESTIONS TO ASK THE CLIENT

As I suggested earlier, first ask yourself, "What do I think I need to know about this patient's family in order to be helpful? Why?" Then as you approach the patient to determine what he or she thinks you need to know, try to approach the patient from a stance of "not knowing" what is best for him or her.

You may ask the open-ended question, "What do you think is important for me to know about your family?" Or you may ask the following questions with the respectful permission of the patient. (I might say, "I'd like to ask you some questions about your family. Please feel free to decline to answer or to ask me why I'm asking that question." This, again, is a narrative therapy approach designed to unbalance the unequal power differential between social worker and patient, which can reinforce the stigmatized position of the patient as "other," or "them," compared to "us.")

- Whom do you consider to be your family, that is, who are the people with whom you have mutually caring relationships?
- Who knows about your diagnosis?
- Have you told anyone in your family of origin?
- If so, whom have you told?
- What were their responses?
- Have the people you have told been able to talk about it with anyone else? (*Note:* It is important to encourage people to give anyone they tell permission to share the news with at least one other person so that they are not isolated with such a painful secret. Also, if parents have told no one in their extended families or none of their friends, it can be an indication of their need for help to deal with the stigma and shame).
- If you have not told your family of origin, why is that? (*Note:* Proceed gently, with respect for people's right to choose whom and when they tell, but also listen for indications of underlying shame and/or fear of rejection.) You might ask questions such as the following:

—What could you tell me about your family that would help me understand why you're reluctant to tell them? (*Note:* This is where you might get some history of abuse, if the patient feels safe enough to share it.)

—Have you thought of telling anyone in your family in the future? Whom have you thought of telling? (*Note:* It is not unusual for a patient to tell the sibling(s) he or she feels closest with first.) Under what circumstances? (*Note:* If the patient says, "When I get sicker," and you know they may not have much time left, you may want to "reframe" the patient's desire to protect the family from pain by suggesting, "It can be a real gift for families to have time to adjust to the shock of the diagnosis—remember how long that took you?—so that they can get the support they need to be there for you.")

- If you are dealing with a parent who does not want to tell his or her children (even though he or she may be telling you incidents that reveal how distressed the children are), you may want to offer help with how to talk with children of different ages about illness and death. (*Note:* This is one of the most difficult issues to face. Most parents find it so unimaginable to contemplate not only the possibility of dying but also of leaving their children fatherless or motherless that they find it next to impossible to consider facing the task of helping to prepare their children for this eventuality. Unless you have a background that has prepared you for dealing with this painful dilemma, you may need to encourage the parents to seek the help of other professionals with expertise in helping children prepare for the loss of a parent. I remember one such child psychiatrist stating emphatically that "parents must not be let off the hook even though they are dying." Talking with their children about what is happening can make a critical difference to the children's life-long mental health.)

CULTURAL COMPETENCY CONSIDERATIONS

I like to acknowledge obvious sociocultural differences—age, race, gender, ethnicity—and to check with people about whether they think I can be helpful to them, given the obvious differences between us. This puts the issue on the table and lets the person know that you want to be sensitive to his or her needs. This needs to be done gently and respectfully. I am letting others know that I do not assume that I can understand where they are coming from, but that I am interested in trying to understand by inviting them to share whatever they feel comfortable sharing of their stories and their concerns. (*Note:* Again, I cannot emphasize how important this stance of "not knowing" has become to me in this work. Even when we think we are dealing with someone from a background similar to our own, we can never presume to know where they have been on their life's journey! Being curious, respectful, and nonjudgmental results in such enriching exchanges.)

- Try to identify the person(s) with whom the patient would feel most comfortable talking about such sensitive issues.
- Would the patient like to bring in his or her partner, a family member, a clergyperson, or other helping person to be included in the discussion of how and when to tell various members of the family?
- Consult with someone, if possible, from the patient's sociocultural background who can help you understand what the particularly sensi-

tive issues might be. (*Note:* For example, some of the people of color I have worked with from a variety of backgrounds have preferred to get both their health care and their support services from our "dominant culture" setting because they did not want anyone from their own communities to find out about their diagnosis. This can be a major issue for people who live in small towns as well. They may travel long distances to get their care elsewhere, which becomes increasingly complicated as they become more ill. Or they may prefer treatment in their own community, regardless of limitations this may impose.

ACTION STEPS FOR SUCCESSFUL INTERVENTION

As hospital social workers, we can build bridges between the patient (and perhaps his or her family of choice) and the patient's family of origin. By listening respectfully to all stories, we model the kind of non-judgmental acceptance so necessary for all parties involved to decrease the isolation that comes from anger, stigma, and shame.

One intervention I have found particularly helpful is to introduce the idea that the secret of the patient's diagnosis is probably not the first family secret his or her parents have encountered. For the patient, this arouses curiosity and relieves some of the pressure. For the parents, and this must be done very cautiously, it can be an invitation for them to reflect back on what they learned from their families about how to deal with "secrets," that is, whatever was considered taboo. It is likely that somewhere in the extended family someone was "cut off" (even disowned) for having a child out of wedlock, marrying outside the faith, not marrying ("living in sin!"), or having an abortion. Often families "shut down" emotionally around these events that are "too terrible to speak about." If parents can reflect upon the effect those "shut downs" had on them, they may be able to see that they would be doing the same thing if they were to treat their son's or daughter's diagnosis of AIDS in the same way. Families can choose to change the family legacy regarding secrets. AIDS is a terrible disease, but the people who get it are not terrible people. Their lives are worthy of praise and celebration, not secrecy and shame.

POTENTIAL BARRIERS TO SUCCESSFUL INTERVENTION

- Our unresolved issues with our own families of origin can hinder intervention. To the extent that we do not feel accepted as we are by our families, we are vulnerable to joining the protection game, that is, protecting the patients from possible rejection by being a "better parent" who accepts them as they are, thus subtly discouraging the patient from working through the issues with his or her own parents.

- Our lack of knowledge and experience in working with people affected by HIV/AIDS can actually be an asset if we invite people to share their stories and if we listen for statements that clarify what they want for their lives. By reflecting back what we hear, checking to make sure we heard it correctly, we can help with the process of clarification and empowerment.

INFORMATION THE CLIENT SHOULD KNOW BEFORE TAKING ACTION

1. Patients need to know that we will respect their definition of "family," and that we will respect their decision about when to tell their families of origin, including with whatever conditions we need to add. (*Note:* We can make it clear that although the patient is our primary client, we are concerned about the welfare of those who care about him or her as well.)
2. Most families do not reject their children when they learn of this diagnosis, but they may need help coming to terms with what such a diagnosis means. Many parents experience profound guilt for not having protected a child (even an adult child) from harm. This guilt may come out in such disguises that one would never imagine it was guilt, for example, "Why weren't you protecting yourself?"
3. Patients often hesitate to tell their families because they have been the primary emotional, if not physical, caretakers in the family. They need to know that they do not have to take on the burden of providing the education and support their families will need. We can help them identify other options.
4. I sometimes remind gay men how long it took them to "come out" and to come to terms with their diagnosis. I then draw a parallel to the need for their parents to have time to absorb the news and to prepare for their "coming out" as parents of a child with HIV/AIDS.

POLICY IMPLICATIONS AND RELATED ACTIONS

- Because of our legal system's definition of "next of kin," people who have not disclosed their diagnosis to parents (or spouse) should be urged to name someone as his or her health care proxy or power of attorney, which includes the right to make health care decisions.

- Because in most states there is no legal recognition of long-term, committed relationships (either same sex or opposite sex) outside of marriage, the rights of such a partner can be challenged by the parents after the patient's death.
- We can encourage patients to find an AIDS-sensitive lawyer and to attend to these legal matters as early as possible.
- We can also appeal to the basic decency of parents to respect the wishes of their son or daughter regardless of how they may have felt about the person's lifestyle.
- And finally, we can advocate for support services that take seriously the needs of the "family," for example, assisted living arrangements that allow patients to have their partners or children with them.

Bereavement Work in the Acute Care Setting

Judith Hanson Babcock

WHY DO THIS?
STATEMENT OF THE PROBLEM AND ISSUES

When I began working with people with AIDS in an acute care setting ten years ago, most of our patients died in the hospital, most frequently, it seemed, from PCP (pneumocystis carinii pneumonia). There was, at that time, no effective prophylaxis to prevent this devastating infection. In those early years, I often met families who had flown in from all parts of the country and learned that their son was gay, had AIDS, and was dying. Bereavement work was done in a crisis of numbing shock. All I could hope to do was to let the grief-stricken families know what a very special person I thought their son (brother, nephew, etc.) was and to facilitate the process of answering their questions about their son's life, death, and funeral arrangements.

Over the years, treatments and prophylaxis have developed for nearly all of the opportunistic infections. Hospital stays are few and brief, usually just a few days to diagnose some new infection. Then the patient returns home with a visiting nurse or hospice referral, or to a chronic care (skilled nursing) facility or inpatient hospice to die. Treatments that required two- to three-week acute hospital stays (with plenty of time to get to know the patient, partner, family, and friends) are now often done at home. Also, with treatments available for nearly all the opportunistic infections, it is becoming common for patients to receive all of their care in outpatient settings—perhaps including visiting nurses at home—until their final months, when the body can no longer keep up the fight, even with the help of all the available drugs. Then we are likely to see several admissions—one after another—usually very brief—until the patient dies.

In the present context, most patients choose to remain on multiple drug therapies (a combination of treatment and prophylaxis for the multiple infections that accompany the final stages of AIDS). This means they are less likely to have a prolonged period of hospice care. They are more likely to keep fighting until the very end, with more hope that if they live a little longer, new treatments for extending their lives, if not a cure, will be found. That has been their experience. Unlike "the early days" when patients expected to die of PCP in six to eighteen months, patients who have survived the past five to ten years have seen the development of one new life-prolonging treatment after another, giving them more reason to remain hopeful.

This shift can be problematic for the social worker attempting to do bereavement work. In "the early days," it was not unusual to have patients ask for help with making their wills and planning their funerals soon after you met them. Now they may postpone such considerations until it is too late, leaving partners with incomplete, unsigned wills and families distraught at having learned very late that a son, daughter, or parent had known for eight to ten years that he or she was HIV positive, but had not told them until near the end.

Thus, it is again not unusual to meet families who have only recently learned about the diagnosis. Helping those families prepare for the loss of the person who is dying is made much more complicated by the secret-keeping (if some family members do not know the true diagnosis) and the shock of disbelief if they have just been told. The stress on the staff—including the social worker—is enormous when the patient is still insisting upon not disclosing the diagnosis while family members are preparing to provide the patient's terminal care at home.

Other bereavement issues include concerns for the families who, because of the stigma surrounding AIDS, are less likely to turn to their extended families, friends, and churches for support. This leaves them isolated and at risk for retreating into possible feelings of shame for lying about the diagnosis, or for having ambilivalent feelings about the person who died, feelings they did not have the time or opportunity to deal with prior to the death. Furthermore, it is my belief that if family members cannot speak truthfully about the diagnosis, no one can appreciate the depth of their pain. And another painful secret enters the family system to be passed on—unnamed, too awful to be spoken of—to succeeding generations.

In addition, for the partners that are left behind, those who are HIV positive may wonder who will be there to provide for them the exhausting care they have just provided for their partners. Those who are HIV negative may experience the debilitating depression of "survivor's guilt." (*Note:* There are instances when the patient's family of origin and family of choice form a team and work together to provide the necessary support. I remember one set of parents who flew to Boston from the midwest to provide one-week-per-month respite for the family of choice. I have also known families who provided the care needed by the surviving partner when he or she, in turn, became ill, just as any other in-laws might be expected to do.)

EXAMPLES OF HOW THE ISSUE MAY PRESENT

Case Study 1

A patient is admitted to the hospital with a diagnosis suggestive of end-stage AIDS, for example, PML (progressive myelo-leukoencephalopathy), an infection of the brain for which there is no treatment. The social worker has never met the patient or his family because he has only recently returned to his parents' home for care. The PML has affected the patient's balance and coordination so that he cannot walk without assistance. The patient has learned from his former physician and his own research that the course of PML is likely to be rapid, with unrelenting deterioration, and loss of one bodily function after another, ending with his death. He is still clear enough in his thinking to be terrified of what lies ahead and worried about how his parents will cope with such a devastating decline. He asks for your assistance in finding resources to help provide the care he knows he will need. His parents do not yet comprehend the magnitude of their undertaking when they insist upon providing his care at home.

Your exploration of existing resources finds no one who has even heard of PML, and none of the other health care facilities within one hundred miles have had any experience with a person with AIDS. You finally find one facility connected with the nearest major medical center, 150 miles away, that is willing to take this patient when his care becomes more than his parents can handle. It is winter in your northern state, and you patient's parents cannot afford to leave their jobs and move to the area where their son could receive the best care. The most they could hope for would be one visit each weekend.

You learn that if your patient were to return to the major urban area where he was living previously, he would have an extensive support network of friends, as well as facilities able to provide any level of care he may need.

Case Study 2

An African-American woman with a past history of IV drug use has been "clean and sober" for seven years. She has four children, two of whom still live in a foster home where they were placed ten years ago when she was actively using. Two children she has had since she has been in recovery (ages four and six) live with her. She has worked hard to remain in recovery and make a good home for herself and her younger children. The children do not know that their mother has AIDS, but they know she is very ill because she keeps having to go to the hospital. People from the church come to take care of them when this happens, but no one has yet offered to take responsibility for the children when the mother dies.

The patient's mother lives in another state and cannot afford to take an extended leave from her job to care for her daughter. In addition, she has two other children with AIDS, one of whom lives near her in a halfway house for recovering addicts. She is responsible for the three children of that son, whose wife already died of AIDS.

FACTS THE SOCIAL WORKER NEEDS TO KNOW
BEFORE PROCEEDING

In case study 1, the social worker would need to know some basic medical information about PML, for example, that a patient often presents looking like someone who has had a stroke, with similar symptoms depending upon the area of the brain affected (one-sided weakness, loss of speech, partial paralysis). It can progress very quickly—a few weeks to a few months—with loss of one function after another occurring daily to weekly. It can be one of the most devastating ways for persons with AIDS to die because they may not "look" sick when the symptoms begin. Such patients may have been well enough to work, and they are often alert enough to be aware of the deterioration as it happens. (*Note:* Other final infections can also progress rapidly, for example, a lymphoma or the widespread dissemination of a long-standing CMV infection.)

Given these circumstances, time is of the essence. Contingency plans need to be made in anticipation of a possibly rapid deterioration. The patient may leave the hospital following diagnosis needing no more care than the parents can easily provide, but one week later, he may not be able to walk. Two to four weeks later he may need total twenty-four-hour assistance for all activities of daily living. (*Note:* This is a worst-case end-stage AIDS diagnosis, but it highlights the importance of our role as planners of continuing care.)

Thus the social worker needs to know the following:

1. What care will be needed?
2. What "natural supports" does the family have, for example, how many family members and friends can be counted on to help out, and what specifically can those people provide?
   - Hands on care, for example, helping move the patient for bed changes
   - Respite care, for example, sitting with the patient while other family members take a break
   - Meal preparation, grocery shopping, laundry, etc.

   Are the family members and/or friends aware of the patient's diagnosis? Do they need basic AIDS education, especially including infection precautions that will need to be taken? Patients and/or family members are often trained to give intravenous medications at home, including helping to monitor a morphine drip to relieve pain, if that is an issue.
3. What "formal supports" are available?
   - Visiting nurse/home health aides/ in-home hospice
   - Inpatient facilities, for example, chronic care hospital, skilled nursing facility, nursing home (Are they prepared to take someone with AIDS, or might they need AIDS education for the staff?)
   - Inpatient hospice (Some home hospice programs have contracts with their local hospitals to provide short-term in-patient respite care or pain management evaluation.)
4. What will the patient's insurance cover? (With some managed care providers, that is the first and only question. They determine what the patient's options are. In other cases, insurance companies have HIV case managers who will negotiate with the company to provide the care you [the medical team] recommend. If there is no HIV case manager, you may be able to advocate with the insurance provider to support the preferences of the patient/family/care team especially if no less-expensive options are available. [For example, some patients have little or no coverage for home care, but, if the only option is an extended hospital stay, insurance companies may make exceptions.])

Another issue it is helpful to keep in mind is the loss of a child. Losing a child is one of the most devastating losses parents can suffer. Parents are not supposed to outlive their own children. They are supposed to be able to protect their children from harm. When you add the stigma of AIDS, these parents may be surrounded by people—including their own family and friends—who believe that their son or daughter deserves this fate. They may even have believed this themselves—or continue to believe it—due to such strong social reinforcement.

When considering case study 2, it would be helpful for the social worker to know as much as possible about African-American families. Since workers from the dominant white/Anglican culture may have had limited opportunities to work with and learn from people of color, as well as people from a variety of other sociocultural backgrounds, it is important for us to acknowledge those limitations and to assess our own assumptions before we proceed. For example, in this case I indicated that the woman had her own history of IV drug use, accounting for the placement of her children. However, many women of color have been infected by partners who were either IV drug users or who had had sex with other men. Some of these women are middle-class professionals. You simply cannot make assumptions when working with people with HIV/AIDS.

The worker would also want to find out what resources are available for helping this mother make plans for her children's care. (See Lori Weiner's chapters in this book for valuable information and suggestions for working with this type of mother and her children).

Finally, the social worker needs to be aware that in the context of HIV/AIDS, bereavement issues are present throughout the course of the disease, from diagnosis—with the loss of expectation of "a long and healthy life"—to the multitude of other losses that occur over time. Examples of these losses include the following:

- loss of ability to work, which can lead to multiple other losses, for example, dramatic changes in the standard of living, often necessitating moving to subsidizied housing; loss of social contacts with fellow workers; loss of a sense of role in society, which can, in turn, cause loss of self-esteem
- loss of energy to do those things that had been pleasurable, including traveling, going out with friends, having sex, and even eating (many medications cause nausea)
- loss of familiar body image, from obvious KS (Kaposi's sarcoma) lesions, weight loss ("I don't recognize myself when I look in the mirror"), or the insertion of a permanent central line (usually under the skin in the upper chest) if long-term daily IV fluids or medications are required

- threatened loss of eyesight from CMV (cytomegalovirus) retinitis, a fairly common infection in later stages of HIV/AIDS that can cause blindness if not treated

People respond in amazingly different ways to these losses, depending upon the resources (emotional, spiritual, financial, and social supports) they have to draw on. We know that every new loss can stir up every previous loss we have experienced, and many people with HIV/AIDS have also suffered the loss of close friends or partners to AIDS. Having witnessed firsthand the devastation AIDS can cause, people commonly say, "I know I'd never be able to go through . . . [whatever they fear most]." Many people say they would rather die than go blind, for example. But the human spirit (or fear of dying) usually prevails, and what has been "unthinkable" becomes tolerable when the time comes to face it.

On the other hand, what has impressed me most over the years is the determination I have witnessed by so many people to find their own ways not to allow AIDS to take over their lives. They choose instead to find ways to live their lives as fully as possible by "taking it a day at a time," and by continuing to celebrate life in the face of death.

KEY QUESTIONS TO ASK THE CLIENT

Because of the factors outlined earlier, it is very possible that you may not have had a chance to form a relationship over time with a patient who now presents at a very late stage of his or her illness. Obviously, the following questions are easier in some ways if you have had a long-term relationship with the person. However, it can be terribly difficult for the social worker who has known someone for five to ten years (or even five to ten months) to think of preparing for the loss of that person with whom you have shared a deep and meaningful relationship.

So I think it is helpful to begin with an acknowledgement to the patient of how difficult this conversation about preparing for the end of his or her life may be. Also keep in mind that this subject is so painful that others may be avoiding it altogether; thus, your willingness to talk about it can be a gift.

Again, I would start with gently asking how I can be of help. Are there specific questions or concerns the patient may want to express? "What would it be helpful for me to know about your situation?" If the person is very ill, you might ask him or her, "Who would be the best person to fill me in on what I need to know about what you want for your care?"

If the person gives me permission to proceed, some of the questions I might ask are as follows:

- What are the things you want me to pay particular attention to? (What is it important for us to talk about?)
- What resources do you have to draw on—inner strengths as well as other people?
- How would you like for things to be for whatever time is left before you die?
- Do you want to die at home?
- If so, whom do you want to be there?
- What would you like to have done with your body (that is, cremation or burial)?
- Who knows about what you want to have happen?
- Do you have any unfinished business you would like to attend to?
- Is there anyone you want to see?
- Is there anyone with whom you would like to make peace?
- What are your spiritual beliefs? (*Note:* Most people will respond by talking about their religious/church upbringings from which many people with AIDS have been alienated. I draw a careful distinction between this and the person's spirituality, their beliefs about themselves, and the meaning they give to their lives.

However, I also ask whether the person would be interested in talking with an AIDS-sensitive representative of his or her particular religious tradition to discuss and perhaps resolve what may have resulted in a painful cutoff from what could now provide a source of blessing. I have seen some remarkable healing of old anger and hurt from such a nonjudgmental, AIDS-sensitive reconnection.)

In addition, patients will often express strong feelings about not wanting a traditional funeral or burial. I may explore with them whether they might not consider honoring the wishes of those who will be left behind for whom those things may be a great source of comfort. This sometimes softens the anger that may be underlying this final "acting out" against one's parents, if that is what it is about.

CULTURAL COMPETENCY CONSIDERATIONS

Going back again to the importance of acknowledging how limited is our knowledge of any sociocultural context of which we have not been a part—including not only race and gender but also class, religious background, and sexual orientation—we need to turn once again to our "consultants." Books, articles, and other professionals more knowledgeable than ourselves may provide helpful background information, but only "the people who come to consult with us," that is, our clients, really know what has been their experience within the cultural context from which they come. Therefore, we can respectfully inquire about what we need to know about people's beliefs about death and dying, what happens at the time of death, what if anything happens to the person after death.

Case Study

> I was recently privileged to be part of the dying process of a man from South America. His girlfriend was terrified of staying in the room with him. I asked her what ideas she had about what happens when people die, and she said she had heard that "they cry." I described some of the deaths I had witnessed and acknowledged that each is different and that no one can predict exactly what will happen, which gave her permission to talk more about her fears. I explored with her the preference of either staying at the bedside of her dying partner or returning home to await the news of his death. Neither option seemed acceptable, so I asked what would help her feel safer if she were to stay. She said she could stay if her partner's mother stayed with her, and she also wanted the nurses to let her know—wherever she was—when the end was near so that she could decide where to be at the time of the actual death. This respectful process enabled that young woman to ask for what she needed.

I had heard and read about the sterotype of the "emotional" response of "Latin peoples" to death, but having never experienced this, I was less than helpful in making advanced arrangements for providing an appropriate setting. (The patient's room was at the opposite end of the hallway from any conference room where the family might have gone.) However, I was present at the time of the death and was swept up into what felt like a "dance of mourning" that followed. I felt privileged to be included, and I came away from that experience having even more questions about the dominant culture's tradition of "keeping a stiff upper lip." In the face of the death of a son or lover, weeping and wailing felt much more appropriate! I had also felt caught in the "clash of cultures" between the "hospital's culture" and the family's culture. I found myself acting as a spokesperson and advocate for the family's need to be able to respond in what was to them a culturally acceptable manner.

ACTION STEPS FOR SUCCESSFUL INTERVENTION

It is easy to feel helpless when confronted with a person who is about to die—or entering the final stage of life. Again, you can let the patient be your guide. Only he or she knows whether he or she wants your assistance with continuing the fight to stay alive, or with having permission (from herself or himself, from family, and/or from medical providers who have fought so hard to keep him or her alive) to give up the battle, or however the person views this stage. I often choose to acknowledge the courage I have witnessed over the months or years and the reality that AIDS wins in the end, regardless of how noble the battle has been. This often helps to reframe what others may see as "giving up," and brings the focus back to the fight with which the patient has been engaged, the life he or she has lived. When I am meeting with the patient alone, I may ask him or her if he or she has witnessed the dying of any friends or former lovers to AIDS. If so, it is not unusual for people to have flashbacks of those scenes. It can be very reassuring for the person to know that the flashbacks are normal and that how those other people died may not indicate what lies ahead for him or her. This can open up a chance for the person to share what they are afraid of—being alone, being in pain, or becoming incontinent or demented. Once the fear is named, it can be addressed, for example, the patient's physician can reassure the patient that his or her comfort will be the primary focus of care.

It may also be helpful to explore gently what the patient would consider "intolerable" and to ask whether the person has considered ending his or her own life at some point. (*Note:* In my expeience most people living with HIV have witnessed what devastation AIDS can bring about, and for many of them the knowledge that they could choose to end their own lives before "the intolerable" occurs is a source of comfort, not an indication of pathology. However, it is also important, in the context of such suicidal thoughts, to consider the possibility of a treatable clinical depression, that is, not to assume that "of course the person is depressed, they have AIDS and are dying."

If the person's symptoms are suggestive of a clinical depression, I will suggest that they consider a consultation with a psychiatrist with AIDS experience, to explore whether an antidepressant could improve his or her quality of life, perhaps freeing energy for the process of saying good-bye, or for continuing the fight, if that is his or her preference.

Sometimes people just need to be reassured that providing their care will not overburden their caregivers or that other options for care exist. For example, a professional woman who is the sole parent of a young adult son was greatly relieved to hear about an inpatient hospice she will be able to go to when she needs the care she would not want her son to provide.

When I am sitting beside the bedside with family members present, I speak to the patient of how much knowing him or her has meant to me. Sometimes I also model soothing ways to touch a patient who may be restless or uncomfortable so that hesitant family members get the message that it is safe to touch their loved one. I have also encouraged parents who have not reached a point where they feel comfortable disclosing the diagnosis in the obituary to write their own obituary that celebrates the life of that son or daughter in any way they want to remember him or her. Then, I invite them to share this with me and other staff members who knew their child.

I have also found it helpful, when the patient is dying, to ask whoever (family, friends) could be called to come in and comfort them. I also ask whether they'd like a priest or rabbi or chaplain to be called. Some of the most healing moments in this work have occurred when the family and staff gathered around the bedside while a chaplain prayed for everyone involved. Suddenly, the burden is shared. No one is isolated in his or her task.

If the person is going home to die, a predischarge meeting can provide many levels of support. The patient's physician may be able to explain that everything possible has been done and that the patient's comfort will continue to be the primary concern. (Most people fear pain more than any other aspect of dying.) The patient's nurse can outline all of the kinds of assistance the patient will need, and help write up daily schedules for medications, etc. If the patient is receiving physical therapy, the therapist can outline the exercise program to be continued at home. (*Note:* A physical therapy referral can send a powerful message to a patient that concern about his or her future quality of life is continuing.) Including someone from the home care agency can let the patient and caregiver(s) know that continuity of care is also a major goal.

The social worker at such a meeting can create a space where any concerns the caregiver(s) may have can be addressed. He or she can encourage the asking of any questions, regardless of how "stupid" they may seem to the caregiver(s), by reminding them that this is "uncharted territory" for them, and there is no reason why they would have all the answers! We can also encourage caregiver(s) to set limits on what they can do and to ask for and accept whatever help is available. We can also educate them about resources for support that may be available to them. Most of all, we can try to decrease the isolation that so often accompanies this diagnosis by giving caregivers the opportunity to talk about what this is like for them. If they can be helped to face the situation with less judgment and guilt and more love and acceptance, they will be more likely to be able to accept the outside help they will need.

If you are involved in a support group that includes friends and family, allowing them to continue to attend after their loved one dies is helpful. They can be an inspiration to others (including people living with HIV) that people who die are not forgotten and that those who cared about them can survive and even continue to reach out to others affected by HIV. If no support group or bereavement group is available, try to connect the people who are grieving with at least one other person in their situation. This helps decrease the isolation that places people at risk for a more complicated bereavement.

POTENTIAL BARRIERS TO SUCCESSFUL INTERVENTION

The interventions described in the last section may sound appealing, but they may also sound next-to-impossible with the current demands of shortened lengths of stay often coupled with increased caseloads. While you are trying to spend time with a dying patient and his or her caregivers, you may be getting paged constantly about the other twenty to thirty patients for whose discharge planning you are responsible. Additionally, your hospital administration may have limited awareness of how time-consuming the discharge planning process can be for a person with AIDS, given the scenarios suggested earlier.

We must also deal with our own lack of training and experience and our discomfort with issues concerning death and dying. We may not want to be there when the patient dies, nor to sit with the family at the bedside just after the patient has died (when we may be called to provide comfort and to help with the process of contacting other family members and/or the funeral home).

This is a time to remember that we do not have to be alone in these final tasks. I often take the hospital chaplain along when I get such a call. We can all "touch base" with whoever we feel safe with (a colleague, a supervisor, someone on the staff—perhaps the patient's nurse—anyone who can say its okay to have whatever feelings we are experiencing) so that we can go to the waiting family and be there for them.

Again, it is not about knowing all the right things to say. A simple "I'm sorry this had to happen to your loved one" goes a long way. We can check in to see if there are any final questions about contacting the funeral home. One very important detail is to let the family know if the person is eligible for subsidized funeral expenses, or at least to suggest that they ask the funeral director about that. (In Massachusetts, if a person is on Medicaid, $1,100 of a $1,500 basic funeral will be reimbursed, but only if the family pays no more than the $400 difference.) For many poor families, funeral costs could otherwise be impossible. I have sometimes contacted churches for help with expenses for people who were not legal residents.

The most important gift we have to offer is our ability to be there and to care about what is happening in contrast to a society that often seems to turn its back on people with HIV/AIDS.

INFORMATION THE CLIENT SHOULD KNOW
BEFORE TAKING ACTION

If you are able to meet the patient before he or she is at the very end of his or her life, it can be very helpful to suggest that the person consult with a lawyer (many AIDS service organizations have volunteers who do this work pro bono) about making sure their final wishes will be carried out. An AIDS-sensitive lawyer can help the person make a will and to arrange for someone to be power of attorney, and/or health care proxy (to make medical decisions in the event that the person is unable to make his or her wishes known). In addition, the person can make a living will designating what he or she would and would not want for treatment in later stages of the illness. Although living wills are not legally binding in many states, their intent is often honored by the courts and by families as a clear indication of the person's wishes.

The patient also has the right to know what options exist for care when he or she becomes unable to care for him or herself. (These options have been outlined earlier in this chapter.)

In addition, the patient needs to know what your role will be as the disease progresses and he or she deteriorates; for example, would you be able to continue to see the person if he or she went to another facility or home to die?

And finally, those who are left behind—family, lover, friends—need to know what bereavement resources are available to them. Can they come to see you? Are there bereavement groups in the area where they live? I encourage people to contact their nearest AIDS service organization to inquire about groups. If they are not interested in a group, I try to help them connect with at least one other person in their situation, that is, another father, mother, sister, brother, friend, or lover who has also lost someone to AIDS, so that they can at least have telephone contact with someone who knows what they are going through.

POLICY IMPLICATIONS AND RELATED ACTIONS

Hospital administrators are faced with daily threats of cutbacks in Medicare and Medicaid, and they are confronted by the need to downsize inpatient facilities as more of the provision of health care shifts to the outpatient or "sub-acute" setting. In this context, they do not want to hear about the greater complexity of providing care to people with HIV. Sadly, it appears that the situation for hospitals will continue to get worse. You may already have had your job redefined from "clinical social worker" to "case manager." You may be reporting to a nurse instead of receiving supervision from a senior social worker. You may feel that if you complain about this situation, you will lose your job.

In this context, it can be difficult if not impossible to find the time or energy to advocate for the needs of your HIV patients. You can easily feel like "the voice crying in the wilderness." But that is our professional mandate—to advocate for those who are most vulnerable in our society.

What I have learned over the years is that there can never be "enough" help for the awesome burdens imposed by AIDS, especially in a society in which many choose to make AIDS a moral issue and feel free to judge those who are infected as having deserved their fate. What we can do is speak out against this stance with each person we meet. We can accept people with HIV/AIDS without judgment and encourage their families and caregivers to do the same.

We can also learn a lot from the people who consult with us (our clients and those who care for them). We can learn to move from isolation to sharing our lives with others. (Support groups for AIDS professionals can also be very helpful.)

We can learn to take the very best care of ourselves that we know how—rest, exercise, take vacations, hang out with friends, meditate, go on retreats—whatever we need to refresh body, mind, and spirit so that we can do this challenging work. In short, we can learn from our clients how precious life is, and we can celebrate life every chance we get!

Involving Families
in Hospice and Home Care

David J. Brennan

WHY DO THIS?
STATEMENT OF THE PROBLEM AND ISSUES

At some point in the course of their illness, most people with AIDS require a home care agency's involvement in providing support in their primary home. This chapter will examine how to involve families in providing home care and hospice care to people with AIDS (PWAs).

Nowadays, managed care encourages us to keep people out of the hospital and to provide less expensive care. This care is often provided at home both for cost-efficiency and for the client's comfort. Also, we commonly use infusion equipment and other high-tech medical management to provide care for people at home. Access to and the quality of home care services to PWAs had been improving over the last decade because more and more resources had been pouring into the provision of home care services. For instance, federal monies from the Ryan White Care Act have been used all across the nation to supplement the kinds of services that regular home care agencies have been able to provide for PWAs. In today's health care and federal financial struggle knowing where the funding may go in the future is difficult.

When we think about involving the family in the decisions, and discussions regarding home care, we should note that PWAs have challenged health care agencies to look differently at our concepts of family. We have begun to think about what comprises a family, whom the members are, how we define a family, and what a family is to us.

All families include both families of origin and families of choice. The family of origin is the biological family: mother, father, and siblings. The family of choice includes those to whom the client chooses to be close, including a partner, a legally married husband or wife, children, neighbors, friends, or others. The term "family" is currently being used in its broadest sense to include family of origin and family of choice.

People with AIDS often have very limited families of origin or, if they do have families, these families are stressed out and dealing with a number of issues that I will discuss later. It may be that a family of a PWA consists only of a case manager or volunteer from an AIDS service organization or members of a twelve-step support program. As providers, we must look at the issues of understanding the family dynamics in order to prepare our client for receiving home care and hospice services.

Home care services provide medical care for someone at home and may include nursing services, home health aide services, IV infusion, physical and occupational therapy, and sometimes psychiatric and/or social work support.

Hospice is a type of home care that focuses on caring for clients during the final phase of their illness. In addition to the other services home care can provide, hospice home care can provide regular psychosocial support, chaplain services, volunteer assistance, and bereavement support for families after the death of a client.

Providing hospice care for someone at home is often very complicated to introduce into a family system because, for many people, hospice means the end of the line. Hospice care may signify that someone has given up or that someone is not worthy of getting continual aggressive treatment. Because hospice care can provide some increased services to families, including social work and bereavement support, it can be beneficial for most families of PWAs.

Knowing the difference between home care and hospice care is also important. Home care and hospice have many similarities; in fact, home care agencies often have a hospice component as part of their continuum of care. Home care provides skilled nursing services, home health aides, homemaker services, and the ability to provide infusions for patients at home.

Hospice care is focused on palliative and comfort care. Clients generally must have a six-month or less prognosis documented by their physician in order to obtain a hospice benefit. Once receiving the hospice benefit, they are provided palliative care, which means they are provided care for any symptoms including pain. Hospice care provides a team approach, including nurses, home health aides, social workers, chaplains, homemakers, and volunteers who meet on a regular basis to discuss concerns regarding the patient's care. Hospice has a family-centered approach that includes bereavement services for the family for at least one year after the PWAs' death. Hospice is reimbursed on a per diem rate; because of this reimbursement structure, many hospices have been reluctant to provide care to PWAs. Home care services are generally reimbursed on a per visit rate; therefore, each service that a home care agency provides is reimbursed at a particular set rate.

It is also important to note that there are an increasing number of inpatient hospice facilities. Each program runs differently, setting up its own admission criteria and other protocols. Some inpatient programs are acute facilities, with twenty-four-hour staffing; some are residential programs, which are essentially housing, with the hospice providing the services to the clients in the residence. Some are units in hospitals or nursing facilities, some are free-standing programs. Again, knowing the resources in your area is helpful.

Hospice was essentially the nation's first managed care program because hospices are expected to maintain the cost of providing care to clients at approximately one hundred dollars per day (1995 rate). When clients are on very expensive medications, as people with AIDS often are, providing care at that cost is very difficult. Knowing where in your geographical area your clients are being served and where their other needed services are located in order to make sure that a unified system of care for that person exists.

In order for someone to remain at home, usually there needs to be someone else present who can assist in the coordination of services in and out of the home. This person is called a primary caregiver. Although a primary caregiver is generally not required for someone to be admitted to hospice, assigning this role to someone—be it family of origin or choice, a friend, neighbor, etc.—is usually helpful. Some family members may be reluctant to provide support to someone at home. Family members might have some fears regarding transmission; they might also have fears regarding issues of substance abuse, medications, or high-tech equipment. Perhaps the stigma associated with HIV concerns the caregivers. Therefore, involving family members in getting proper care for the client at home may prove difficult.

Often, insurance issues such as coverage of services and other financial matters will be issues that families need to think about in order to make sure the PWA receives the services she or he needs. The systems of insurance coverage are very complicated and vary from insurance to insurance as to what would be provided for someone at home. Families may be dealing with a great deal of anxiety regarding these issues and will need some support and assistance. It will be helpful to be familiar with the various policies and to have some contact with a case manager so they are familiar with you and your role with the family. Because policies and procedures are very complicated, families will require your support and patience in explaining the various rules and terms.

Feelings of helplessness are common among family members providing support to someone who is extremely ill, particularly when he or she is at home. They feel helpless because there are a lot of opportunistic infections that we can not treat curatively, and therefore it feels as though there is "nothing to be done." This is far from the truth. To address this helplessness, it is useful to assist the family in focusing on what they *can* do and *are* doing. This will decrease the overall feeling of helplessness.

EXAMPLES OF HOW THE ISSUE MAY PRESENT

The most common time for the issues concerning hospice and/or home care for a patient to present is when a patient is discharged from the hospital. In hospital settings, home care services are generally arranged through the physician and the social work/discharge planning department of the hospital. The discharge planners are under tremendous pressure to get the individual out of the acute care setting as soon as possible. Therefore, having a clear understanding of what the family is already capable of managing at home is important.

Clients may already be at home, experiencing changes in their physical and emotional status that require the intervention of home care or hospice service organization. The client may be not able to prepare her or his meals or take care of household chores, and she or he may be getting weaker and need some support. The client may not be in a crisis or emergency situation, requiring hospital admission, but rather, may be experiencing a slow deterioration.

Home Care and Hospice

- Families might already be involved in providing home care to someone, but may begin to need extra help as the PWAs' needs increase (e.g., as families in which someone is working or situations where someone has very limited family support).
- Families that are completely isolated from support systems are going to have a very difficult time in accessing home care services and will need extra support from social workers who are aware of the available resources.
- Various family members may have different ideas about how to proceed with the care at any point in time. One may feel someone is not safe to return home while another feels capable of providing care at home if more family members helped or if more support were available.
- Identifying all the people involved in the care at any given point in time may be difficult. Therefore, it is imperative to assist the client in identi-

fying one person in the system who could be a primary caregiver and who might be able to understand what the PWAs' needs are and help facilitate communication with other members of the system. This may require legal documentation such as health care proxies or powers of attorney.
- The care of PWAs is often provided by various agencies that may or may not communicate with each other. Knowing the other players who are involved in the care and having contact with them regarding the needs of the patient is important so that we can provide a smooth transition to home care services.

When various opinions about how to proceed with the care for a patient exist, consider gathering the members of the team together in a family meeting or team meeting to address the concerns.

Hospice-Specific Issues

After people are hospitalized and receive numerous treatments to fight off various opportunistic infections, there often comes a point when the medical providers can offer very little acute intervention. It is important to note that a lot of people with AIDS have great difficulty thinking about hospice care for many reasons, such as the following:

- Many PWAs are young and may associate hospice care with elderly patients.
- Health care providers often have a difficult time assessing when it is appropriate to address the issue of hospice care with a patient for fear that the patient might think the health care provider is assuming that the patient will die soon or that they are giving up on the patient.

Health care providers would do well to think about our own comfort level when talking with our patients about hospice and issues of death and dying. Often patients have already considered that, at some point, they may die from HIV. They may or may not have verbalized it, but on some level, they have probably thought about it. In some cases, a patient feels great relief that one health care provider is willing and open to talk about his or her needs, particularly hospice or death and dying issues. In one of my cases, the referring visiting nurse told the wife of a patient that she should not talk to hospice providers because they will tell the patient he is dying and force him to think about it. The woman met me outside of the patient's apartment for fear I would discuss his dying with him. She was reluctant to allow me to meet with him. This patient was very ill, and I gently convinced her it was important that I meet him to see if he had any questions regarding hospice before we began services. I met with the woman and her husband, who stated very clearly to me with no prompting, "I know I am dying. I think my wife doesn't realize this; can you help her?" Over the next week as he started hospice care, they both opened up tremendously about his dying and their needs and resolved a number of issues. He died six weeks later. Clearly, they just needed a hospice worker who was able to let them talk about his dying instead of maintaining their denial.

FACTS THE SOCIAL WORKER NEEDS TO KNOW
BEFORE PROCEEDING

Resources

Social workers must be aware of the resources available to any patient. These resources include various home care and hospice programs, their specialties, their availability within certain geographical areas or within various cultural populations, community resource agencies, AIDS service organizations, volunteer service agencies, meal delivery systems, and financial assistance programs. It is important to contact your local public health department to find out if they have a listing of resources available to PWAs in your area.

Insurance

You must also know how to deal with insurance. Insurance companies are influenced by the marketplace and have various plans to cover services. It is helpful to understand what someone's insurance is, how the insurance system operates, and who the case manager is who might be involved in the care of this person. You should develop a working relationship with the insurance companies to understand how they may be able to provide the services your client needs.

Referrals

Before proceeding with a referral, you should learn the history of the disease and the history of the patient's and family's understanding of the illness. Given the diverse cultures affected by HIV, you must be certain that the family and the client understand the implications of HIV disease and you should determine their needs regarding care. Developing a connection with at least one family member who can help make decisions is important.

Legal Concerns

At this point in time, if you have not yet done so, it is critical to be able to discuss with a client the issues regarding living wills, advanced directives, and guardianship/adoption if children are involved. Encourage the client to appoint someone to make decisions in the event that he or she is not capable of making decisions. Provide this information to the medical team who is providing care. Find out if the family has the ability or the willingness to provide the patient with care at home. Often, family members are reluctant to consider the possibility until they understand fully the implications of that care and have their questions answered.

KEY QUESTIONS TO ASK THE CLIENT

Many people with AIDS have been through various intake processes and have been answering the same questions over and over again. Take advantage of any opportunity that you have to collaborate with other providers to relieve the stress on clients.

- *Physical Needs.* What are the patient's needs? Can the individual ambulate, verbally express him or herself, prepare his or her meals or take care of household tasks or activities of daily living? Is the person bed bound? Can he or she get up and out, and/or drive?
- *Emotional Needs.* Assessing how someone has been coping is very important. Does he or she have some sort of psychiatric history? Do the client and family members have difficulty expressing feelings about what is happening to them? Do the client and family members have a clear sense of what is happening? Can they talk openly about the illness? Do they have support available? Do the family members and client have friends or other people who understand HIV that can listen and support them?
- *Spiritual Needs.* Do the family members and client have relationships in the spiritual community that can support their needs?
- *Social Needs.* Is the family system isolated? Are there family members or friends nearby who are supportive and available who might be able to assist in providing care?
- *Legal Needs.* Has the client drawn up a will, living will, health care proxy, declaration concerning remains, and financial durable power of attorney? Have arrangements been made for custody or guardianship of children if needed? Is the family aware of the legal issues? Are there complicated concerns between a family of origin and a family of choice?

These issues can be legally complex and should be addressed while the patient's mental status is clear.

- *Medical Needs.* Does the family system have an understanding of the illness? Ask clients what they understand of the medical system, and determine what is covered for their care and what is not, financially. Do the patient and family members understand the role of the various players in their home care needs. If a home care program is to be used, will there be any added expenses to the patient and family? Is there a primary contact person in the agency that is providing home care? Is there a primary nurse? If hospice is going to be used, do the client and family members have an understanding of what the prognosis is?
- *Primary Contact.* Ask the client if he or she has one key significant person who will be able to assist in making decisions. This would be considered a primary caregiver for hospice and home care agencies.
- *Interagency Communication.* In order to establish clear lines of communication, ask the client what other agencies are already involved, and who the key contact people are from those agencies. Ask clients if they have already had contact with a home care agency or hospice program that they are familiar with and would like to utilize. Most PWAs have been through the process of dealing with someone else who has died of AIDS or has required health care, and they may be familiar with a certain program or agency that they would like to work with for themselves.

CULTURAL COMPETENCY CONSIDERATIONS

Because of the diverse cultures affected by HIV, you should determine the resources that provide home care services and hospice services for PWAs as well as their ability to meet the needs of your client and your client's culture. In other words, familiarize yourself with the agencies to which you are referring and their ability to match the needs of your client.

Make an effort to understand the diversity of the team providing care. Is this agency flexible enough to meet the needs of someone who has a different cultural understanding of AIDS or HIV or a different understanding of health care or how systems work? Literature and community resources should be made available immediately so that the family can understand and access services as soon as possible.

Multicultural Concerns

- *Communication.* Is language, literacy, or disability a block to accessing services?

- *Family.* How does this person's culture define family? Is there a large network of family or a small tight-knit nuclear family? Is there severe discrimination against nontraditional families? How does the family and its culture deal with feelings and illness?
- *Meaning of Illness.* How does this culture view illness? How is illness treated? Are there deep-rooted issues regarding shame, illness, treatment, and beliefs?
- *Meaning of Dying.* How does this culture and family cope with death and dying? Are these subjects to be avoided? Is there a desire to avoid the issue? Are certain roles for certain family members at the time of dying culturally designated?
- *Access.* Does the family and culture avoid having "strangers" in the home, especially people from another culture or background?

Respecting the various and unique cultural needs of a family is very important, especially as illness progresses.

ACTION STEPS FOR SUCCESSFUL INTERVENTION

Assessment

We must have excellent assessment skills to understand the client's and family members' needs. This can be accomplished through one-on-one interviews, telephone calls, discussions with other service providers, and/or a family meeting. Through this assessment process, we should identify the resources available to a patient or a family at any given time. If we understand where the family lacks support, we can then help them make some choices regarding their needs. Having family members choose from a variety of options helps provide excellent quality home care services.

Assessing a family's needs is simply a way of understanding the situation in the home.

- Is the client going to be alone for hours during the day? Will he or she have someone available to check in with a phone call or a visit on a regular basis? Will there be someone with him or her twenty-four hours a day? Does he or she have the support needed? Does the family have a clear understanding of the progression of the illness and what could be next—that there may be episodic events and opportunistic infections which might require hospitalization?

Evaluating the care plan for the patient and family is the next crucial step. For PWAs, because the illness can consist of episodic opportunistic infections, monitoring how things are at home can be very difficult until a crisis situation occurs. Creating a plan that can be modified according to the changing needs of the patient and family provides optimum care.

Once you have compiled all this information, contact the most appropriate home care or hospice agency, based on where the client lives, what her or his needs are, what the agency can offer, and often, how unproblemmatic the insurance and managed care relationships are. The agency will generally need to know much of the information previously described.

POTENTIAL BARRIERS TO SUCCESSFUL INTERVENTION

Communication

If the client's needs are not clearly stated and communicated to the family and the agency that will provide the home care or hospice services, the services will most likely not be provided in a consistent manner.

Limited Resources

Another major barrier is the limited resources available to PWAs, particularly in rural areas. For many home health care agencies, stigmatization of and discrimination against PWAs still exists. Some home health or hospice agencies might not be willing to deal with people with HIV because of the costs they may incur. Certain staff members, nurses, home health aides, and social workers might be unwilling to work with PWAs for fear of transmission or being stigmatized themselves. Because no one agency should be expected to be the sole provider of HIV services, the creation of AIDS consortiums that include home health and hospice agencies will encourage education, training, and support among care providers.

Cultural Competency

As discussed earlier, another barrier is an agency that is not culturally competent in caring for PWAs. The concept of cultural competency does not just focus on issues of someone's race or ethnic background; it also includes issues of language, class, age, and sexual orientation. If any agency is not capable of providing culturally competent care to a client, the quality of care provided will decrease. If staff members are unable to communicate because of language barriers or are unable to comprehend the religious or spiritual beliefs of the culture of the client, then they cannot adequately meet the needs of the client.

Accessibility

Another barrier is that many clients are inaccessible. Many PWAs are homeless, have very limited resources and supports, or have very little or no insurance assistance. Therefore, they may get "lost between the cracks." Social workers must advocate for the underserved and disenfranchised clients who are not currently receiving care.

Finances

Finances are often a potential barrier as some insurance companies will not cover certain components of home or hospice care, or they will limit their services in order to manage their care. (See Jay Laudato's chapter, "Economic Supports and Advocacy.")

Geographic

Of course, geographically many barriers often exist if agencies are not willing to work in certain areas. Inner city areas may be considered dangerous for home health care agencies to serve, and because of the epidemiology of HIV, there are often many inner-city clients who are people of color, have long histories of substance abuse, or who require extra care. Many agencies have found ways around this by using taxicab services or other kinds of security services to provide care. Be certain that any agency you refer to is willing to access the clients "where they are."

INFORMATION THE CLIENT SHOULD KNOW BEFORE TAKING ACTION

Home health agency and hospice care referrals often do not directly involve the client because they take place when the client is very ill or there are many stressors on the family system. We somehow manage to forget that the client is at the center of the system and is the person who should be, if capable, making decisions regarding his or her care.

Clients should know ahead of time the issues regarding their finances and legal concerns involved in receiving care at home. They should also know what is and is not covered, and if any unexpected fees may be involved. Specifically, clients should know what services are going to made available to them. Some issues to consider include the following:

- Are they going to receive a nurse's visit? If so, how often, and what will the nurse be expected to do?
- Will a social worker visit, and if so, what will the social worker be providing?
- Will the person have a home health aide and for how many hours?
- What other services are included in their care?
- Often, the person will assume that because they have "good" insurance they will get twenty-four-hour coverage at home. At this time, under managed care, the system is too stressed to provide twenty-four-hour care for most people at home. Therefore, the client should have a clear understanding and expectation of what the home care and hospice services will be.

POLICY IMPLICATIONS AND RELATED ACTIONS

Social workers must get actively involved in the health care reform movement. Managed care, as it is coming to be seen, is beginning to define how we will provide home care. At this point in time, because home care is seen as less expensive, it will be continuously utilized by managed care companies. However, managed care is going to continue to attempt to lessen the cost of providing care, even for people at home. Therefore, it is important that we are involved in actively advocating to ensure that PWAs receive quality home care—including the supports and systems that they need wherever their home might be, whether that means living with their family, in a shelter, in a prison, or in a group or single room occupancy home.

RECOMMENDED READINGS

Macklin, Eleanor (ed.) (1992). *AIDS and families*. Binghamton, NY: The Haworth Press.

Rosen, Elliot J. (1990). *Families facing death: Family dynamics of terminal illness*, New York: Macmillan/Lexington Books.

von Gunten, Charles, Martinez, Jeanne, Weitzman, Sigmund A., and Von Roenin, Jamie (1991). AIDS and hospice. *The American Journal of Hospice and Palliative Care*, July/August.

Walker, Gillian (1991). *In the midst of winter: Systemic therapy with families, couples, and individuals with AIDS infection*. New York: Norton.

Bereavement Work
in Hospice and Home Care

David J. Brennan

WHY DO THIS?
STATEMENT OF THE PROBLEM AND ISSUES

Current psychological literature often reminds us that the effects of grief on human coping are profound. If we do not have the opportunity to express our grief and receive support concerning our grief, long-term implications for our mental health may ensue.

People who have lost someone to AIDS are experiencing many profound issues. These range from dealing with multiple losses, which is in effect dealing with trauma, to being consumed by the overwhelming nature of the grief process, to being isolated from appropriate supports. Most agencies that provide care to people with AIDS (PWAs) do not provide follow-up after a death. In fact, people who are dealing with the death of someone with AIDS often find themselves in complete isolation without much support at all. Often, even the professional caregivers are no longer involved. Therefore, we as social workers must think about ways we can provide quality care to people who are grieving the loss of someone to AIDS.

EXAMPLES OF HOW THE ISSUE MAY PRESENT

Literature demonstrates that people who are grieving often have the following symptoms similar to depression:

- increased confusion or disorganization
- periods of intense emotional feelings such as crying or anger
- interruptions in eating and sleeping patterns
- feelings of extreme hopelessness

Someone who is grieving may seek assistance because of the above-named symptoms. Therefore, people may present in a medical, mental health, or therapeutic setting with symptoms indicating depression or other types of acute reactions. If we are not aware of someone's history of loss, we may not be aware that their physical illness might be a normal manifestation of the grieving process. Someone may present with what looks like an unexplained depression until we look further and identify a loss (or several losses) that may be related to their current depression.

Because most human beings have extreme fears about their own deaths or the deaths of those close to them, sitting with someone who is experiencing a significant loss or death is painful for us. Therefore, unfortunately, in our society, grieving people are frequently isolated and do not have an opportunity to talk or be open about their pain because those around them have a difficult time understanding it. Experience has shown that prompting people to tell their stories of loss and to talk openly about their grief-related feelings is very helpful. These feelings include the following:

- anger
- abandonment
- jealousy
- relief
- joy
- deep pain
- deep sorrow

Grief is a pervasive part of the human experience, and our losses are many and varied. When working with someone who is experiencing symptoms of depression, be certain to ascertain their history of loss, by exploring deaths (recent and historical) as well as other losses, such as divorce, significant changes in relationships, health, or career.

FACTS THE SOCIAL WORKER NEEDS TO KNOW
BEFORE PROCEEDING

Grief and bereavement are a part of every human being's experience. All of us have experienced various types of loss in our lives, whether from death, divorce, jobs, or money; therefore, we can all relate to loss at some level. Grieving is considered by most experts in the field to be a very natural process. Resources on grief and bereavement (see the recommended readings at the end of this chapter) describe various types of developmental paths or stages that someone may go through as well as the issues they may be dealing with during the grieving process.

First and foremost, when you are doing an assessment, particularly of someone you know has had a loss due to AIDS, you must find out about other losses they have had in their life. At the time of death or loss in someone's life, the client often begins to think about these other losses: family members who have died and other important people who are no longer with them. Allowing people to look back at other losses gives them an opportunity to talk about what their needs are at this point in time. They have a chance to reflect on other relationships that have ended due to death, breakup, divorce, or other causes.

The issues for people dealing with an AIDS loss or death are very specific. Often their grief has to be hidden. Because of the stigma associated with this illness, people may say it was a death from cancer or some other terminal illness. Therefore, because isolation is a tremendous issue in dealing with any loss, it can be exponentially compounded because it is an AIDS death and the family has not shared the diagnosis with anyone. This stigma and the accompanying shame and isolation are the most difficult concerns of someone who is grieving a death from AIDS.

We should also take into consideration that, at this point in the epidemic in this country, most people in urban areas who have lost someone to AIDS probably know other people who have died of AIDS and are therefore experiencing more than just this one loss.

The episodic and unpredictable nature and progression of this illness leaves many questions in the minds of those who have lost someone to AIDS as to whether or not the deceased person could have continued to fight the illness or could have continued to get better. This may trigger feelings of guilt and shame attached to the death.

Survival guilt may be a factor when a parent loses a child or an HIV-negative partner or spouse wonders why he or she was not infected, especially if he or she has engaged in any high-risk behaviors.

KEY QUESTIONS TO ASK THE CLIENT

Collecting details regarding the death from the person who is coming to you for bereavement support is useful. This assists people in talking about the death and also gives you information about the series of events.

- Where and how did the death happen?
- Who was present at the death?

- Was the person comfortable?
- Was the patient at a point of acceptance that death was going to happen, or was he or she anxious about and/or terrified with the concept of dying?
- Did the person who died indicate repeatedly that he or she wished the family could have done more?
- What is/was the level of helplessness or hopelessness experienced concerning the death for the person who is coming for bereavement support?

The feelings that arise during the grieving process are natural, yet often we do not allow ourselves to experience these feelings of anger and extreme sadness. When people are given the opportunity to express the intensity and magnitude of what they are feeling, they often cope more effectively with life's day-to-day situations. Expressing intense feeling (by crying, getting verbally angry, or expressing any outward emotion) are often seen as signs of weakness in our culture. When people repress feelings of sadness they are considered "strong." *This misconception is the greatest challenge to a social worker when providing support to someone who is grieving.*

Support Groups

Most bereavement literature encourages people to participate in support groups because one of the key components of bereavement support is preventing isolation from others who are experiencing a similar situation. This is particularly true of people who have had a loss due to AIDS, primarily because of the stigma associated with HIV. One should always ask someone who is interested in bereavement support whether he or she is interested in connecting with a group of people who are experiencing a similar loss (see the support group section of this book) or whether he or she prefers one-on-one support.

The intensity of a support group or the fear of being "known" may keep people from joining a support group. Some bereavement programs do educational and social events or workshops (e.g., fundraisers for a program or workshops on common legal/financial affairs that follow a death) as a means of breaking the ice and encouraging interaction with others who are grieving.

Spiritual/Religious Beliefs

The client's spiritual and/or religious beliefs will have a profound impact on his or her coping. An assessment of a client's spiritual or religious beliefs regarding death and dying will assist in understanding the individual's needs and generate ideas regarding resources for support. Spiritual beliefs can be a source of comfort during the grieving process. Many people with AIDS—given the history of judgment by some religions regarding HIV, homosexuality, drug use, and addiction—often feel completely discouraged from seeking support from their church, temple, or other place of worship. Pastoral and chaplain services are available through AIDS service organizations, hospitals, and hospice programs. Many church and religious groups do provide supportive pastoral care and support, and social workers should know these resources in their area.

Assessing the supports of the client at the time of his or her grief is important. Ask the client who the key people are in his or her life. Who can be allies in coping with grief? Are there some people who can hear this person's pain or hear the story more than once? Are there other people who can allow your client to laugh and be lighthearted? Are there other people who the bereaved can call at any time of day or night when in need of support?

CULTURAL COMPETENCY CONSIDERATIONS

HIV has affected many cultures, and the needs and responses of these groups to death and dying and the grief process are extremely varied. Some people in various cultures and communities are accustomed to extremely limited discussion of the person who has died or any of their feelings. In many cultures, crying or feeling emotionally vulnerable under any circumstances is considered a sign of great weakness, and therefore, people are not encouraged to express their grief. In other cultures, expressing grief in loud and dramatic ways is considered absolutely essential to show the world how extreme your feelings are regarding the death. Furthermore, various families within these cultures deal with the death and dying process very differently.

A bereavement program or grief support program should have a clear sense of the needs of the communities that will be served. Some communities will need a quieter, more reserved space to sort out issues and feelings. Others will need very limited intervention, as the concept of outside support is not relevant: Grief is kept in the family system. Others will need intensive support from professional agencies and social workers to allow families to work through their grief.

Bereavement programs should also be flexible in offering various types of supports including one-on-one support and group support as well as psychoeducational support and social supports. Any bereavement support program should match as closely as possible the cultural needs of the community it is serving and, therefore, should have a built-in flexibility to be able to meet the needs of various communities.

ACTION STEPS FOR SUCCESSFUL INTERVENTION

Services to offer those who are grieving are the following:

- support groups
- individual counseling
- specially trained "bereavement" volunteers
- maintaining a network of bereavement volunteers
- social and educational events on issues such as stress management, financial matters, and legal issues
- Therapeutic services that do not involve talking, such as art, music, and dance therapy

It is imperative that any agency providing bereavement support provide not only psychotherapeutic or emotional support for people who are grieving, but also educational support to family and friends who are grieving. Often, people live under the assumptions of our society that people who are grieving should keep it to themselves, that time will heal everything, and that they just need to meet a new person to be able to resolve their grief. Of course, the grieving process is not that simple; grief is a complex and lifelong process. Providing clear action steps to successfully intervene can become complicated.

The primary method to intervene well is to continually assess the needs of those who are grieving. This can be accomplished by utilizing narrative family treatment theory. This theory provides an understanding that the telling and retelling of an issue or problem allows the grieving person to heal with each retelling. It also allows the practitioner to assess the person's current needs and concerns, including getting an understanding of how the person is coping on a daily basis. Is the client able to get out to various meetings or see other people? Is he or she completely isolated? Can the individual function in a day-to-day routine? Are feelings arising that could use the assistance of counseling, support from friends, or artistic or creative activity?

The assessment of the needs of people who are grieving is the most critical role that the social worker can take in supporting someone through the grieving process, and educating the client about the grieving process.

In providing counseling to bereaved individuals, it is important to remember that grieving people need to tell their story—the story of the person who died and of his or her actual death. The story needs to be told over and over again. In the retelling of this story, grieving people begin to make meaning of the loss and to adjust to a new life without the deceased person.

Second, giving people room to feel their feelings is also important. It may be difficult for us to hear someone repeat their feelings of sadness or loss or anger. We often describe them as being stuck in their feelings instead of encouraging them to retell their story. We often do not allow for the fact that people may need to tell their story over and over in a supportive environment in order to be able to feel their feelings. Therefore, allowing space for people to express their feelings is another key component in intervention. The concepts of narrative treatment theory are particularly helpful in grief work because each time a client tells his or her story, he or she develops a new understanding of the process and gathers new insights.

Third, it is important to give people the opportunity to reflect on their relationship with the deceased person. Therefore, open discussion about both the good and the difficult parts of that relationship is strongly encouraged.

Finally, it is important for people to make connections that allow them to move forward in their life. William Worden's fourth task in *Grief Counseling and Grief Therapy* is investing in new relationships. As people move on in their lives, they need to build stronger and more committed relationships and to begin to reinvest in their life.

Multiple Loss

No definitive time frame for dealing with grief exists, but it is important to note that in the communities most adversely affected by HIV and AIDS, people are dealing with an overwhelming number of deaths. As stated earlier, people dealing with the loss of someone to AIDS have often lost more than one person to this disease. This will continue as time moves on and people with AIDS develop more support groups and support organizations. Therefore, communities dealing with HIV/AIDS are confronting multiple loss and bereavement overload.

This phenomenon is often similar to post-traumatic stress disorder although the "traumatic stress" is recurrent and chronic, not "post." Individuals experiencing this often feel confused by their feelings and overwhelmed by the number of deaths they have experienced. They also experience symptoms similar to post-traumatic stress disorder, including numbness, depression, and potentially self-destructive behavior.

Again, providing opportunities for people to feel all their emotions as part of the grieving process is also important. We must provide the opportunity for clients and to think clearly about what we need as a community to move forward and to have opportunities to be playful and lighthearted about our grief. In some support groups the focus is very intense at times, but at other times, a sense of lightness can help people remember that there are good things about life and good things about the person who has left them.

Most agencies do not have a clearly delineated bereavement program. Hospices are required to have a bereavement component to their care. AIDS service organizations and some mental health programs also have a bereavement component. It is important to be familiar with the resources available to you as a provider if your agency does not provide bereavement services.

POTENTIAL BARRIERS TO SUCCESSFUL INTERVENTION

One of the most obvious barriers to successful intervention is that grieving people are often isolated and may feel they need to keep their grief to themselves, because if they share their grief with others, they might be considered weak or be shamed. Therefore, we have learned to be creative about the ways in which we provide opportunities for people to do their grief work. Support groups and individual counseling are ways to facilitate this process, but we can also create rituals that allow us to think about how we are coping with our losses. The Names Project AIDS Memorial Quilt is one clear example of a creative response to the overwhelming grief. Certainly, music concerts, memorial services, theatrical productions, and other kinds of rituals have been very beneficial in helping people heal their losses. Political action and volunteering are often key components for people who are trying to heal their grief. Many opportunities exist for people to get politically involved in HIV work and to volunteer to provide support for other people who are dealing with HIV. Each of these interventions has the added benefit of successfully decreasing isolation.

Other obstacles to successful intervention are cultural barriers and resource barriers. Bereavement services are often considered secondary and not primary care. If people do not get to do all the work they need to in order to grieve, they may internalize their feelings of shame and isolation. This can result in depression or other situations in which clients do not take good care of themselves, including relapses into substance use or unsafe sex.

We must think of grief work as preventative work to assist people who are struggling with overwhelming loss from decompensating into difficult life situations, which would make them unable to move forward in their life. Because bereavement work is often considered secondary, limited resources are put into the needs of our grieving communities.

INFORMATION THE CLIENT SHOULD KNOW
BEFORE TAKING ACTION

Clients must be aware that no magical cure for grief work exists and many myths concerning grief prevail. One of the myths is that time will heal everything: if you just repress your feelings for awhile, the feelings will go away. We need to be able to express our feelings and to think about what we can do to move our lives forward.

Clients should also be aware that people grieve distinctively and differently. Some people can talk about their grief; others cannot. Some people can cry about their grief; others cannot. Therefore, when getting involved in any kind of bereavement support work, know that people are going to respond to grief work very differently. This variation in response requires flexibility on the part of someone entering any kind of bereavement group or bereavement social setting.

Another myth is that when we are grieving, we should do it alone and not burden other people with it because other people do not want to hear too much about our loss. It is, of course, extremely healing to go through the grieving process with other people providing support to you.

An important thing for clients to note regarding the grief process is that, for people with AIDS, the family makeup is often different than for people with other illnesses.

Families facing an AIDS death may be experiencing many other losses, such as poverty, violence, and other inner-city issues. AIDS may just be, to quote a client, "one more thing."

A situation may occur in which the patient who has died had a lover and a family of origin who were not aware of each other, or the family of origin was not aware that the patient's roommate was also a lover. Because these things are not always clearly understood by all involved parties, the grieving process becomes confusing and complicated. If the family members are not aware of the relationship of the surviving partner, they might not be able to be as supportive of that partner. Also, families may have a difficult time accepting the partner even when it is clear that the person was their child's partner.

Providers must be aware that sometimes the grieving process of the family of origin and family of choice may need to be very separate processes. Often the lover or significant other of the person who has died needs different supports and different types of care than the family of origin. Tensions between the family of origin and the family of choice may exist—but not always. Literature has pointed out that when the family of origin and family of choice are aware of each other and supportive of one another, the grieving process tends to go better for both parties. Therefore, it is important to encourage people to have some opportunity to resolve some of these issues before the death. If they are not resolved before the death, it may be necessary to provide separate support so that they may be able to do their grief work in their own manner.

POLICY IMPLICATIONS AND RELATED ACTIONS

The clearest policy implication is that if people do not have opportunities to grieve, they can very easily become trapped in compulsive or anxiety-reducing behaviors that may put them at risk for HIV transmission or other concerns, including substance abuse. The long-term mental health effects of communities grieving are documented in stories of Holocaust survivors and other situations of post-traumatic stress disorder.

RECOMMENDED READINGS

Froman, Paul Kent. (1992). *After you say goodbye: When someone you love dies of AIDS.* San Francisco: Chronicle Books.

Walker, Gillian. (1991). *In the midst of winter: Systemic therapy with families, couples and individuals with AIDS infection.* New York: Norton.

Worden, William (1982). *Grief counseling and grief therapy.* New York: Springer Publishing Co.

Helping a Person with HIV/AIDS Get into Clinical Trials

Fred F. Boykin

WHY DO THIS?
STATEMENT OF THE PROBLEM AND ISSUES

Today medical treatments for a person who is infected with HIV abound. Along with antiretrovirals (such as the drug AZT), a number of treatments for opportunistic infections (such as Pentamidine or Bactrim for pneumocystis pneumonia) exist. For the true usefulness of these drugs to be known and for them to become widely available, they must first be tested in a strict scientific manner. We call these tests clinical trials.

Most clinical trials begin as experiments done in a laboratory environment. The drugs are first tested in cell cultures and then in animals before they are given to human beings. If the findings in the lab are positive, the experimenter attempts to formulate the most safe and effective treatment for study in human beings. However, even though years of research may have occurred in the laboratory, there is no guarantee that a drug will be effective or free of major side effects until it is tested in people.

Human clinical trials have been in existence in the United States for many years. In order for any drug to be approved and widely available for treatment, it must first undergo extensive clinical trials to prove its usefulness as a treatment. Many times these trials compare the new treatment with standard treatments that have already been proven to be effective. Several years may pass before a particular treatment is finally approved by the Food and Drug Administration (FDA) and becomes available for general use by physicians. Therefore, some persons choose to get involved in clinical trials before they are sure of a drug's efficacy.

A person with HIV/AIDS can get involved in a clinical trial in many ways. He or she may get involved with a study supported by an individual drug company or by a government agency. The clinical trial site may be local (a patient's primary care doctor may even be involved with a particular study) or may be located in a different area of the state or the country. Clinical trials supported by the National Institutes of Health (NIH) are protocols sponsored by the federal government and conducted at their facility located in Bethesda, Maryland. The NIH recruits people from all over the continental United States to participate in HIV/AIDS clinical trials.

There are three levels of clinical trials for most HIV/AIDS drug studies:

1. *Phase I Trial:* This is the first setting in which an experimental drug is given to humans. These trials are designed to answer initial questions about a drug's safety. Researchers look for information about the drug's side effects, safest dose to give a patient, and the body's ability to handle the drug. Such information can usually be gathered in less than one year. Phase I trials are conducted on a small number of people, usually less that fifty, and all participants receive the experimental drug.

2. *Phase II Trial:* If results from Phase I trials show that a drug is safe, it can enter the second phase of testing. Phase II studies enroll larger numbers of patients, as many as a few hundred. In these studies, researchers attempt to establish solid evidence of the drug's effectiveness against HIV infection, AIDS-related immune deficiency, or opportunistic infections. Phase II trials may take from one to two years to complete. For example, if a new antiretroviral drug is being tested, clinicians will do extensive testing on viral load, T-cell counts, and other HIV-related parameters. At the same time, the researchers will examine toxicities that may occur in the liver, kidneys, lungs, heart, and other organs.

3. *Phase III Trial:* These trials seek to prove with certainty the value of the new drug compared to other available therapy or placebo (see the following section). Clinicians also look for long-term side effects that may not have appeared in earlier testing. For that reason, these tests may take up to four years to complete. Phase III clinical trials often enroll several hundred to a few thousand individuals and are controlled and blinded (see the following section). When Phase III clinical trials are complete, drug sponsors present results from all laboratory, animal, and human studies to the FDA for review in the form of a new drug application for approval to market the drug.

BENEFITS AND RISKS

Some of the reasons why an HIV-infected person would be interested in HIV/AIDS clinical trials are as follows:

- The patient would be one of the first to receive a promising new treatment. A successful new treatment may prolong life or improve the quality of life.
- A person who participates in a clinical trial is helping others with HIV/AIDS by assisting in research. Many patients in clinical trials obtain great satisfaction by knowing that they have helped further progress toward greater understanding of HIV/AIDS and perhaps eventually the creation of a vaccine or even a cure.
- The patient receives some medical benefits from enrolling in a clinical trial. The costs of the experimental medications, the physical exam, and much of the ongoing monitoring of the patient's general health are all incurred by the drug company or the sponsor of the experiment. Although such tests are not a substitute for a primary health care team, having another group of providers who are available for input into a patient's physical needs can be helpful.
- Patients who wish to be proactive in their healthcare decision making may find increased self-esteem and psychological strength in knowing they have the most up-to-date treatments available for HIV disease.

It is also important that a person interested in HIV/AIDS clinical trials be aware of the potential drawbacks of participation, which include the following:

- A drug or particular treatment may cause discomfort or unpleasant side effects. These are most often temporary, but they may be substantial or severe. A person who has a significant sense of fear and trepidation about possible side effects should be especially careful in determining if a clinical trial is the proper choice for treatment.
- An experimental treatment may not work, or it may work no better than treatments already available. A risk of any protocol using untested medications or treatments is that there may be no medical benefit to the patient.
- Patients may enroll in protocols thinking they will receive experimental treatments, but this is not always the case. The study may involve randomization, a process that assigns patients to different groups. Some groups may receive the new treatment while others may receive a standard treatment or a placebo, which is an inactive substance given to measure the psychological effects of taking a medication.

- In some studies, patients may be randomized into a control group, or a group that receives only standard treatments or a placebo. The best way to study the efficacy of a new drug is to "control" conditions of one of the groups while giving the experimental treatment to others. Although the patient may be randomized into the control group, he or she will still receive the most effective treatments known. For example, if an antiretroviral drug is being tested, the control group would receive standard retrovirals (AZT, ddI, ddC, etc.) while the experimental group would receive the new treatment.
- Protocols sometimes employ a procedure called blinding. In a single-blinded study, the patient does not know whether he or she is receiving the controlled or the experimental treatment. In a double-blinded study, neither the patient nor the health care professionals know which treatment the patient is receiving. However, if the patient begins to have significant side effects, the health care workers can use a coding system to find out what treatment he or she is receiving.
- Clinical trials can be burdensome due to their extensive time and financial demands. A few HIV/AIDS clinical trials offer some reimbursement for participation, but often it is not enough to cover transportation costs, food, and other incidental expenses that may be incurred by the patient. If the study requires frequent visits to the clinic or hospital, the patient may experience stress due to separation from their families, friends, job, and support networks.
- Finally, a patient who is considering a clinical trial may be hesitant because he or she may feel like a "guinea pig," or that he or she is merely being used in a medical experiment with no possibile direct benefit. This is an important reason for the social worker and other health care workers to be comfortable with the basic tenets of medical research. Also, social workers should become familiar with a patient's rights as a protocol participant, including his or her option to withdraw from a study anytime during the clinical trials process.

EXAMPLES OF HOW THE ISSUE MAY PRESENT

You may receive an inquiry from a patient who has heard about HIV/AIDS clinical trials in a newsletter or newspaper, on radio or television, or through informal sources such as friends. The request may come from another service provider, such as a physician or a nurse, who may speak to the patient about clinical trials. Additionally, a patient who has taken standard treatments and has either had severe side effects or has become resistant to the therapy may be interested in trying a new experimental treatment for his or her HIV disease.

FACTS THE SOCIAL WORKER NEEDS TO KNOW
BEFORE PROCEEDING

The following resources are available for obtaining information concerning clinical trials:

- The National AIDS Clearinghouse (800-458-5231) is a service that provides general information on HIV/AIDS clinical trials. The Clearing House will send the patient information on clinical trials that are occurring within his or her local area. It also acts as a general information source for questions concerning HIV/AIDS.
- Another source of information for HIV/AIDS clinical trials is the National AIDS Clinical Trial Information Service at 800-TRIALS-A or 800-874-2572 (for teletype service, 800-AIDS-TTY or 800-243-7889; for Spanish service, 800-344-SIDA or 800-344-7432). This service will give you information about clinical trials in your area, or any other trial nationwide.
- The AIDS/HIV Experimental Treatment Directory (212-719-0033) is produced quarterly by the American Foundation for AIDS Research (AmFAR) and describes clinical trials in the United States. This directory details the protocol and the treatment being studied, the inclusion/exclusion criteria for the individual trial, and phone contacts for each clinical trial site.
- Information on HIV/AIDS clinical trials at the National Institutes of Health (NIH) can be obtained at 800-AIDS-NIH (800-243-7644) and 800-4-CANCER (800-422-6237). These services recruit nationally for HIV/AIDS clinical trials conducted at the NIH Clinical Center in Bethesda, Maryland. If a patient qualifies for participation after the initial screening visit, a stipend for travel and food/lodging may be available to defray the costs of getting to and from the Clinical Center. There is also a twenty-four-hour fax service at 1-800-772-5464, extension 94, which will fax information about HIV/AIDS trials conducted at the Clinical Center by the National Institute of Allergy and Infectious Disease (NIAID) and the National Cancer Institute (NCI). The fax service gives details of trials for which patients are currently being recruited and can send you information on those trials. The caller must have access to a fax machine in order to receive the information.
- There is also an online HIV/AIDS database service offered by the National Library of Medicine in Bethesda, Maryland. AIDSTRIALS

provides information on clinical trials approved by the Food and Drug Administration. AIDSDRUGS is another service that provides information on treatments being used in HIV/AIDS clinical trials. To obtain a free information packet, call 1-800-638-8480.

KEY QUESTIONS TO ASK THE CLIENT

The social worker should explore the reasons a patient is interested in clinical trials. It is important that the patient understand both the benefits and risks of participation. The patient may have unrealistic expectations of a "cure" from the experimental treatment, or conversely, fear that the treatment may harm him or her significantly.

Other questions should address the requirements of the clinical trial and its potential impact upon the patient's employment and home life. Some clinical trials require only a brief visit to a local trial site on a periodic basis. Other trials may be extremely time-intensive, requiring several days or weeks spent in an inpatient hospital setting many times a year. Most trials are somewhere in-between, requiring approximately one visit per month after the first few visits. The patient should explore the frequency and amount of time required for protocol visits with the clinical trial contact person at the time of initial contact.

The social worker can determine if the HIV/AIDS patient is aware of potential side effects from the treatment. Experimental medications can have side effects that range from very mild (such as fatigue, dry mouth, occasional diarrhea, etc.) to extremely severe (such as high fevers, shaking chills, severe diarrhea, sharp stomach pain, etc.). People who have very low tolerance for pain or have a great deal of anxiety should be cautioned about this aspect of participation in a study, and they should be sure to read the protocol carefully for the reported or expected side effects of the medication.

ACTION STEPS FOR SUCCESSFUL INTERVENTION

1. Have the patient obtain information on clinical trials that may interest him or her. Be sure to discuss the information with the patient, to ensure that he or she is clear of the benefits and risks of enrolling in the trial.
2. Encourage the patient to discuss the possibility of enrolling in a clinical trial with his or her primary physician. In most cases, participation in a clinical trial requires the assistance and cooperation of the patient's primary physician. The physician should also be given information about the clinical trial to help inform and assist the patient in making the

decision, and in identifying possible problems that could occur with the experimental treatment and the patient's current medication regimen.

3. The HIV/AIDS patient should talk with his or her significant others about becoming involved in a study. Ssignificant others should be part of the decision-making process in order to provide support and encouragement to the patient.

4. After the patient has discussed the possibility of enrollment with the primary physician, significant others, and his or her support system, he or she should directly contact the clinical trial site. The social worker may be able to assist the patient in obtaining the original information packet, but it is advisable for the patient or patient's parents to speak to a contact at the site if at all possible. After initial information about the prospective participant is obtained by the clinical trial site, an appointment may be made by the clinical trial study coordinator for an initial screening visit. Be sure the patient knows what he or she needs to bring to the appointment (e.g., medical records, living will, identification, etc.)

5. At the screening visit, the patient will likely undergo an extensive physical and psychosocial evaluation. This initial visit may take three to four hours or more. As soon as all of the results of the tests are reviewed, the patient will be informed of his or her eligibility for the clinical trial. If not eligible for this particular trial, the clinical trial specialist may suggest other clinical trials or alternatives that the patient could pursue.

6. If the patient is accepted into the trial after the screening visit, he or she will be asked to sign an informed consent form. The informed consent form is a document describing the study and defining the potential benefits and risks of participation in the particular trial. If unsure about any point, the patient should be encouraged to ask questions or to seek clarification. Even if a patient signs an informed consent, he or she is free to leave the trial at any time during the study. If the patient entering the study is a child, a parent or legal guardian must sign the consent form.

7. Ideally, the patient's employer should be informed of the patient's decision to participate in the clinical trial process. Since most trials require visits to the clinic/hospital during working hours, the patient will be taking time off from work responsibilities. If the employer is well-informed, possible future problems (e.g., multiple absences during the day) may be avoided. The patient may want to call the employer's personnel or human resources department to request advice or suggestions on how to discuss this situation with the employer. The social worker can be of assistance to a patient who is having questions or problems about speaking to his or her employer, and can help determine the personal risks of the decision to disclose this information.

POTENTIAL BARRIERS TO SUCCESSFUL INTERVENTION

As previously stated, a patient must be able to meet the schedule for visits to the clinical trial site. The protocol may require numerous visits, and some may even include one or more days as an inpatient. Persons entering a trial must often be willing to take time off from their jobs or maybe even postpone vacations or trips in order to go to the clinic for a scheduled visit.

The possibility of receiving blinded treatment regimens and other unfamiliar experiences may cause stress and anxiety in a patient who is considering enrolling in a clinical trial. The potential for side effects and the effects of clinical trial participation on significant others must be considered before a patient enrolls. The social worker should become knowledgeable about the particular trial in order to assist with the patient's concerns or fears. The social worker should inform the patient that he or she can withdraw from the study at any time in order to alleviate unacceptable levels of anxiety or stress.

Some patients may be anxious about enrolling in a particular trial because they have received negative "word of mouth" information about a treatment. Nonscientific articles appear frequently in the national, state, or local media and may dampen a person's interest in getting into a particular experimental trial. Since developments in the treatment of HIV/AIDS are moving so rapidly, misinformation may be spread before reliable scientific results are accrued and published. Social workers should explore the reasons behind a patient's interest in clinical trials, and if possible, research information that may seem incongruous or decisions that appear to be hastily made.

Finally, the cost associated with participating in a clinical trial may be prohibitive for some patients. Since many clinical trials sites do not offer child care or transportation reimbursement, a person with children or one who has a modest income may not be able to afford to participate. In some clinical trials, a small stipend may be offered, but even then, the payment may not be made until the person has completed the trial. The social worker can assist a patient with access to financial assistance, transportation tokens, childcare resources, etc., in order to facilitate protocol participation.

INFORMATION THE CLIENT SHOULD KNOW
BEFORE TAKING ACTION

HIV/AIDS clinical trials are tests to see if a new treatment can be given safely or if it is better than other treatments already approved and readily available. Certainly, there is good reason to believe that the new medication or treatment will benefit the patient, but this cannot be assured until it has been tested carefully. Unfortunately, no one fully knows what the long-term side effects of new medications will be.

The clinical trial is not a substitute for primary health care for the HIV/AIDS patient, even though some of the benefits of participation in such trials include frequent physical exams, blood and other lab tests, and some free medications. Unless the study is conducted in the patient's primary care setting, the person with HIV/AIDS should not rely on the clinical trial site for his or her main source of treatment. Thus, HIV/AIDS patients should continue to maintain their current health insurance. When the clinical trial is over, the patient will be referred back to his or her primary care provider for all future care. For this reason, the patient's primary physician should be updated constantly on the progress of the clinical trial.

The social worker may find that a patient becomes discouraged or frustrated about the trial if he or she is not obtaining the desired results. The patient may have doubts about whether to terminate participation in the study, or may seek to find another trial that he or she thinks may be more beneficial. The social worker can support these actions through the patient's rights of self-determination, but should also be available to remind the patient that he or she will affect the trial's results by withdrawing prematurely. Social workers can assist the patient in contrasting his or her responsibilities regarding participation in the trial and his or her own personal health needs.

POLICY IMPLICATIONS AND RELATED ACTIONS

Social workers can advocate for their patients by informing them of the potential risks and benefits of a clinical trial, and making sure they understand the possible barriers to entering and remaining in the trial.

Social workers can speak with a patient's family or employer to help explain why a patient with HIV/AIDS wishes to participate in a clinical trial or to address concerns or fears. Be sure to have the patient sign a release of information form before speaking to anyone.

Social workers can assist primary care physicians and other members of the health care team by advocating for their patients to participate in a clinical trial.

Social workers can advocate for their patients by assisting them with the information provided to them concerning the trial. In this way, the social worker can also gain understanding of the treatment being offered, the amount of the patient's time the trial will consume, and other concerns that may not be apparent to the patient.

Social workers should advocate that all clinical trial sites be universally accessible to patients with HIV/AIDS. Issues such as child care, meal vouchers, and transportation vouchers at clinical trials sites should be available to assist those with children or those who need financial assistance in order to remain on a clinical trial.

Social workers can become involved in local, state, and national HIV/AIDS forums in order to become more politically active in HIV/AIDS issues. Each local chapter of National Association of Social Workers (NASW) has an HIV/AIDS liaison who keeps local social workers informed about HIV/AIDS clinical trials. About 15 National HIV/AIDS advocacy organizations (e.g., ACT UP) have subgroups for monitoring clinical trials.

TO LEARN MORE ABOUT CLINICAL TRIALS

Call the AIDS Clinical Trial Information Service at 800-TRIALS-A (800-874-2572) and ask for the AIDS/HIV Treatment Directory to be sent to you. You may also ask to speak with a specialist to ask questions or to get information.

Call the CDC National AIDS Clearinghouse at 800-458-5231. This is a voice mail service; you should choose the option that refers to the HIV/AIDS Clinical Trials services. You may request two pamphlets explaining the HIV/AIDS clinical trial process titled, "AIDS Clinical Trials: Talking it Over" and "AIDS: Finding Better Treatments with Your Help" from a clinical trials specialist. You may request a video on clinical trials titled "Know Your Options."

There are resources on the internet for social workers who have access and are interested in HIV/AIDS clinical trials. The internet services at the CDC National AIDS Clearinghouse includes a directory of AIDS-related news, including clinical trials. To correspond with the Clearinghouse, send e-mail to aidsinfo@cdcnac.aspensys.com.

Helping a Person with HIV/AIDS Prepare a Power of Attorney and a Living Will

Fred F. Boykin

WHY DO THIS?
STATEMENT OF THE PROBLEM AND ISSUES

At times in the disease process, the HIV/AIDS patient may have to make difficult or painful choices concerning his or her medical treatment. If the patient is unable for reasons of severity of illness or dementia to make such decisions, it is important that he or she have previously executed documents, known as advance directives, that designate someone to speak for the patient or identify specific treatments and/or procedures that he or she may or may not want. Two important advance directive documents are the "living will" and "durable power of attorney for health care." A living will informs doctors and other health care providers of the person's wishes concerning life-sustaining procedures or treatments when the patient has become critically ill. States have different requirements concerning the procedures and treatments a patient can address in this document. The patient must understand that the living will is a statement of wishes and desires that can be changed at any time. However, the living will is a valuable tool to help physicians, other health care workers, and significant others make appropriate decisions about medical treatment when the patient cannot.

The durable power of attorney for health care designates another person, typically a family member or friend, whom the patient wishes to make medical decisions if he or she becomes unable to do so. The designated person (known as a health care proxy) should be someone the patient knows well and trusts implicitly to make informed decisions based on what he or she would want. It is therefore crucial for the patient to discuss all of his or her preferences of various options concerning treatments, pain management, extraordinary medical procedures, etc., with the health care proxy.

A number of reasons explain why a person with HIV/AIDS should complete advance directives. They are as follows:

• Advance directives can provide the patient with considerable peace of mind that his or her wishes concerning medical procedures are known, and that he or she will have some input in the decision-making process, even if he or she becomes unable to make autonomous decisions due to the severity of illness. For example, the patient may wish to withhold certain painful and/or life-sustaining treatments that would only delay an imminent and/or inevitable death.

• Advance directives allow family members and significant others to understand more clearly the opinions and wishes of the person for whom decisions regarding treatment must be made. This documentation can help family members and significant others feel more assured that they are acting in the patient's interests if it becomes necessary to make these choices. Thus, advance directives relieve a good deal of stress on the family and significant others during a very difficult period of time. For example, it can be greatly reassuring for the family members and significant others to know the wishes of HIV/AIDS patients who are unconscious in the intensive care unit (ICU) at a hospital and need tubes to be inserted for breathing.

• Advance directives guide the health care team in identifying the person who should be contacted to make certain health care decisions and the specific procedures and treatments the patient may want. If the advance directives have been discussed with various members of the health care team (e.g., primary care physician, social worker, nurse, etc.), then decisions regarding his or her treatments will be much easier to make. Copies of the advance directives should be distributed to all of those responsible for the care of the patient to ensure that his or her wishes are carried out.

• The process of completing advance directives may give the patient a sense of control over the disease, especially at a time when the patient's life frequently is being dictated by the medical system. When a patient is forced to comply with multiple requests of doctors, nurses, social workers, hospitals, etc., to make his or her own wishes known and to have a "voice" in certain medical decisions can be quite empowering.

Some points to consider before the HIV/AIDS patient executes advance directives are as follows:

• Completing advance directives may bring up difficult and painful issues for the patient. For example, the HIV/AIDS patient may be thinking about the pain and suffering that may be in his or her future. Also, he or she may be contemplating the dying process for the first time. The issues of funerals, burial versus cremation, and similar topics can be unnerving for the patient. The social worker should be prepared to validate the patient's feelings and explore any distress that he or she may incur in the process of preparing advanced directives.

• The patient will probably have to speak to family members, his or her significant other, health care providers, and support systems about the advance directives. This may be difficult, especially if the patient has not told family members or friends about his or her HIV infection. The patient may need to be prepared to address these issues with the significant persons in his or her life. Social workers should make the HIV/AIDS patient aware of these consequences of completing advance directives, especially if the patient has withheld significant information from loved ones regarding the illness. Social workers should also be prepared to use such methods as role-plays to assist the patient in the process of revealing his or her intentions for medical treatment.

• The actual execution of these documents will vary from state to state and may be more difficult in some states than in others since states have individual advance directive laws. For example, if an HIV/AIDS patient living in New York moves to South Carolina to be with his or her family, the advance directives completed in New York may not be legally binding in South Carolina. Therefore the patient's family and/or partner should pursue preparing an advanced directive in the state to which he or she has moved. As a general rule, however, advanced directives for one state can serve as a guideline of the patient's wishes in other states.

EXAMPLES OF HOW THE ISSUE MAY PRESENT

HIV/AIDS patients may be asked about advance directives through a hospital admissions office. The Patient Self-Determination Act of 1990 states that all persons entering medical facilities (hospitals, nursing homes, etc.) that accept federal funding (e.g., Medicare or Medicaid) must be informed about their right to have advance directives. These facilities may ask whether a patient has an advance directive and must be able to provide a patient with the advance directive information if someone requests it.

A patient may also be approached about advance directives when he or she visits his or her doctor, nurse, social worker, or other health care provider. A friend or family member may ask the patient about his or her wishes concerning medical procedures. Finally, the patient may have had a recent crisis in his or her life, (e.g., the death of a close friend or family member) that stimulated his or her thinking about this subject.

FACTS THE SOCIAL WORKER NEEDS TO KNOW
BEFORE PROCEEDING

Each state has its own laws and regulations concerning advance directives and their appropriate use. It is vital that the social worker know how to access information on the regulations for advance directives in the patient's state of residence and the state where the patient's medical facilities are located. This is especially important since some patients who can no longer independently manage their own needs choose to move to another state to be cared for by a family member. Choice in Dying, 200 Varcik St./10th Floor, New York, NY 10014-4810 (800-989-WILL), is a nonprofit organization that provides information on advance directives in every state and answers questions concerning end-of-life medical care. The social worker should request an informational packet from all applicable states.

States vary widely on the information they require in the living will and durable power of attorney for health care forms. For example, some states do not allow family members or health care workers to be proxies or witnesses on advance directive documents. Each state has specific definitions about when the advance directives take effect, which medical procedures they cover, and who can be the designated proxy for the power of attorney for health care.

KEY QUESTIONS TO ASK THE CLIENT

Determine the motivation for the HIV/AIDS patient's interest in advance directives. Has a recent death in the patient's family or friendship network prompted this action? Has the person just learned that he or she is HIV positive and is having a panic reaction to the news, feeling he or she has to get his or her "affairs in order" immediately? Or has the patient decided to pursue this after some contemplation and discussion with others?

Many important issues can be pursued by the social worker and the HIV/AIDS patient when the discussion focuses on advance directives. Thoughts concerning "unfinished business" that the patient may have with a family member, significant other, or friend may be a topic that arises during this discussion. The feeling of needing to leave a lasting legacy or contribution to society may be an important issue to some patients. The social worker should willing to explore these and other life-review issues with a patient if they should arise during preparation of these documents.

Has the patient thought about life-sustaining medical procedures (ventilator or breathing support, resuscitation orders, palliative/comfort care versus aggressive medical treatment, etc.) that he or she would or would not want if the disease became life-threatening? Has he or she discussed these matters openly with his or her family members and significant other?

Some of the most common issues that a patient should think about concerning life-sustaining medical procedures are listed below. The following is not meant to be an exhaustive list; however, these are issues that persons most commonly address in their durable power of attorney for health care:

Artificial Nutrition and/or Hydration: If a patient cannot eat or drink, does he or she want nutrition and fluids provided by tubes or other devices?

Cardiopulmonary Resuscitation (CPR): Does the patient want treatment to restart his or her heart if it has stopped beating? CPR can be performed by drugs, electric shock, pushing on the chest, or putting a breathing tube down the throat. In many states, a patient can designate which, if any, of these procedures he or she may or may not want.

Comfort Measures (Palliative Care): Does the patient wish to be kept as comfortable and pain-free as possible without having any life-sustaining treatments? In other words, would the patient prefer to only have sedatives or pain-relieving medications, rather than antibiotic medications that may help with the illness, but may only serve to prolong a terminal condition?

Do Not Resuscitate (DNR): Does the patient want a DNR order in their advance directives, which states to the physician and the health care team that he or she does not wish to have any CPR procedures performed if his or her heart stops beating?

Intensive Care Unit (ICU): Would the patient want to be transferred to the ICU if his or her condition deteriorates?

Life-Sustaining Treatments: Many medical procedures, drugs, blood products, and medical devices can prolong life when death is otherwise imminent. Some are innocuous, but many can be painful and/or mood-altering. Does the patient want such treatments, and if so, how far should the health care team go to prolong life?

Quality of Life: From the patient's individual value perspective, what is it that makes life worth living? These values can be very difficult to determine, and must be discussed with significant others. Some of the quality-of-life issues most often discussed are activities of living such as eating and personal hygiene, being as pain-free as possible, being able to understand and talk to others, and so on.

Ventilator Support: Does the patient want to be placed on a breathing machine (known as a respirator or ventilator) if he or she cannot breathe without assistance?

ACTION STEPS FOR SUCCESSFUL INTERVENTION

1. Call Choice in Dying at 1-800-989-WILL and ask for advance directives information for the patient's state of residence (*Note:* If the patient's health care facilities are located in a state other than the state of residence, the patient should ask for advanced directive information from both states). Choice in Dying will mail a packet of information that includes a brochure answering basic questions concerning advance directives.
2. When the patient receives the packet from Choice in Dying, have him or her bring the information to the social worker. Be sure to go over the information thoroughly with the patient. If needed, have the patient speak to his or her physician about some of the medical interventions that are used in life-threatening conditions such as ventilator support, cardiopulmonary resuscitation, etc. (Refer to the previous section for guidelines of questions that should be addressed.)
3. Encourage the HIV/AIDS patient to speak to a number of his or her family members and friends about the advance directives. He or she should clearly state to them which treatments should or should not be given if a life-threatening event occurs.
4. The patient should also choose one person or one person and an alternate to be the durable power of attorney for health care decisions. There are many options concerning the choice of proxy or proxies. Sometimes the closest family member, significant other, or close friend is an obvious choice. However, some HIV/AIDS patients have more confidence that decisions based upon their wishes will be carried out by individuals less emotionally involved, and therefore will choose a proxy outside their intimate family or closest friends. In either case, the person chosen as the proxy and the alternate should have an in-depth discussion with the HIV/AIDS patient about his or her wishes. The patient should be very honest and clear about his or her preferences, including life-sustaining treatments. Of course, no one can anticipate every potential medical scenario. Therefore, the discussion should con-

vey the overall intent of the patient regarding these types of treatments. The health care proxy should have a general understanding of the patient's values and how they relate to his or her wishes concerning the prolongation of life. Conversely, the patient should be aware of the basic moral and ethical values of the proxy to ensure that there are no unacceptable conflicts between them regarding any of these issues.

5. Once all of these discussions have taken place, the HIV/AIDS patient should complete the advance directive forms. Most hospitals and clinics have standard advance directives forms that can be completed with the assistance of the social worker or other health care professional trained in advance directives. It is suggested that the patient complete both the living will, which discusses treatment preferences, and the durable power of attorney for health care, which designates a proxy. By completing both forms, the HIV/AIDS patient will have greater assurance that his or her wishes will be honored if he or she cannot make independent decisions.

   If the health care agency does not have the appropriate forms, the social worker should contact the local community AIDS service organization (ASO) for referral to attorneys or others who can help prepare them at no cost or at a sliding scale fee. Some larger ASOs have legal clinics where HIV/AIDS patients can obtain these documents and have informed persons assist with their completion.

   The forms should be completed as thoroughly as possible and witnessed according to state requirements. For example, some states do not allow health care workers or anyone who may benefit from a patient's estate to be witnesses on advance directives forms.

6. Have the HIV/AIDS patient give copies of these forms to the designated proxy and the alternate proxy, all important health care providers (primary physician, social worker, etc.), and his or her attorney, if applicable. Ideally, the HIV/AIDS patient should arrange a meeting with his or her primary doctor to discuss any issues or questions concerning the advance directives. The more informed the health care team is, the more the patient can be assured that the advance directives will be followed in accordance with his or her wishes.

7. If the patient is hospitalized, he or she should bring a copy of the advance directives to the admissions office or emergency room. The admissions office will file these forms in the patient's chart for future reference. The HIV/AIDS patient should also keep a copy of these documents to help inform the attending health care team of his or her wishes if necessary. If the patient is not able to take the advance directives documents to the hospital, the proxy or other loved one should be certain to bing them and give them to the appropriate health care staff.

POTENTIAL BARRIERS TO SUCCESSFUL INTERVENTION

The social worker should be informed of the state's advance directive statutes so as to be fully aware of the documentation required. Good intentions on the part of the social worker could become disastrous for the patient if proper procedures are not followed.

The HIV/AIDS patient may want to complete advance directives, but may be hesitant to speak to significant others about end-of-life issues. This is difficult for everyone, and the patient should be empowered to think about the consequences for loved ones if no advance directives are completed. It is another burden on family members when they must make these difficult decisions with no prior guidance or understanding of the patient's desires. The patient can feel less anxious knowing that he or she has completed documents that address these issues, relieving the significant others from making these decisions without any input.

Even though advance directive forms are completed according to state guidelines, there is no absolute assurance that all of the patient's wishes will be honored. It is often a medical decision when treatments are no longer effective and when discussions about advance directives should take place. For example, a patient's advance directives may state that he or she does not want intubation unless life expectancy is less than a 50 percent possibility. The physician may be convinced that there is a 70 percent chance that the patient will recover, and therefore will order that the breathing tubes be placed. This is why is it vital that the family and significant others remain in close contact with the physician to keep communication open. Each hospital/health care facility should have a bioethics department or ethics committee that can be consulted if a conflict occurs regarding the patient's health status.

The designated proxy on a durable power of attorney should be aware that family members or significant others are also invested in the HIV/AIDS patient's treatment. Conflicts may arise among intimates concerning which medical procedures should or should not be performed on the patient. The proxy should be aware that emotions are very intense when people deal with decisions concerning the life and death of a loved one, and that open discussions among all interested parties are important in order to air these feelings. Although the proxy must eventually make the final determination of the patient's wishes regarding treatment, harsh feelings can be avoided by including as many people as possible in these discussions. The social worker can assist the loved ones in reaching consensus about decisions and/or ventilation of difficult feelings if he or she observes conflict.

Sometimes a family member or significant other is in direct opposition to the treatment decisions made and attempts to block or thwart any actions of the proxy. Difficult and painful emotions may be expressed during this already stressful time for the loved ones. The social worker should assist the family members and significant others with a discussion of any disagreement with the proxy, and mediate if needed to gain a more positive outcome for all concerned parties.

INFORMATION THE CLIENT SHOULD KNOW BEFORE TAKING ACTION

Two other important documents that a patient with HIV/AIDS should consider completing that are related to his or her advance directives are known as a durable power of attorney for health care and a living will.

The living will and the durable power of attorney for health care pertain only to medical situations that the patient may face. If the patient is interested in designating a proxy for financial matters, he or she should talk with a lawyer or other person trained in legal matters about completing a form called a power of attorney. (This document concerns primarily financial decisions while the durable power of attorney for health care addresses health-related issues.) This document gives a person certain fiduciary rights (paying bills, writing checks, etc.) while the HIV/AIDS patient is alive. After death, the power of attorney is no longer valid.

The will is another important document for a person with HIV/AIDS. The will takes effect after a person's death. The will often names an executor—a person who is responsible for the distribution of the assets of the person's estate, decisions regarding burial/cremation, etc. This document often lists the specific beneficiaries of the estate and addresses the deceased person's preferences for funeral preparations. It is recommended that the will be completed with the assistance of an attorney or legal specialist to ensure that is properly executed.

Assistance in completing both of these documents can often be obtained from the local ASO, which may refer the patients to local attorneys or legal specialists in the area who will complete the forms for little or no fee. If there are no ASOs in the area, the social worker should call a local university's law school to attempt to find volunteer attorneys, legal clinic members, or student attorneys who could help.

POLICY IMPLICATIONS AND RELATED ACTIONS

Social workers should continue to advocate for appropriate action and implementation of advance directive legislation on the state and federal levels.

Social workers who are employed in hospitals and similar health care facilities can advocate for social work involvement in bioethics committees. Social workers can be invaluable in representing the needs of the patients and significant others when appointed to such committees.

Social workers can assist primary care providers in hospitals, hospices, etc., by advocating for their patients about any concerns regarding patients' advance directives.

Social workers should fully explore the patient's wishes regarding health care decisions. The social worker should be able to explain in general terms why advance directives are important, and be versed in the particular requirements of the state(s) in which he or she practices.

Social workers can work with the health care proxy to advocate for the patient's rights. As mentioned previously, significant others or family members may be strongly opposed to measures specifically agreed upon by the patient and the health care team and/or the proxy. Social workers can assist the proxy in the difficult task of advocating on the patient's behalf.

Social workers can speak with a patient's family or significant others concerning the advance directives. If the worker has a good understanding of the patient and his or her wishes, the social worker can advocate for the patient by addressing any questions or fears that may arise from the advance directives.

To Learn More About Advance Directives

Call Choice in Dying 1-800-989-WILL (1-800-989-9455) and request an advance directive packet for your state(s).

Call the American Hospital Association (1-800-242-2626) and ask for pamphlet #166909, "Put It in Writing: Questions and Answers on Advance Directives." There is a cost for the pamphlets, but they are quite helpful in explaining the basics of advance directives.

RECOMMENDED READINGS

Kortlandt, C.E.M. (1990). AIDS and living wills. *AIDS and Public Policy Journal*, 5(4), 157-166.
Dimond, E. P. (1992). The oncology nurse's role in patient advance directives. *Oncology Nurses Forum*, 19(6), 891-896.

PART B:
SERVICES IN MENTAL HEALTH SETTINGS

Individual Clinical Issues

Patricia U. Giulino

WHY DO THIS?
STATEMENT OF THE PROBLEM AND ISSUES

A patient of mine once said that "one of the worst things is feeling trapped, emotionally, physically, and medically. Only about fifty percent of the problem is medical in nature. The emotional and psychological pain is the worst part." That AIDS is a medical disease is a well-known fact; that it has profound psychological and sociological ramifications is less acknowledged. Mental health services are not a luxury in this epidemic; they are a necessity. HIV infection yields an overlay of neuropsychiatric problems, thus making differential diagnosis a complex process.

An HIV-positive diagnosis creates a time of crisis, which often leaves people feeling anxious, overwhelmed, depressed, and/or emotionally numb—all very normal responses. Despite the fact that HIV has been in our lives for over a decade, a diagnosis continues to strike a note of terror to the individual receiving it. No known cure exists, and one is forced to live with a great deal of uncertainty and ambiguity. In addition, such a diagnosis is not always met with compassion by family members and society, which affects an individual's ability to adapt.

HIV-positive individuals live with a high degree of stress and a possibly complicated treatment process. An uncertain journey awaits. The experience of HIV is ongoing and changing over the course of living with it. The illness has an unpredictable course and medically affects patients in different ways; thus, determining the timing or the severity of the symptom is difficult. This is an inherent source of stress as it means that individuals must tolerate high levels of uncertainty that extend over a long period of time. Emotional levels constantly shift.

A diagnosis is disruptive and fragmenting to the self and frequently reawakens developmental needs and traumas, exacerbating underlying issues. Psychotherapy can help people regain some stability and equilibrium, as it helps contain and modulate the affects so that the trauma can be addressed in the treatment. Therapy can help people return to a previous level of coping, decrease anxiety and depression, and improve interpersonal relationships (Nichols, 1986). Treatment provides a place for people to address their fears, to enhance problem-solving skills, and to obtain information that will give them options and a sense of control. It provides a place for the client to feel humanly connected, which is vital in the ongoing maintenance of the self. With the help of therapy, people can begin to take charge of their life and accept responsibility for it.

EXAMPLES OF HOW THE ISSUE MAY PRESENT

A client may be referred by his or her primary care physician. The reasons for the referral will vary. Someone may have recently received a positive antibody test and feel anxious and overwhelmed; someone else may have been living with asymptotic HIV for several years and only recently began to develop symptoms, thus causing them to feel anxious and depressed. It is imperative for the social worker to do a careful psycho-social assessment to determine what services and other interventions a client may need. Assume nothing and start with the client. The reason they are meeting with you may be different from that of the referring person.

Common presenting symptoms, anxiety and depression may manifest in many ways. Individuals may report feeling sad, lonely, unattractive, and despairingly hopeless and helpless. It is not uncommon to see someone who has been previously functioning autonomously and doing well in many aspects of his or her life now feeling emotionally regressed, dependent, and needy. People with HIV/AIDS often speak of feeling incredibly fatigued, with a loss of energy, a decreased libido, and even interrupted sleep patterns that result in sleep deprivation. They may be apathetic, unmotivated to pursue interests, socially isolated, or experiencing marked changes in appetite. On the other hand, they may be highly agitated and anxious with highly obsessive thinking patterns that interfere with their everyday functions and relationships.

One should consider whether this is an adjustment reaction to coping with a life-threatening illness, a major depression, or an organic mental disorder, known as AIDS dementia complex (ADC), which is also frequently referred to as HIV cognitive/motor complex, HIV encephalopathy, or AIDS dementia. The frequency of HIV dementia parallels the progression of systemic HIV disease. Such dementia affects less than 5 percent of patients with asymptotic HIV infection, but 15 to 66 percent of patients with AIDS-defining illnesses.

Symptoms may be slow in onset or abrupt and severe, particularly if no antiretroviral therapy is involved. In the early stages of HIV infection, these cognitive symptoms may manifest as the following: shortness of attention span, i.e., inability to read a book or a newspaper or follow a conversation or a TV show; short-term memory loss; decreased ability to concentrate; and difficulty in planning complex activities. Behavioral symptoms include apathy, depressed mood, fatigue, social withdrawal, and insomnia. Motor symptoms may include gait disturbance, clumsiness, and changes in handwriting. As the disease progresses, a client may experience seizures; difficulty with gait; mania; and psychosis. As many of the early symptoms resemble depression, an inclusive premorbid psychosocial history will help to delineate and tease out the etiology of some of the symptoms. This is complicated and not always possible. Some of the changes we witness early in the diagnosis are subtle and barely discernible; however, medications are available to treat the symptoms, and a referral to a psychiatrist for psychopharmacological intervention is important. In addition, the client may require consultation with a neurologist for further evaluation of the symptoms.

Clients may also present with a need for concrete services, i.e., information about health insurance, Medicaid, housing, and legal services. While they are not seeking mental health services per se, this is an active way to engage individuals who might not otherwise have considered the benefits of treatment.

Individuals may present as suicidal although this is not a frequent initial presentation. A past history of suicide attempts should be obtained to determine whether or not the patient is experiencing a major depressive episode, dementia, delirium, or a substance abuse problem. They may need psychiatric hospitalization.

FACTS THE SOCIAL WORKER NEEDS TO KNOW BEFORE PROCEEDING

Having some understanding about the medical aspects of HIV/AIDS is important. You should not become overwhelmed with feeling you need to know all the facts before proceeding. Our clients are often the best teachers. It is useful, however, to know some of the common symptoms, treatment applications, medications, and their side effects, and to recognize that individuals with HIV also have colds and flus—not every symptom is an HIV-defining illness.

One must also be sensitive to cultural issues and accept patients as they are. You need to be aware of your prejudices, your judgments, your homophobia, and your addictophobia, and to have colleagues and supervisors available for ongoing consultation to address these issues as they arise.

Over the course of this illness, individuals need a wide range of services that may include a medical provider, insurance, legal consultation, housing, alternative medicines including Chinese herbs and acupuncture, and nutritional counseling, to name a few. You need to know about the availability of resources in the community in order to refer clients as necessary.

Some understanding of death and dying issues and the nature of dealing with anticipatory grief is very helpful. People often describe that living with HIV is like living with a time bomb and never knowing when it will go off. Living with this high degree of uncertainty over an extended period of time is stressful.

KEY QUESTIONS TO ASK THE CLIENT

An initial psychosocial assessment may take one or two sessions. First of all, you should determine with the client why he or she is there, as well as what he or she is looking for and hoping to achieve. In other words, what are his or her needs? As stated earlier, the client's needs may be different from the referral source, if he or she is not self-referred. Components of this evaluation should include referral source, reason for referral, chief complaint of client, history of present illness, family history, social history, medical history, psychiatric history, current and past medications, and a substance abuse history.

A mental status exam will help determine the presence of any neurocognitive impairments. It will be useful to ask them when they tested positive for HIV, why they got tested (i.e., what were the circumstances that prompted them to receive the antibody test), and what, if any, symptoms they have experienced. Ask for their current CD-4 count; viral load; medications, including antiviral treatment protocols and protease inhibitors; and any side effects experienced from these medications. Many of the medications used in treatment are highly toxic, and it is not unusual for someone to have experienced difficulty in tolerating them.

Given the stigma and discrimination attached to HIV/AIDS, individuals often struggle with the issue of revealing their positive antibody status to others. Inquiring as to who they have told, both within their immediate biological family and any extended network of family and friends, is useful. What was the response they received? Was it supportive or not? Ask whether or not people at their worksite know, including their boss or supervisor. Find out who is in their support network.

Ask about previous losses of friends or family members to HIV/AIDS and/or number of friends they may know who are currently infected and living with HIV. Many individuals are coping with multiple losses due to AIDS, including the loss of a former partner or spouse. The magnitude of the loss can be overwhelming and can affect individuals' ability to manage effectively. Getting a sense of how they have coped with these losses and how they subsequently deal with stress is useful in assessing their coping methods.

For individuals with a substance abuse history, you should ask about the substance used, length of time they used, detoxes they have undergone, their current substance use, and their attendance at support groups including Narcotics Anonymous and/or Alcoholics Anonymous. It is important to note that individuals who may have been clean and sober for an extended period of time may start to use again upon learning they are positive for HIV.

In addition to individual treatment the client may also need referrals to other treatment modalities, such as psychopharmacology, group psychotherapy, family and couples therapy, neuropsychological testing, substance abuse treatment, and case management. Given the complexity of this disease, the psychosocial ramifications, and its impact on the person, it is not at all uncommon to be treating someone who is also involved in many treatment modalities with a host of different providers.

At the end of the assessment period, it is important to respond to the referral source, if they are part of the health care team, informing them of the treatment plan. This is helpful in establishing a sense of cohesion in the overall treatment of the client.

CULTURAL COMPETENCY CONSIDERATIONS

Cultural background and lifestyles are important. Being culturally sensitive means listening to the diversity of and understanding the realities of people's lives. They need to be understood within their social, ethnic, and cultural complex. As psychotherapists, we do not have to be members of a specific culture in order to understand someone's experience. Our clients will tell us if we accept them for who they are and provide them with a supportive environment.

Language

For individuals for whom English is not the primary language, find a clinician who speaks that person's language, whenever possible.

Location

Given the stigma of HIV/AIDS, individuals may be reluctant to seek services in their neighborhood health center out of fear they will be seen by a neighbor or friend, resulting in a loss of confidentiality.

In some cultures a stigma exists regarding mental health services and psychotherapy specifically. People may need reassurance when accessing these services.

ACTION STEPS FOR SUCCESSFUL INTERVENTION

A diagnosis of AIDS or of being seropositive for HIV is a trauma that threatens an individual's sense of cohesion and overall functioning. It is a time of crisis. People often feel fragmented and damaged, and they are at high risk for anxiety and depressive disorders. Even relatively healthy individuals may decompensate.

AIDS is an acronym for acquired immune deficiency syndrome, which implies that it is not a singular disease entity but rather a composition of infections occurring over a spectrum of time. In the initial phases of the disease, the immune system is able to effectively fight off infections; however, with each new infection, the immune system becomes more compromised and is less able to do so. Over the course of time of living with HIV, people cycle through many periods of medical relapses and remissions.

There is an emotional accompaniment to all of this. People often feel as though they have no control over either their life or the disease process, particularly because they can feel quite healthy and symptom-free one day and seriously ill and impaired the next. Given this, we must recognize that there may be recurring crises along the disease continuum.

The experience of living with HIV infection is ongoing and changing, and it challenges the most resilient self. Despite the narcissistic injury that accompanies an HIV diagnosis, negotiating the course of living with the virus often is marked by tremendous psychological growth. The work done in psychotherapy can be reparative of the many underlying issues that surface as a result of the diagnosis. Neither the disease course of HIV nor the course of psychotherapy is linear in its progression, but rather each passes through subtle phases. One moves from the initial crisis toward achieving a sense of balance while integrating HIV into the overall functioning of the self. However, as relapses occur, treatment may be marked by the patient's diminished capacity to function as he or she is forced to cope with new infections and the accompanying medical treatments. An opportunity for growth occurs as the patient negotiates the cycles of relapses and remissions.

It is useful to think of the psychotherapeutic process as being comprised of four interweaving threads: (1) HIV; (2) the patient's response to HIV; (3) the response of the patient's care and support matrix, including friends, family, health care providers, etc.; and (4) transference. All of these factor into the ongoing treatment process to varying degrees at varying times. The treatment helps individuals to experience, integrate, and adapt to HIV-related events. The emotional response to such events is often intense. The transference provides for a relationship that helps organize and contain intense emotions within the context of a holding environment where one can be heard, supported, and understood. Being understood is an essential part of healing, and when patients feel understood in their helplessness, it often helps them to move on.

This is exemplified in the crisis of a patient first learning of his or her seropositive status. Initially, there is a lost sense of the future and a profound sense of hopelessness. You may witness increased destructive behavior—e.g., substance abuse, sexual acting out, or suicidal ideation—to defend against the intense affect that is aroused. Ongoing relationships are often disrupted, and individuals lose sight of their goals, dreams, plans, and even life's meaning.

Case Example 1

Mr. T's initial diagnosis of being positive for HIV created major chaos in his life. At the time this occurred, he had been working for a major computer company with a good salary and living with his wife and three children. His sexual contact with men was limited to anonymous encounters at roadside rest areas on his way home from work.

His coming out was perilous. It occurred at work when he "came on" to a fellow employee, who then disclosed the incident to Mr. T's boss and colleagues. Mr. T then began to experience verbal harassment from his colleagues. With this he became increasingly paranoid and depressed, quit his job precipitously, and was hospitalized for a psychotic depression. During this admission, he was tested and found to be positive for HIV.

His seropositive diagnosis also marked the initial stage of his coming out as a gay man, all within the environment of an inpatient psychiatric unit. At the time he initiated outpatient treatment, he was separated from his wife, had lost his job, was partially blind as a result of a virus that had infected his eye, and was living on disability in a third-floor room in the home of his elderly parents. His contact with his three children was limited to a few hours on the weekend.

His world literally fell apart. He had lost his job, his marriage, and his role as a father as he had known it. He was not sure what it meant to be seropositive, gay, and legally blind. What it did mean was that he could not work, support himself or his children, or drive a car and that he felt powerless and out of control over most of his life.

The therapist becomes a sustaining and organizing person and provider of a safe holding environment that facilitates the containing and modulation of the intense affects and helps the patient achieve a sense of control. The focus of the treatment is to help patients stabilize and achieve some sense of control over their life. In our capacity as psychotherapists, we both listen to our patients as well as assist them in concrete ways. We may obtain a primary medical provider, provide education and information about the disease and its transmission, or help them to access other resources of care and social support. All of this enhances the developing treatment alliance.

You may find that once they have achieved some sense of stabilization from the initial trauma of diagnosis, some patients choose to discontinue treatment. As clinicians we may feel they have more issues concerning the diagnosis that need to be addressed; however, we need to respect a "healthy denial" and allow them to terminate treatment. Healthy denial does not prohibit the person from accessing appropriate mental health and medical services, but rather allows the person to move on with his or her life within the context of living with HIV. Frequently, at a later point in the disease course, or as either medical or psychological symptoms arise, individuals will reenter treatment.

Once having negotiated the initial trauma, people move, albeit slowly, toward integrating HIV into their sense of self. How well one adapts depends on previous levels of coping and the degree of or lack of support they experience from their support network. This initial trauma reawakens past narcissistic traumas that add to the affective intensity of the diagnosis. Consequently, patients may be emotionally labile with many feelings of self-blame, guilt, anger, and self-pity, with common symptoms of anxiety and depression. At this time a psychopharmacological consultation is important, as medication can diminish symptoms and allow people to address the underlying dynamic issues in the psychotherapy.

A significant part of the treatment is developing a sense of meaning out of what seems so meaningless. Viktor Frankl tells us in his book *The Unheard Cry for Meaning: Psychotherapy and Humanism* (1978) that there is a healing force in meaning. He speaks of persons in death camps, and says that what upheld them was that life has meaning to be fulfilled, albeit in the future. People often seek out help because they cannot make sense out of their life. Treatment is a vehicle for people to organize and understand their experience. Gaining a sense of understanding of one's life provides cohesion, balance, and a sense of mastery and control.

A case vignette may illustrate the existential nature of HIV psychotherapy.

Case Example 2

Mr. G was a bright and articulate gay man in his thirties who was referred to me for treatment by a colleague who was leaving town. Mr. G had been in treatment since his diagnosis of Kaposi's sarcoma (KS) two years prior. Spirited and friendly, he quickly engaged in the treatment process with me. He had been quite fond of his former therapist, but very matter-of-factly and without apparent remorse, he accepted the termination of that treatment.

What stands out in his history is the suicidal death of his father by hanging when Mr. G was only four years old. The family history was replete with losses. Mr. G, the fourth of five children, was only one of three living. A brother and a sister, who were twins, died in separate car accidents several years apart. The mother was described as strong and loving, and someone who had worked hard to keep the family together. Although she lived in another part of the country, Mr. G maintained close contact with her and knew he could always turn to her for help.

Living on Social Security Disability Income (SSDI) and Medicaid, he felt beholden to a system that was dehumanizing and denigrating. He was losing his hair as a result of chemotherapy for his KS lesions. His living situation was a source of stress in that his roommate, also infected, was becoming selfish, manipulative, and very dependent. An uncle who lived at some distance in another state and was Mr. G's only living relative on his father's side of the family was kind and caring toward him, but he also sent him explicit seductive messages through cards and gifts. Within the context of discussing these events, he began to disclose a long history of childhood sexual abuse that had extended over his latency years.

What he began to express in the therapeutic hour was that the "pain of AIDS equals the pain of abuse—it never goes away. I feel like a victim of this disease. AIDS is just one more perpetrator." When he was abused as a child, he could distance himself. "They can have my body but not my soul. Now I can't get away. The abuse is inside me. I can feel its presence all the time." All of this was expressed with blinding rage in our sessions, followed by a subsequent session in which the subject of abuse would not come up and the hour would be filled discussing any one of another set of issues.

I began to notice myself often feeling sleepy during our sessions and at times feeling as though I was being lulled into a hypnotic trance. This had not gone on for long when Mr. G presented to his primary care physician that he wanted a new therapist. His current one was falling asleep on the job.

His physician called in a psychiatric consultant. What was revealed was that Mr. G was feeling very close to me and he was afraid I would leave him like his former therapist. He was frightened by the intensity of his affect, and he wanted to protect me. He was unsure whether or not he would destroy me with it. He was able to draw the parallel with me to his mother. He felt the need to protect her, and he never wanted her to know the pain he had inside.

Mr. G returned to the treatment and the therapeutic task was to offer reconstructive interpretations that would put the rage into its transferential context. He needed to protect me from himself for fear he would destroy me and then he would not be able to do the work he needed to do. Therein lay the paradox of the treatment. He could not both protect me and do the work. As I acknowledged his fear of losing me, his rage, and his sense of victimization, he felt listened to and understood. His feelings, reactivated from childhood, were given legitimacy, and he could begin to give expression to them without fear of loss. As the abused child, he had suppressed all the anger and rage he felt out of a sense of shame and guilt that he was somehow responsible. Now with AIDS it was clear to him that he was not responsible for the virus that was abusing his body. He was not seeking it. AIDS was allowing him full reign to the anger and rage he had suppressed for years.

As he was able to understand the meaning and motivation for his anger and rage, he began to gain control over these feelings. He also became clear and unambivalent about not allowing himself to be victimized by the "system" on which he was dependent for all of his benefits. He also began to recognize that my apparent sleepiness had completely disappeared and that it was a part of the way he protected me and himself from his rage. He would defend against it by lulling both of us into a trance. My withstanding his anger and his challenges allowed for his further development and growth. The transference relationship helped him organize and contain his emotions and ultimately provided him with an interpretation of the problem.

Individuals seek out experiences that help restore cohesion and facilitate integration. What the diagnosis means, how it is experienced, and how the patient works to regain and maintain equilibrium becomes the work of treatment. It is important to note that this is a treatment progression that is often disrupted by medical symptoms, crises, and hospitalizations. It parallels the roller coaster ride of the disease course as one cycles through relapses and remissions. A central question is "How does one maintain a semblance of normal life in the abnormal presence of a life-threatening illness, when the only certainty is uncertainty?"

During the end stage of living with HIV, it is common for people to reminisce about their life. They often know they are "living on borrowed time" and may want to complete unfinished business. It is important to leave room for hope while facilitating a letting-go process. We need to inquire if there are final conversations they wish to have with family members and friends. Within this context you need to reassure your patients that it is normal and expectable to have a myriad of different feelings toward different people, including family members. They may need to be reassured that all relationships entail a degree of ambivalence. In working through the *separation* process, the experience of both positive and negative affects is necessary. This may not always feel safe for people so we need to appreciate with them the resentments that may have accrued over the years. Remember that each individual in this process is engaged in saying good-bye—both the patient who is dying and the family members/friends who will remain.

In this final stage of life, the patient usually turns inward. This withdrawal is normal and expectable behavior. As patients are preparing to lose everyone and everything, they begin to disengage and distance themselves. You need to respect this behavior and not ask more of the patient than he or she can give. You may need to give them permission to die.

CENTRAL THEMES IN THE TREATMENT

Within the context of psychotherapy, many themes become central to the treatment. Some issues force us to pose difficult questions to our patients and questions for which there often are not absolute and clear answers. You may find the following summary of the key issues that emerge in treatment useful.

Loss

Treatment is framed by issues of separation and loss: independence, control, friends, family, jobs, financial security, home, the ability to make choices, lifestyle, changing body image, mobility, a sense of future, etc. (the list is endless). One of the tasks of treatment is facilitating movement through these losses through negotiation, grieving, letting go, and moving on.

Self-Blame and Guilt

There is often a lot of self-blame and guilt concerning a lifestyle and behaviors that may have led to becoming infected. A seropositive diagnosis exacerbates many unresolved issues in these areas and treatment provides the opportunity to work toward some resolution.

Revelation of HIV Status

Given the highly stigmatized nature of this illness, individuals appropriately struggle with who to reveal their diagnosis to out of fear of retaliation or rejection. AIDS is not an illness that is always met with compassion. Individuals fear being rejected, isolated, and abandoned by those they need most.

These fears also surface as individuals attempt to negotiate friendships and intimate relationships. Frequent questions asked are the following: "Do I tell someone about my HIV-positive status?"; "When do I tell them?"; and "How do I tell them?"

They need to weigh the pros and cons of informing someone. Part of the desire to inform someone may be the wish to receive support, care, and understanding, and this wish may be met with rejection, anger, and disappointment. Many times the patient may be in the position of educating the other person and providing reassurance that he or she is going to be alright.

Ambiguity and Uncertainty

Individuals may be healthy and asymptomatic for many years following their HIV-positive diagnosis; however, they are forced to live with the ongoing uncertainty of not knowing when they might become symptomatic. They wish for answers, particularly from the medical community, often using their CD-4/viral load count as a measure of health or non-health. Individuals are looking for absolutes and certainty, and a CD-4/viral load count is sometimes the only thing that feels real or certain.

Fear of Symptoms

Many patients have witnessed someone who had died of AIDS so the fear of symptoms is not abstract but real—very real. This virus manifests itself with a variety of different symptoms depending on each individual's immune system. People wonder which symptoms will affect them and how the disease will manifest for them. The greatest identified fears are the following: fear of pain, fear of losing one's mind, and fear of losing control of one's body. You should never deny your patient's fears, but acknowledge how frightening they are and facilitate a discussion about them. This will help to diminish their affective intensity.

Despair versus Hope

The challenge for our patients and ourselves is to negotiate that fine line between despair and hope. Given the scientific breakthroughs of the past decade and the promises held forth by the scientific community, people are living longer with the virus and there is reason to be hopeful. Yet, we need to recognize that there is still no cure and infected people live with a life-threatening virus. As clinicians you need to help your patients find a balance so they do not become so despairing that they either give up or deny what is going on to the point that it interferes with their care.

Sex

Sex is always a highly charged topic and particularly if it has been the transmission route for HIV for someone. This topic leads to discussion about underlying conflicts about sexuality and sexual conduct. It raises issues around intimacy and closeness. Questions arise such as the following: "Should I or should I not have sex?"; "Should I have anonymous sex?"; "Do I inform my partner?"; "If so, when and how?"; "What is safe?"; and "Is anything safe?" As a clinician, you also need to consider how you might feel and react when an HIV-infected patient tells you he or she is having unprotected sex with someone—particularly if you learn that the other person does not know about your patient's positive antibody status.

Many medications are used to treat this disease, particularly antidepressants, which diminish sexual functioning. Patients may decide to discontinue medications for this reason. It may be helpful to weigh the pros and cons with them concerning their decision.

Fear of Transmission

When people receive the news they are seropositive for HIV, they may have already transmitted the virus unknowingly to a partner. The complicated guilt accompanying this fear will take time to work through. The patient may also fear infecting someone in the future. Thus, your patient may need information about sexual behavior and transmission.

Financial Concerns

Individuals fear losing their job, which in turn has many implications secondary to loss of income, i.e., loss of home, possible loss of health insurance, and loss of a lifestyle. This can often start a sequence of events that are anxiety-producing and stressful for the patient. For example, patients first lose job and health insurance and while waiting to see if they qualify for public assistance, they may lose or need to change their health care providers. In addition they may not be able to purchase their medications. They may have a health insurance plan that only reimburses them for medications after they have paid for them. Consequently, patients are frequently required to raise large sums of money to pay for their medication, which may create undue hardship. They are then in a position of negotiating a complicated and not always sympathetic public assistance system during a time when they are feeling physically and medically compromised.

No matter where they begin, for the most part, individuals with HIV eventually become poor. This leads to issues of decreased self-esteem, a diminished sense of self-worth, and a poor self-image.

Shame

For many, a profound sense of shame is attached to a diagnosis that is associated with having defects and flaws. This feeling is frequently compounded by earlier affective experiences of feeling flawed, often leading to feelings of self-blame for being infected. For example, patients may say, "If only I weren't gay," or "If only I'd been more careful." The stigma attached to HIV only complicates the issue and leads to shame-induced concealment, self-loathing, and condemnation.

POTENTIAL BARRIERS TO SUCCESSFUL INTERVENTION

In 1947, a psychoanalyst named Dr. Paula Heimann defined therapy as a "relationship between two persons and what distinguishes the relationship from others is not the presence of feelings in one person and their absence in the other, the therapist, but above all the degree of the feelings experienced and the use made of them" (1981). As mental health providers, many of the issues we struggle with parallel the issues the patient is going through. Treatment is a relationship. How do we sustain those feelings that arise in us? Only to the degree to which we can acknowledge, confront, and understand the feelings of sadness, hopelessness, despair, rage, disgust, etc., will we be able to help.

This is stressful work. The risks for stress are not equal in all types of health work. Adler (1984) points out that individuals working with the terminally ill are especially vulnerable to stress. Research done by Beehr and Bhagut (1985) concludes that factors contributing to stress are situations characterized by high levels of uncertainty, associated with important outcomes, and extending over a long duration. Stress can lead to burnout, which is characterized by physical, emotional, and mental exhaustion. Ineffective coping strategies include emotional detachment from the patient, withdrawal, cynicism, and rigidity.

The following are some of the challenges we face as mental health providers.

Helplessness, Powerlessness, and Frustration

In the face of no cure, treatment is palliative, yet we need to maintain calm and remain a stabilizing influence for our patients. Our feelings of helplessness, powerlessness, and frustration mirrors our patients' feelings. We are working with a disease that is highly stigmatized and is usually not met with compassion. As providers working with infected individuals, we also may experience discrimination by family, friends, and institutions. We, like our patients, are looking for certainty in the face of uncertainty and ambiguity. We are also continually confronting the existential reality of our own limitations as healers.

Loss

As therapists we continually deal with inevitable loss, as well as repeated attachment and loss. For every patient who leaves us through death, another one awaits us in the waiting room. Sometimes it feels as though we have no chance to recover from a death before we must take on a new patient. The volume of loss is high, and there is a sense of relentlessness of the collected grief that we absorb.

Deterioration of Body and Personality

We bear witness to mental and physical deterioration as the disease progresses and our patients' bodies become so ravaged that they sometimes only bear a slight resemblance to their former self. Our patients often evoke feelings of familiarity in us, yet they remain strangers to us in their appearance.

Death through HIV is long-suffering and disfiguring. Cognitive, behavioral, and personality changes are often precipitated by infections in the brain. The loss of dignity with which our patients suffer is very difficult to watch and may produce its own kind of countertransference.

Withdrawal

Often we may wish to withdraw from all this pain and suffering. As caregivers we cannot always withdraw; however, we need to choose boundaries in the service of better meeting our patients' needs. It is easy to lose perspective with either too much intimacy or too much distance. The extremes are the inhibited empathizer who is afraid to get involved and afraid to feel the affects versus the uncontrolled empathizer who tends to become intensely involved (see the chapters by Kitsy Schoen and Jay Warren, which discuss caregivers' needs).

Overidentification

This is a disease that affects people who are young- to middle-age adults. They are in the prime of their life and facing end-of-life issues. AIDS throws the assumed sequence of life's events out of order. We identify with our patients, and this sense of sameness is challenging. It can lead to overprotectedness or being overconcerned.

The affective component of the empathic work is intense, which intensifies the relationship. There is a high probability of severe regression due to the following: trauma, neurological complications, and the patient's premorbid level of functioning. It is a treatment process that deals with life's most primitive issues: sex and death.

As therapists we provide support; show interest; express care, understanding, and guidance; provide a source of strength and calmness; help to recognize disappointments and fears; facilitate discussions to help our patients achieve a sense of mastery; and provide emotional sustenance and validation of feelings. We provide containment and opportunities for growth and do reparative work concerning a basic narcissistic injury, i.e., a diagnosis for HIV. Therapy provides our patients with a vehicle to attach meaning out of something that seems so meaningless.

REFERENCES

Adler G. (1984). Special problems for the therapist. *Int J Psychiatry Med* 16:91-98.

Beehr T.A., Bhagat R.S. (1985). Introduction to human stress and cognition in organizations. In *Human Stress Cognition in Organizations: An Integrated Perspective*. Beehr TA, Bhagat RS (Eds.). New York: Wiley, pp. 3-19.

Frankl V.E. (1978). *The Unheard Cry for Meaning: Psychotherapy and Humanism*. New York: Simon and Schuster.

Heimann P. (1981). *On Counter-Transference in Classics in Psychoanalytic Technique*. Langs R. (Ed.). New York: Jason Aronson, Inc., pp. 139-142.

Nichols S. (1986). Psychotherapy and AIDS. In *Contemporary Perspectives on Psychotherapy with Lesbians and Gay Men*. Stein TS, Cohen CJ (Eds.). New York: Plenum, pp. 209-239.

Disrupted Dialogues:
Working with Couples

R. Dennis Shelby

WHY DO THIS? STATEMENT OF PROBLEM AND ISSUES

Theoretical and practice models for couples and family intervention are numerous and can often be applied to work with people in an ongoing relationship impacted by HIV infection. The psychological challenges to couples are considerable; they often change over the course of the infection and are colored by the unique characteristics of the relationship and the two individuals. The social worker working with HIV will encounter a wide range of issues and problematic situations within the context of couples' work. In this chapter I will outline the framework I use with couples and point out some of the more frequent issues I have encountered over my years of work with HIV. Though the cases used to illustrate work with couples are gay couples, many of the basic concepts also apply to heterosexual couples.

RELATIONSHIPS AS DIALOGUES

In an effort to elucidate the complexity of relationships I use the term "dialogue":

Dialogue refers to the area of shared experience and its many components that exists between two people in an ongoing intimate and sexual relationship. As each relationship is comprised of two unique individuals, each relationship will have its own unique dialogue. Some aspects of the dialogue may change and evolve over the course of the relationship; others will endure throughout the lives of the individuals and their shared experience. The components include the love-object relationship in particular, the self-object functions each

183

partner experiences, and the collective and individual hopes, dreams, fears, triumphs, and frustrations encountered in an ongoing relationship. Ultimately, the dialogue is the sense that another person is an integral part of one's daily experience—that two people are participating in life together. (Shelby, 1992, p. 49)

To this definition we must also add the dimension of shared affect experiences (Shane and Shane, 1993), a more conscious level of communicating in which affective experiences of a range of intensity can be acknowledged, tolerated, and perhaps most important, talked about between the two people in the dialogue.

In my work with couples, I tend to focus on the selfobject dimension and the related aspects of affect modulation and responsiveness. In this perspective, periodic or chronic failures of responsiveness to one or both partners' needs are seen as the problematic aspects of the dialogue of the relationship.

Kohut (1977) pointed out the following: "I know of no mature love in which the love object is not also a selfobject, or, to put this depth psychological formulation into a psychosocial context, there is no love relationship without mutual self-esteem enhancing, mirroring, and idealization" (p. 141). As we have often observed in work with couples and in our own personal lives, when a relationship is functioning well, the psychological status of the individuals is often enhanced. When there is a disruption, indicated by tension, disappointment, or conflict, individual psychological status often declines, and varying degrees of anger, sadness, and loneliness can dominate. When the couple is facing an HIV-related problem, another layer of complicated and often intense affects is added to the dialogue.

When the dialogue is disrupted, affects related to HIV often flood one or both members of the couple, creating a confusing and more disorganized situation. The dialogue is often capable of quietly modulating a great deal of affect in the face of HIV. When there is a disruption, both members are often surprised at the intensity of their reactions, fears, and anxieties. At times, one or both members of the relationship may act and respond in ways that further exacerbate the disruption and instability. During these times of disruption, we are called upon to intervene. Depending on the practice setting and the needs of the couple, either a long-term approach or several sessions exploring a specific transition point may be indicated.

Wolf (1994) asserted the following:

Spouses are used by each other for a variety of selfobject functions. Intimacy facilitates controlled regression to primitive merger without fear of irreversibly losing the autonomy of the self. Expansion of self boundaries to include the spouse allows for participation in the self-sustaining selfobject experience of the other as if it were the self. On the other hand, frustrations and disappointments in the expected and needed selfobject experiences threaten the cohesion of the self and may lead to behaviors that threaten the marriage. (pp. 78-79)

One must keep in mind that relationships are ultimately born of hope, the hope that individual lives will be enriched through a relationship with another human being. Indeed, perhaps no greater joy exists than that experienced by new couples who have found each other and are in the throes of what has been termed "limerance" (McWhirter and Mattison, 1985). In sharp contrast, we observe the rage, despair, and often deep sense of betrayal in the wake of a partner's failure to respond in times of distress. Similar emotions arise when we are pushed away, our love is rebuffed, or in a more general sense, as is the case with HIV, the dialogue is threatened by an infectious and often terminal illness.

HIV infection is often experienced as an ongoing assault on the cohesiveness and integrity of the self. While the diagnosis of HIV infection often brings with it an initial fragmentation, research (Shelby, 1995) indicates that the experience of HIV infection is an ongoing, transforming process, that while it may lead to greater coherence over time, it is a coherence within the context of chronic illness and many destabilizing events occur throughout out the course of the infection. Abramowitz and Cohen (1994) and Cohen and Abramowitz (1990) have outlined the impact of AIDS on the self. The authors point to disruptions in the most basic sense of self, the body self, the disruptions in self object bonds that come via losses of supportive individuals, and disruptions in the tripartite self: mirroring, alter-ego bonds, and idealized bonds. The authors also point out that AIDS can recapitulate preexisting self issues: "As selfobject ties are disrupted, which in turn destabilizes the self, the PWA [person with AIDS] may experience his current situation as a recapitulation of an earlier inadequate selfobject milieu" (p. 215).

Taking this individual depth perspective into the context of a relationship offers a framework for understanding potential disruptions in the couples' dialogue. The destabilization of self in one partner often engenders the need for enhanced responsiveness from the other partner/spouse. Preexisting self-deficits are often enhanced by the impact of HIV infection; consequently, if the partner is unable to meet the need for enhanced responsiveness, then he may be viewed as yet another disappointing selfobject. On the other hand, the diagnosis or progression of HIV infection in the partner is often destabilizing for the uninfected (or "well") partner, due to the threatened loss of the dialogue and the disruption in the sense of the ongoing sustaining aspects of the relationship. Thus, in the context of a relationship, we have two people whose sense of coherence is disrupted and threatened on a number of levels, both individually and collectively. (See Shelby [1992, 1995] for a more thorough narrative account of these processes.)

Any illness is disruptive to the self and to a relationship. To this disruption, we must add the additional burden of the psychological horror of the illness as terminal and as being—or potentially being—sexually transmitted. Yet another burden is the greatly enhanced social stigma that accompanies HIV infection and AIDS. Any relationship faces the possibility of events and crises that push the couple beyond their capacity to modulate and respond. AIDS and HIV infection are often a constant strain, with periodic peaks that generate considerably intense states of affect, thus testing and straining the relationship's capacity to modulate and respond.

The work of McWhirter and Mattison (1985) suggests that relationships between two men have a developmental life as well; that is, the needs of the two men and the general characteristics of the relationship change and evolve over time. The authors detail six developmental stages and their characteristics: blending, nesting, maintaining, building, releasing, and renewing. My experience has been that in addition to disruptions in the psychological life of the relationship, the development of the relationship is often disrupted by HIV infection and AIDS. While one partner may want to push forward with new projects or ideas, the other partner may want to—and need to—maintain the status quo in order to minimize any disruption in a life that is already threatened with disruption.

While the paradigm of the self and relationship as a dialogue and the paradigm of stages of development are radically different ways of conceptualizing relationships, and not always compatible, they offer alternative lenses from which to view the relationship and the particular difficulties of the couple presenting for our help. At times these paradigms may provide us with metaphors for describing to a couple what we see as happening in the relationship that is so confusing, disruptive, disappointing, and alienating.

From my perspective, the ultimate goal of couples work is to help the two individuals talk to each other, and consequently, be more empathic toward each other. While this may seem simple, and indeed it is deceptively simple, time and time again in consultations, students and professionals alike seem to have overlooked this simple but incredibly helpful activity. I am equally delighted when I hear that a good conversation has occurred outside of my consulting room as in it. We must remember that oftentimes we will be asking couples to put into words private thoughts and fears that may seem unspeakable.

When a couple seeks our help, we become a third person invited into the dialogue. Our role is to modulate affect and to establish a rapport that conveys our interest in both peoples' thoughts, concerns, fears, and affects. As we establish rapport, hopefully both people feel safer to feel and to express concerns and issues that are often perceived as threatening to the relationship. In the case of couples work with HIV, phrases such as: "I get afraid during sex that you will infect me," "I am afraid you are going to get sick and die soon," "Sometimes I get angry and envious that you are negative, and I have AIDS," or "Last night I dreamed that you died, and the doctors told me that I had AIDS too" are common.

KEY QUESTIONS TO ASK THE CLIENT

The initial aspect of any clinical work is the assessment, which includes obtaining a general idea of what is going on that has led the couple to seek outside help. I tend to ask myself the following general questions as I listen to and ask the couple about their experience as partners and individuals.

Medical

- What is the nature of the HIV-related problem?
- Who is infected, and how long have they individually and collectively known of the infection?
- What stage of infection is one or both of the individuals in, and have any changes in medical status occurred?
- What currently is being done medically: antivirals, prophylaxis, or more intensive treatments such as infusions?
- Have any concrete hardships been brought on by medical intervention or disease progression?

The Dialogue

- What was the individual and collective initial response to the knowledge of infection?
- Have their been any recent changes in the medical status of one or both of the individuals?
- What has been the history of the relationship, what has worked well, and what has not?

- What are the general characteristics of the relationship, and what stands out as being uniquely helpful and sustaining as well as unhelpful and destabilizing?
- Is there a discrepancy between the reported stage of infection and individual or collective psychological experience of the stage of infection?
- What are the reported frustrations and concerns?
- What are the dominant affect(s) (anger, sadness, anxiety, etc.)—both individually and collectively—and how do affects change over the course of the session?
- What are the patterns of responsiveness and lack of responsiveness as the couple relate concerns, conflicts, frustrations, and accompanying emotional states?
- What is not being spoken about both generally and HIV-specifically?

CONSTELLATIONS OF RELATIONSHIPS AND HIV/AIDS

Any clinical work tests our assumptions about human nature, what is and is not "moral," the way things should and should not be in general, and evokes our own disappointments, struggles, hopes, and fears. Perhaps the most daunting task in any clinical work is not to apply our personal ideals of how people should be, but rather to work with what is presented to us, respect the dialogue, and attempt to move forward. I have picked up the pieces, so to speak, far too many times when a therapist (for whatever reason) told the couple that they should break up, that there was no point in them staying together. Perhaps the therapist was baffled or frustrated by the complexity of the unhappiness, could not tolerate the affect states generated by the couple, or was embarrassed that two gay men should behave in such an unpleasant manner.

Just as hope can bind two people, so can misery. Behind the misery is often the hope that things can or will get better. When both partners have lost a number of people to AIDS, despite the misery in the relationship, there is often the profound fear that one or both people cannot bear to face yet another loss. While much is made of the concept of "intimacy" in the clinical literature, I have yet to come across a satisfactory definition. If we look at what has actually occurred in the gay community in the face of AIDS over the past fifteen years, we see far more loyalty than abandonment. In the case of some couples, the misery that binds is enhanced by the sense that to leave the relationship would be intensely disloyal.

In working with couples, we are faced with the assumption that HIV infection is a disease of promiscuous or drug-injecting individuals and that infected people should politely refrain from sexual contact. In fact, HIV infection occurs at a substantial rate within the context of established relationships. In the late 1980s I asked two physicians—one in San Francisco, the other in Chicago—to look at the relationship status in their caseloads of AIDS patients. Both found that approximately 60 percent of their gay male patients with AIDS considered themselves partnered (Shelby, 1992). As AIDS moves more into the heterosexual communities of various ethnic groups, we will see more and more couples and their children facing the complexities of HIV infection and AIDS.

A wide variety of constellations are evident in couples facing HIV infection. One individual may be HIV negative, the other positive; both may be infected, with one partner more advanced in the infection than the other. The relationship may have begun with knowledge of differing or same HIV status, or the status may have been determined as the relationship evolved; that is, the couple may have made a commitment to each other and as part of that commitment decided to get tested. HIV status may change over the course of the relationship, with a previously negative partner testing positive. Some relationships may begin after a diagnosis of full-blown AIDS. And of course, given the progressive nature of the disease, the stage of infection with its consequent medical and emotional needs will transform as well.

Despite the disruptions that HIV infection brings to individual psyches, the need for life to continue to unfold and evolve is often present. Part of this forward-moving tendency is to attempt to establish relationships. Infected people often date, and they frequently are looking for and available to new relationships. It is not at all unusual for HIV-negative people to establish a relationship with someone who is infected. As for the infectious nature of the disease, in the gay community men have had to believe in the concept of safe or safer sex in order to pursue their sexual lives. In the earlier limerant stages of a new relationship, the HIV infection and its consequences may be, and often is, minimized by the negative partner. Clinicians not experienced with HIV may be baffled by an HIV-negative person entering a sexual relationship with someone who is infected. A wise mentor once pointed out to me that we have far less conscious control of the attachments we make than we think we do. Once the attachment to another is mobilized, we also see mobilized the complex meanings of attachment for that particular person.

Couples often seek our help concerning transitions or progressions in the infection. They may also seek or help when spoken or unspoken concerns about AIDS result in the feeling that the relationship has stopped evolving. In actual clinical work, things are rarely as neat and tidy as the written word and the conceptualizations that lie within. Let's look at a couple that found out one partner was positive in the early stages of the relationship and another couple for which the problem revolved around a significant change in medical status. A couple that knows of early HIV infection and that things are stable medically will have very different needs than a couple facing a change in medical status and the hardships of advanced HIV infection.

NEW RELATIONSHIPS AND HIV INFECTION

As AIDS has become an ever-increasing aspect of life in the gay community, the antibody status of the people involved in new relationships surfaces as an issue with which to be dealt. Indeed, in the country as a whole, pregnant women are now being advised to be tested for HIV infection, and in Illinois, for example, testing for HIV was required for several years to obtain a marriage license. So a couple may find themselves falling in love, wanting to build a life together, but having HIV hovering in the foreground or background. It is not uncommon at all for new couples to voluntarily be tested for HIV as part of their process of coming together. For some couples there will be relief, for others great shock and hardship.

BRIAN AND CAL

Brian and Cal were both in their early thirties when they entered treatment. Brian is a lean, rather constricted, obsessive-compulsive man. He holds an MBA and is meticulous about budgeting money, housekeeping, and any other task he takes on. Cal is a rather large, warm, and friendly kind of guy. Not as formally educated as his partner, but very adept and respected in his line of work, Cal is very likable, spontaneous, at times impulsive, and very quick to identify with people he perceives as "victims." Several months into their new relationship, the two men decided to be tested together. Cal was positive; Brian, negative.

Several months after being tested, Brian called, requesting couples' treatment due to "problems Cal was having with being positive." He went into great detail about how Cal was showing all the signs of someone having difficulty with being positive that he had read in an article. Cal had refused to join a support group, but had agreed to couples work.

During the initial session, both men presented the history of their relationship, their deep feelings each other, and their plans for a Holy Union or commitment ceremony. However, since Cal tested positive the couple had had numerous arguments. Cal was feeling increasingly depressed and out of control, was experiencing mood swings, and was having periodic anxiety attacks. Brian kept repeating that he had no problems with Cal being positive, that he fully intended to remain in the relationship, but he was very concerned about Cal's emotional state and wanted to know what could be done to help him.

At this point Cal began to cry. He related how Brian only made him feel worse. Since the testing, Brian had been reluctant to kiss him; sex had fallen off to nothing. Brian always seemed to have an excuse for not engaging in sexual activity; Cal found himself feeling like a leper and enraged with the man he had been so deeply in love with several months earlier. Sex was very important to Cal; he tended to enjoy passive anal intercourse and "wild and free," spirited sex. They had great sex before the testing, which was safe, but also spontaneous and exciting. As Cal was relating his sexual desires, I observed Brian cringe. With little prompting, Brian went into an elaborate, anxious, and constricted monologue about safer sex and about how no one knew what was really safe. He wanted to know what should be done with Cal's semen. Should it go on a towel? What if he had a rash or a break in his skin . . . what then? After several minutes of Brian's anxious concerns, Cal became acutely upset, relating how bad he felt—the longer Brian talked, the worse he felt. Cal thought that perhaps it would be easier to terminate the relationship. Cal wanted to "forget" about testing positive, to just shelve the whole thing, and get on with life, get things back to normal—the way they used to be—but Brian's anxious concerns kept his HIV status in the forefront of his mind.

Over the next few sessions, I pushed each man to talk about his individual fears about Cal being positive. With a good deal of support and structure, Cal related his intense fears of becoming ill, as well as how he felt damaged, diminished, and dirty. He tended to experience himself as the least successful member of his family, always messing up. He felt that he had really messed up with this one because on top of everything else, he was going to get AIDS. Brian was shocked, but interested and empathic; he moved closer, taking Cal's hand as he related the extent of his distress. Brian continued to deny having any difficulty on his part other than anxious concerns over sex. With some very provocative maneuvering by myself ("Are you telling us that you have no fears, or sadness, or anger over this?"), Brian began to relate the extent of his concerns—his fear of losing Cal, his devastation that the only man he felt he had ever loved may become ill, his own intense fear of diseases and illness. Cal was shocked. He had increasingly viewed Brian as cold and rejecting, not devastated in his own right.

As the work progressed, Cal related how he had taken care of his father as he slowly died of brain cancer. He knew firsthand how hard it was to care for an acutely ill person. As is often the case, there were times when Cal was so exhausted that he wished his father would hurry up and die. He had tended to view Brian as very steady and together, but now he wondered if Brian could really handle taking care of him should he become ill. Each experience of feeling rejected further eroded his confidence in Brian and accentuated his guilt over wishing his father would die. Brian was shocked by the degree of Cal's disillusionment with the relationship, his past history with terminal illness, and the depth of his pain. Again, Brian moved closer to Cal.

DISCUSSION

In thinking about this case, we observe a number of potentially problematic dynamics: the stance/response of the negative partner to the positive partner's distress; the difficulty of the positive partner in obtaining independent help with the impact of HIV and hoping/expecting the negative partner to modulate his distress; the fear of infection and its experience as an injury to an already vulnerable self; and the infected partner's application of what I call the "deathbed template"—that is, rather than asking "Can we create the house with the picket fence together?" he asks "Can this person sustain me in illness?" to interactions in the present.

In positive/negative constellations, one often observes the negative partner taking a stance similar to the well partner when the other partner is acutely ill (Shelby, 1992). The negative partner tends to adopt a steadying stance, feeling that he needs to be strong and organizing in the face of his partner's distress. In some cases, this may also be a defense against the intensity of the affects in the dialogue. At times though, the positive partner may feel that his distress is being minimized if not negated and that he is all alone in the face of his anxiety and fear. The negative partner may also fear that by sharing the extent of his distress that he will only be further burdening his already burdened partner. Helping both individuals relate their sadness, fear, and anxiety actually tends to bring the couple together, and it causes them to realize that they both are saddened and scared that this horrible thing has happened to them, not just to one of them. The couple is then better able to respond to affect states and thus feels more confident in their ability to manage the complexity of what they are individually and collectively feeling. Again, with enhanced responsiveness between the two people, affects are modulated rather than accentuated, and the dialogue operates more smoothly. Perhaps most important, the danger of viewing the well partner as an unresponsive, disappointing, and unreliable transference figure diminishes.

Often we will encounter a tendency on the positive partner's part to want/hope/expect the negative partner to modulate and respond to distress rather than tend to it on an individual basis through support groups or psychotherapy. The negative partner may pull back in the face of such pressure, leaving the positive partner feeling abandoned in the face of his distress. In this case, part of the couple's work may be pointing out this dynamic and working through the positive partner's anxiety about becoming involved in a support group or, depending on the severity of the distress, individual treatment. In a number of cases, I have observed the relationship to settle down considerably as the positive partner tends to his distress in the context of an HIV support group. When the couple is further stabilized, a support group for positive/negative couples may also be suggested.

In observing sexual dialogues between people for whom HIV is present or potentially present, several dynamics consistently appear. For many people there is considerable psychological difference between having sex with someone who may be positive and having sex with someone known to be positive. Most efforts in the area of sexuality have been aimed at informing people of safer sex guidelines and convincing them to follow such guidelines in order to avoid infection. This is the behavioral dimension. As for the psychological dimension, we are actually instilling anxiety into sexual acts and sexual fantasy. That is, one does not need to be anxious about mutual masturbation, hugging, etc., one should be somewhat anxious about fellatio, and one should be very anxious if not terrified about anal or vaginal intercourse without a condom. The presence of HIV in a cultural group such as the gay community also extends into the realm of modulating the intrusion of HIV and the fear of infection into one's sexual fantasy life. Thus, while we are faced with having to believe in the concept of safer sex in order to maintain a sexual life, we are also faced with the constant, and at times highly disruptive, intrusion of the horror of HIV into fantasies that are often highly charged with excitement, vitality, and the desire to connect with another person. Again, observation indicates that people generally are more able to minimize the intrusion of HIV when the partner's status is unknown than when it is known. As we heard in Cal's account, the sexual dialogue shifted dramatically once the infection was identified. Safer sex guidelines did little to modulate Brian's anxiety. I usually take the stance that with or without guidelines, the fear is there, and that ultimately, the two people need to negotiate what is comfortable for both of them. In the case of Brian and Cal, Cal was very comfortable with anal intercourse with a condom, but Brian was terrified. The issue of sex surfaced repeatedly between the two men, with Cal experiencing Brian's anxiety as a self-injury with consequent rage and disappointment. Cal would bring in guidelines and attempt to point out Brian's folly, which got us nowhere. Gradually, Cal accepted that it was easier to negotiate and stay within the realm of Brian's comfort rather to be repeatedly frustrated and disappointed.

A second dynamic regarding sexual activity and fear of transmission is that it is not a steady state; rather, the level of anxiety often ebbs and flows in both the infected and uninfected partners. Just as a person with HIV finds the degree to which he or she feels infectious and damaged highly variable—with times of relatively little anxiety, contrasted by times of higher anxiety—the negative partner often finds his or her fears of being infected fluctuating as well. Fear of transmission may increase in response to a change in medical status, a new medication regime, the death of a friend, or an AIDS-related item on a newscast. The negative partner may react by pulling away from the sexual dialogue, and often feels guilty and confused as well. It is often helpful to point out that this is just the human mind at work; the individual and collective experience of HIV infection is constantly changing and evolving, and feeling infectious or at risk of being infected fluctuates as well. No one is intentionally being rejecting or disloyal; it is just one more part of the complexity, the challenge, of living with HIV.

The third dynamic is the specter of the "deathbed template." By this I am referring of the tendency of both partners to fantasize about the deathbed scene and the affects that accompany it. In new relationships, both people often fantasize about reaching a sense of fulfillment with the other person—what the two people can create or experience together. However, when HIV is involved, the specter of illness and death is often commingled with joyous fulfillment. For the infected partner, this often reflects the longing to be surrounded by loving, supporting, and modulating others, tending to him at a time of great vulnerability. He longs to make a peaceful transition to death surrounded by a sustaining matrix of loving people rather than alone, wretched, and terrified. The problem becomes that some people will apply this template to new relationships, or they will compare conflicts with their partner to this template.

In new relationships this template places a great deal of pressure on the other individual, as well as a sense of desperation on the infected person's part. Infected people may consciously feel or unconsciously sense a great need to get the relationship solidified so that they will not die alone. In the case of a conflict, it can heighten affect states as the partner is viewed as not being reliable enough to be there until the end. The fear of being abandoned and dying alone rushes in, adding to the intensity of the infected partner's distress. In working with men whose attempts at dating have failed, many times it appeared that the boyfriend who terminated the relationship was not so much afraid of the possibility of forming a relationship with a man who may die, as he was fleeing the intense pressure and expectation to be there and to not disappoint at a time of great need. Thus, the "deathbed template" hindered his feeling the excitement of the possibilities of what the two of them may create together.

For the negative partner, the template may come to represent what is down the road—that the relationship will ultimately end in premature death, rather than blissful retirement. Again, both people are often relieved to talk about this image that can appear so close even though medical indications may be that life-threatening illness is far away in time. The therapist needs to listen for associations and interactions that indicate that it is operating at an unspoken level and fueling affective intensity. While it may be an anxious image for all concerned (including the therapist) again it is present in the dialogue, and by the therapist demonstrating his/her capacity to talk about it and tolerate the affect states, the couple is better able to work with their affects and fantasies, and how they impact the dialogue of the relationship.

DISEASE PROGRESSION AND CHANGING NEEDS

Couples who have dealt with the knowledge of HIV infection in one or both parties often reach an equilibrium in terms of their response and approach to the infection. However, a significant change in medical status is often highly disruptive for the infected individual as well as the relationship. Clinical experience indicates that often depression and anxiety may emerge at these transition periods, reaching levels that require clinical intervention. Now one or both people may feel lost, overwhelmed, and confused, rendering past methods of coping with psychological impact of the disease ineffective.

Fred and Ralph

Fred and Ralph were both in their late forties, and had been together for many years. Both were highly successful in their individual careers, but several years ago had joined forces in a new business venture that required both of them to use their skills and work as a team. They had known of

Ralph's HIV infection for several years; his condition had been quite stable. There had been minimal talk between the two men about the infection and its potential consequences. Ralph tended to be the gatekeeper in this area, and would allow little if any consideration of the fact that he was infected. Fred was referred to me by his physician. He had become increasingly anxious and depressed following Ralph's diagnosis of a life-threatening disease.

In our first meeting, Fred alternated between his anxiety over the severity of Ralph's illness and his fear of losing him, and the exciting business plans that lay ahead. He spent more time relating the business ventures than he did his fear of losing Ralph. As we talked, it seemed to me that although Fred was flooded with fear and anxiety, he did not feel permitted to discuss his concerns. Keeping this in mind, I asked about how the two of them were handling the situation, the change, the severe illness. He went on to say that every time he tried to talk about it, Ralph shot him down and told him he was overreacting. If he tried to talk about business plans that may have to be altered because of the illness, he was told that he was being hysterical. He tearfully mentioned that there was not even a will, and that he was terrified to bring the subject up. He desperately wanted to talk to his partner about all of this, but was afraid not just of the intensity and sadness of the subject content, but of being soundly rebuffed again. I offered to meet with them as a couple. Fred was elated, but also fearful; I talked to the physician with whom Ralph had an excellent relationship, and had him recommend a few couples meetings. Ralph reluctantly consented.

I met Fred and Ralph as a couple several times. Ralph basically held court while Fred and I listened. There was no problem—he was going to lick this thing; this was just a minor inconvenience along the way. This all was basically Fred's problem. He did not know how to handle death or dying, not that death was a problem, that was still far down the road, if at all. If Fred did try to interject a concern, he was quickly dismissed. The first several sessions were much the same, though I heard between the lines that the two men had begun to talk over the course of the week, that business plans were being discussed, and that a meeting with an attorney to draw up wills had been scheduled.

During the fifth meeting, the presentation was quite different. Ralph was furious at Fred for not being sensitive to his feeling ill after a home infusion. It turned out that the infusion nurse had come to the home, administered the infusion, and that Fred had gone about business as usual, which has been the routine in the past. This time however, Ralph felt quite ill, and Fred proceeded to talk business and discuss plans for an upcoming business trip. Later that evening, a fight broke out over a minor detail and escalated into accusations that Fred did not care about anything but money, with Ralph countering that he was sick and tired of all the abuse that had been heaped upon him since the illness. In listening to their account, I assumed that the infusion had evoked considerable anxiety, and that the couple's work had been relaxing defenses so that affect could be expressed. In exploring, this was not the first time that Ralph had felt ill after an infusion, but it was the first time that he felt scared and needy after the experience. Fred on one hand tried to do what he thought Ralph wanted, but always found the infusions upsetting, and would busy himself with details while it was in progress.

Both men were gradually able to talk more directly about their anxiety over the situation. Although Ralph maintained his holding-court posture, he did confess to feeling increasingly sad and scared that he might not make it, his concerns for Fred should he die, and dragging him through the dying process. Fred was elated at hearing something other than minimization, but it was also clear that Ralph could tolerate only so much coddling, and needed to maintain as much sense of control as possible. A quiet acknowledgment that things were rough was as about as much as Ralph could handle, but it was enough, along with the other safeguarding legal activities, to take the pressure off the relationship. The couple soon felt they were over the hump, and terminated their work with me. I learned later that when Ralph did die, he had softened considerably; he was quite warm, responsive, tolerant, and appreciative of Fred's concern, coddling, and sadness at having to say goodbye.

DISCUSSION

There are two important themes in this case that I would like to discuss. The first is respecting the nature of the dialogue and working within the characteristics of the dialogue; the second is thinking in terms of disavowal versus denial.

The dialogue of every relationship has its own unique characteristics, capacities, vulnerabilities, and constraints. In clinical work, we often must work within the constraints of the dialogue; at times we will be able to expand the relationship's capacity to tolerate affects and to change its dynamic characteristics. At other times, the couple can tolerate only minimal intervention, or the practice setting may not provide for more extensive work. The challenge for the clinician may be to work within the constraints, and not to push the couple beyond their capacity. Though both of these men were highly successful in their individual careers, their relationship had what could be called overadequate/underadequate characteristics. That is, one person presents himself as highly adequate, tends to run the show in terms of activity, planning, general direction and affect on life, while the other individual tends to live in the shadow of the spouse, deferring to his judgment, and often minimizing his capacities, talents, and strengths. In such relationships, it is very important to remember that both people have considerable vulnerabilities that must be respected and worked with.

When the overadequate partner becomes ill, it is often a considerable crisis. The underadequate partner is at risk of losing his highly idealized mate, while the overadequate partner risks losing his sense of control, and faces the need to increasingly "surrender" to the caretaking of his partner. Often, given the dynamics of the relationship, both people are unsure of the underadequate partner's ability to take charge, even though he may be quite capable outside of the dynamics of the dialogue. These couples often do well with minimal intervention; change may seem miniscule, but it may be enough to stabilize the relationship.

In clinical writing about work with HIV, there has been a tendency to overemphasize the concept of denial. In many cases, the concept of disavowal is more useful and accurate. Denial is a defense against affect, while disavowal is a defense against meaning. Technically, a person facing a terminal illness can deny the affects of sadness, rage, and anxiety, and/or they may disavow the meaning—that this disease means that death is a high possibility. An integral aspect of long-term adaptation to living with HIV is a form of disavowal that may take on characteristics of what Kohut termed the vertical split (Kohut, 1971), that is, two radically different aspects of self are so split off from each other that they do not communicate with each other. People with HIV often display this mechanism of coping with the illness and its implications. Basically one aspect of self experiences the self as dying, diminished, and is often highly vulnerable and in great pain, while the other aspect experiences the self as vital, living forever, and is highly engaged in his/her world.

In the wake of the loss of a friend or partner to HIV, a change in medical status or a disruption in the dialogue, the experience of self as diminished and dying may flood in and dominate, leaving the person confused, discouraged, and with a pronounced feeling that he has been fooling himself. Clinically, I have been able to achieve more profound and effective work by responding to the discouragement and loss of optimism when the split breaks down, rather than thinking of the person as previously being "in denial" and beginning to feel what he "should be" feeling. When the metaphor of two different aspects of self is presented to people, they are often highly relieved. They have often been aware of these disparities of self states for quite a while, but afraid that acknowledging the fear of dying is also of giving up, and paving the way for a decline in medical status as well.

In the context of a relationship, the well or less ill partner is often more aware of, or may feel more strongly these two different aspects of self and their related affects. At times, it may be helpful to think of one partner as feeling certain affect states for both members of the relationship. In my experience, the well or HIV-negative partner tends to follow the lead of the ill or HIV-positive partner when it comes to acknowledging affect states about the fear of decline and death. In the case of Ralph and Fred, Fred was flooded by fear, but also deferring to Ralph, and becoming increasingly panicked that the affects and concrete needs were not being tended to. A sense of panic and walking on eggshells may dominate when partners feel the need, but the fear of bringing up such highly charged issues may also occur.

Again it is the therapist's role to modulate affect states in the relationship and to help the couple talk about their fears. When it comes to disavowed meaning, timing and empathic attunement to individual and collective affect states and readiness is highly important. By the therapist demonstrating an ability to empathically address painful images and affects, the couple's ability and confidence is often enhanced as well. While Ralph and Fred did not engage in elaborate discussions about their individual and collective experiences with me, we saw evidence of movement and acknowledgment that was within the capacity of the relationship.

SUMMARY

In closing, this chapter has been a cursory overview of the complexity of clinical work with couples facing HIV. Although there are many models for clinical work with couples, I have focused on the realm of affect states, responsiveness, and dynamics that may interfere with responsiveness. Again, the goals of clinical work with couples are to help people talk about their individual and collective experiences, to help restore the sense that they are in this together, and are capable of managing the hardships as well as their worst fears. Hopefully, clinicians who are not familiar with HIV-related problems will have a sense of the general range of problems that couples encounter and will feel more confident in approaching this highly important aspect of clinical work with HIV-related problems.

POLICY

In terms of policy, the obvious approach in the context of couples is to acknowledge and respect relationships between two men as valid, sustaining, and integral to the well-being of infected and/or ill persons. Hospital and agency settings that are familiar with HIV and AIDS often integrate this respect into their approaches—whether it be visiting in the hospital, affording partners the same privileges as married spouses, or agencies incorporating the partner into the treatment/service plan. People facing HIV infection and/or AIDS are often in highly vulnerable states. Refusing to acknowledge a sustaining relationship—either subtly or in a more hostile manner—only adds to the vulnerability and fear. Refusing to acknowledge a sustaining relationship is bad clinical practice that approaches the unethical and should be guarded against.

LESSONS FROM MY WORK WITH HIV

The lessons I have learned from twelve years of clinical and research work with the HIV epidemic concern issues of resiliency and loyalty. The most compelling aspect of working with the infected and dying is observing the often remarkable psychological growth of my clients in the face of a life-threatening illness. This leads to resiliency and the capacity to keep striving for coherence, to keep on living no matter what psychological and physical hardships are encountered. In my clinical work and observations of my social circle, I have seen a great deal of loyalty—of reaching out to and sticking by partners and friends in the face of great need. Abandonment and rejection seem to get far more attention than they deserve—perhaps because they are our worst fears. Loyalty encompasses a quieter, steadier state of supporting and sustaining a partner or friend in need.

RECOMMENDED READINGS

Forstein, Marshall (1994). Psychotherapy with gay male couples: Living in the time of AIDS. In *Therapists on the Front Line: Psychotherapy with Gay Men in the Age of AIDS.* Cadwell, S., Burnham, B., and Forstein, M. (Eds.). Washington, DC: American Psychiatric Press.

Shelby, R.D. (1992). *If a partner has AIDS: Guide to clinical intervention for relationships in crisis.* Binghamton, NY: The Haworth Press.

Shelby, R.D. (1995). *People with HIV and those who help them.* Binghamton, NY: The Haworth Press.

REFERENCES

Abramowitz, S. and Cohen, J. (1994). The psychodynamics of AIDS: A view from self psychology. In S. Cadwell, R. Burnham, and M. Forstein, (Eds.),

Therapists on the front line: Psychotherapy with gay men in the age of AIDS. Washington, DC: American Psychiatric Press.

Basch, M.F. (1983). The perception of reality and the disavowal of meaning. In *Annual of Psychoanalysis* 11:125-154. New York: International Universities Press.

Cohen, J. and Abramowitz, S. (1990). Aids attacks the self: A self psychological exploration of the psychodynamic consequences of AIDS. In *Progress in self-psychology.* A. Goldberg (Ed.), 155-172. Hinsdale, NJ: The Analytic Press.

Kohut, H. (1971). *The analysis of the self.* New York: International Universities Press.

Kohut, H. (1977). *The restoration of the self.* New York: International Universities Press.

McWhirter, D.P. and Mattison, A.M. (1985). *The male couple: How relationships develop.* Englewood Cliffs, NJ: Prentice-Hall.

Shane, E. and Shane, M. (1993). Sex, gender, and sexualization. In *The widening scope of self-psychology: Progress in self-psychology.* Volume 9. Hillsdale, NJ: The Analytic Press.

Shelby, R.D. (1992). *If a partner has AIDS: Guide to clinical intervention for relationships in crisis.* Binghamton, NY: The Haworth Press.

Shelby, R.D. (1995). *People with HIV and those who help them: Challenges, integration, intervention.* Binghamton, NY: The Haworth Press.

Wolf, E. (1994). Selfobject experiences: Development, psychopathology, treatment. In Kramer, S. and Salman, A. (Eds.), *Malher and Kohut: Perspectives on development, psychopathology, and technique.* New York: Jason Aronson.

Clinical Issues in Groups
for HIV-Infected Individuals

Margaret Smith
Amy Curell

It was the first meeting of what came to be called The Thursday Night Group. In the library of a church, with comfortable chairs and couches pulled roughly into a circle, sat nine individuals with AIDS—eight gay men and one straight woman. The leaders, a noninfected gay man who ran the local AIDS service organization and a straight female social worker from a local hospital, nervously asked each group member to speak about their expectations of and goals for the group. One by one, most of the men in the group stated that they had no real expectations and did not really know what to expect. A few said they came for information about this new "thing" they were facing. Then the leaders came to Linda. In a strong but quavering voice she said, "I have great expectations for this group! I just lost my apartment, I can't work, and I'm getting sick!" She then burst into tears. After a long pause, the social worker went over to her and grabbed her hand; she was soon joined by the other group leader and most of the other group members.

INTRODUCTION

Group therapy has been a treatment method in social work practice for many decades. Psychotherapy models of group intervention evolved into support models that build upon shared information, coping strategies, emotional support and empowerment, and common experience. Groups that social workers have led more often than not combine the support model with some aspects of psychodynamic psychotherapy. Since early in the HIV/AIDS epidemic, groups have been an important component in ameliorating the isolation that people dealing with HIV/AIDS experience and in helping them cope with the complex issues that a diagnosis of HIV presents.

This chapter outlines general clinical issues that arise in support groups for people facing HIV, including persons who are asymptomatic (testing positive for HIV but not necessarily ill) and persons with a full diagnosis of AIDS. Using Garland, Jones, and Kolodny's (1978) five stages of group development as a backdrop, we will illustrate some of the clinical issues emerging at each stage. As we discuss each stage, we will address concerns specific to gay men and to women with HIV/AIDS, as well as those persons dealing with issues of alcohol and drug use concurrent with illness. Issues affecting the social work practitioner will also be highlighted whenever appropriate. Though rooted in established social work group theory and practice, we will draw heavily upon our eight years of experience conducting four women's groups and two men's groups to discuss clinical issues in groups.

GENERAL ISSUES

David Aronstein's chapter elsewhere in this volume presents excellent guidelines on how to organize support groups for people with HIV and their social networks. Facts the social worker needs to know before starting a group, key questions to ask a person with HIV/AIDS seeking membership in the group, and group size, cultural, and language considerations all lay the groundwork for beginning a support group.

TYPE OF GROUP

Social workers who desire to organize and colead a group for people with HIV/AIDS need to decide at the outset what type of group it will be. The group may be open-ended or time-limited; it may be psychoeducational or it may provide for open discussion. Membership may be open or closed. Although group members may understand that this is a support group, not a psychotherapy group, issues concerning patients' family of origin, childhood sexual or physical abuse, and relationships with significant others—as well as several other issues that may be seen as "therapeutic"—will emerge during group sessions. Social workers must be prepared for this. Many of these issues will be common to other group members and are appropriate group material. Others may warrant referral of the group member to an additional group or individual practitioner.

LEADERSHIP

We believe that groups should be led by two workers, with at least one clinically trained. Experience has taught us that women's groups are best facilitated by women. Male cotherapists can lead men's groups, but these groups have also been successfully led by two women or a combination of one male and one female therapist. Skill level and comfort with issues concerning sexuality, dying, death and bereavement, sexual and physical abuse, drug or alcohol use, and HIV-related medical information appear to matter more than sex of the worker.

Having some medical knowledge about HIV is very important. Group members feel reassured by the fact that leaders have an understanding of such phenomena as opportunistic infections, significance of CD-4 counts, and medications as it denotes a commitment to understanding ways in which the medical and psychosocial aspects of HIV are interrelated. However, you do *not* need to be an expert. Group members will teach you about their illness. This information sharing educates other group members as well. Care should be taken, however, because some members may express medical opinions not based on facts—another reason for the social worker to have some basic medical knowledge.

SUPERVISION

Group leaders must obtain clinical supervision to deal with the complicated dynamics such groups present as well as for support concerning issues of loss and grief. Leaders may meet weekly at first with a supervisor then move to less frequent meetings later on. Social workers may want to seek support from a clinically based team such as other social workers working in the field as well.

LOCATION/SETTING

When choosing a space for the group to meet, care must be taken to consider physical limitations of members. Group space must be handicapped-accessible, be close to public transportation, and have ample parking. One of our groups met in the evening in the library of a church, a space with overstuffed chairs, couches, and a fireplace that could be used in winter. The door could be locked, and the curtains could be closed. Group leaders had keys to the space, and rarely was anyone associated with the church in the building during the meetings. Churches may not be the best setting in all cases, but in this one, the choice seemed to facilitate the inclusion of lively discussions about issues of religion and spirituality.

Another setting we used was a local family service agency. Many members were also obtaining other types of treatment in this facility and had a positive affiliation with the location. This level of comfort was further enhanced by our ability to provide food and drinks for the group in this setting.

Essential to any location for a group is the ability to maximize confidentiality and privacy for group members. A community-based setting or medical care facility may offer accessibility; however, some clients may experience anxiety at the possibility of being identified by neighbors and friends frequenting the setting.

LEVEL OF ILLNESS

It may be appropriate to set parameters regarding the level of illness as criteria for entering a group. Members who are asymptomatic may fear the presence of someone with a full diagnosis of AIDS. We have had group members leave the group because of this. We have had symptomatic members become protective of asymptomatic members, restricting their own discussion of medical and emotional problems. This restriction led to some anger at times on the part of symptomatic members. On the other hand, these differences can also be of great benefit to the group. Asymptomatic members can learn a great deal about their own ability to cope with HIV when witnessing another group member survive and effectively cope with an opportunistic infection.

One of our groups limited membership to those with a full diagnosis of AIDS. This group lost thirty-six members over a three-year period. Although the continual loss of member after member and the bereavement that accompanied each loss was very difficult for both group members and leaders, not one member permanently left the group as a result of another member's death. Rather, the group drew closer together upon a member's dying and death, shared more deeply their own fear and sadness, and conducted special rituals at the meeting following a member's death. Ultimately, members of this group were better able to confront their own impending death and to picture what would happen in the group when they themselves died.

DRUG/ALCOHOL ISSUES

History of or current use of drugs and alcohol is a source of potential conflict for HIV-infected persons in a group setting. Group members in long-term recovery may not be able to tolerate members who are actively using drugs or alcohol. Even those members who are on methadone maintenance may not be accepted by those who are completely drug- and alcohol-free. Women infected by injection-drug-using partners may have another whole set of issues to grapple with in regard to other members' substance use. Group leaders are likely to find differences in the provider community. Some providers will refer persons who are actively abusing substances while other providers will not consider that type of client appropriate for a support group. We have found substance abuse issues to be very challenging, especially in groups for women. The appropriateness of group treatment for an individual in recent recovery who is facing a life-threatening illness is one of the most difficult decisions for group leaders to make. Learning about the different treatment models and establishing clear criteria for group admission are critical to a successful group.

SEXUAL/PHYSICAL ABUSE

Group members, male or female, may have childhood backgrounds of physical or sexual abuse and/or domestic violence. One study looking at HIV infection and rates of childhood sexual abuse found that half of the women and one-fifth of the men studied reported a history of rape during childhood or adulthood (Zierler et al., 1991, p. 572). Given this data, the social worker will benefit from learning about the dynamics of sexual abuse trauma, particularly in relation to the use of group treatment as an intervention. Individuals may not be ready to join a support group for HIV-infected persons if they are experiencing acute symptoms of sexual abuse trauma (i.e., flashbacks), major depression, or suicidal ideation. Addressing HIV issues may further intensify these symptoms; thus, other treatment options may be more appropriate. However, a combined group for HIV-positive adult survivors may offer a place to reduce feelings of isolation, stigmatization, shame, and low self-esteem. These feelings are frequently associated with a history of abuse and HIV infection. Each client needs to be assessed individually.

STAGES OF GROUP DEVELOPMENT

Although there are many models of group work, the stages of group development presented by Garland, Jones, and Kolodny in Bernstein (1978) provide the structure and guidelines that best describe our clinical experience. The stages are as follows: preaffiliation, power and control, intimacy, differentiation, and separation. As with most models that use developmental stages, no prescribed time or set number of meetings exemplify each stage we describe. Although different clinical issues arise in each stage, a central theme that runs throughout the five stages is the struggle with the issue of closeness. We have found this to be a core clinical issue in our HIV groups. The question "How close do I become to another group member?" is intensified by fear of losing that member to AIDS and examining the possibility of one's own death.

PREAFFILIATION

The preaffiliation stage is where the approach-avoidance dynamic takes place. The ambivalence about identifying oneself as a person with HIV, trusting others, and risking closeness then dealing with loss is present at this stage. Behaviors that exemplify the approach-avoidance phenomena for all types of groups include the following: coming late to group meetings, not attending several meetings then returning, coming to the group intoxicated, leaving the group meeting before it ends, and either being silent or excessively verbal during group. Group members may permanently drop out. We have found this ambivalence to vary with different group compositions. Gay men who join an all gay or predominantly gay group may already feel a sense of community and commonality that facilitates a more rapid movement through the approach-avoidance phenomenon. Paradoxically, gay men may be more hesitant to get close to other gay men with HIV because they have already experienced the deaths of many friends from AIDS. Some gay men may not be fully identified as gay men, nor with the gay community. These issues may complicate the approach-avoidance dynamic in a gay men's group.

A women's group often gets stuck in the approach-avoidance stage. The initial development of trust, a key task in this stage, can be difficult to accomplish. We have found this difficulty to be more common in women's groups than in men's groups and we have frequently wondered why.

One apparent reason is that many HIV-infected women are struggling to meet basic needs such as economic security, housing, child care, and transportation. These struggles may lead to sporadic group attendance and difficulty making a commitment to the group. Another reason involves the many differences between HIV-infected women, including racial, ethnic and cultural diversity; religious affiliation; alcohol and drug use; socioeconomic status; sexual orientation; and history of physical and/or sexual abuse. A member who has been in recovery from drug abuse for two years may have difficulty trusting another member who has been sober for two months. A member who is lesbian may fear being judged in a group that is predominantly heterosexual. Some women have painfully lost their children to child welfare custody while others are struggling with the guilt and tremendous responsibility of caring for an HIV-infected child. Fear of judgment, stigmatization, and rejection can be further intensified if members have a history of physical and/or sexual abuse. Many HIV-positive women have experienced discriminatory treatment and therefore are hesitant to access and trust service providers. Leaders can expect to encounter these differences (and more) when starting a women's group.

Being a woman and being HIV positive may not provide enough initial common ground among group members when challenged by the multiple differences. For this reason, a women's group may more successfully move through this stage of initial trust if the group has a third or fourth common denominator. For example an Hispanic HIV women's group or an HIV women's sexual abuse survivors group may accomplish this goal.

PREAFFILIATION STAGE: PRACTICE GUIDELINES

Addressing basic needs of members at this stage of group development, particularly for women, is essential. Can transportation be provided by a local AIDS service agency? Can a grant be written to pay for child care? Making a commitment to run an HIV group often requires using core social work, case management skills, and creativity.

Group leaders need to establish safety and structure in order for group members to move through the approach-avoidance stage. This begins at the screening process. Assessing potential group members with regard to substance use, support systems, medical and psychological condition, and their general readiness to participate in a group is essential. In-person screening can begin to build a therapeutic alliance that can then help a client work through the anxiety of the preaffiliation stage.

Reviewing group guidelines and rules and obtaining a commitment from each member is important. Key rules include the following: maintaining confidentiality within the group, not coming to group meetings intoxicated or high, discussing conflicts between members outside of group within the group, coming to group on time, and contacting group leaders when not able to participate. A written contract that members sign can reinforce commitment to these guidelines.

What do group leaders do when members exhibit inappropriate behaviors and/or do not abide by established group rules? The leaders at this stage need to take a more directive role than at later stages by educating group members regarding the importance of adhering to the rules as a means of developing trust. Normalizing the dynamics of the preaffiliation stage for group members can also be helpful. All of these issues should be brought up with the whole group. Offering psychoeducational material at this point may serve two purposes. First, it establishes authority and trust in group leaders by demonstrating their knowledge and interest in HIV. Second, the structure it provides may decrease group anxiety by offering a focus other than that of personal disclosure. Group members may also feel a sense of competency by being able to share their own knowledge.

Group leaders may also consider contacting members outside of the group to discuss possible reasons for coming late, leaving early, or skipping meetings. We offer an example to illustrate our experience with clinical issues in this stage of group development.

> Jane came to one of the first meetings of the group after just beginning to take the drug AZT. For her this signified a drop in her CD-4 count, and a new, more acute level of illness. As she openly talked of her feelings concerning this, she became quite tearful. Jane neither appeared at the next group meeting nor contacted group leaders to explain her absence.
>
> Group leaders called Jane and she stated that it was "too scary to come to group" because she was "just learning to deal with HIV." Jane had had no previous contact with HIV-positive individuals nor had she ever had individual counseling. What are the options group leaders might provide for Jane? Group leaders might talk to Jane about how normal her anxiety is at this point and suggest she come to two or three meetings before deciding whether or not she can tolerate the group. Leaders might refer her for individual treatment as a first step toward working through emotional difficulties concerning HIV. It may indeed not be the right time for Jane to be in a group. In any case, leaders need to leave the door open for Jane to return to the group at any time. In this instance, three or four individual sessions might have smoothed the way for Jane to join the group. Another example of issues arising in the preaffiliation stage of the life of a group involve trust.

Near the beginning of the third session of the women's group Susan began to speak angrily about her confidentiality having been broken by a group member when in another group. Other members shared concerns about their confidentiality being broken. One woman talked about running into another member at a grocery store. Both were with friends and did not know what to say. Group leaders used this opportunity to again discuss members' commitment to group rules. The group also discussed different scenarios of interactions outside of the group. What do you do if a friend asks you, "How do you know that person?" How do you say "hello" to someone outside of the group if others are around?

The preaffiliation stage of any support group is marked by the struggle of members with issues involving trust. Persons with HIV often have more pronounced issues involving trust because of the stigma attached to anyone with the illness. Group leaders demonstrate their own trustworthiness by providing ground rules, by establishing behavior parameters, and by demonstrating their own commitment to the group. Preliminary commitment and trust from group members will usually follow.

POWER AND CONTROL

For social workers who colead a support group for persons with HIV disease, the stage of power and control may offer the greatest challenges. This stage, as its name implies, is replete with conflicts over power and control of the group. Power struggles may erupt between members or with the group leaders as to who in the group has the highest status. This is a testing stage in which differences between group members emerge but are not yet accepted. Vying for leaders' favor, splitting, members confronting each other, forming subgroups, and scapegoating are some behaviors associated with this stage of group development. From a clinical perspective, these behaviors can be distractions from addressing painful issues and feelings. For men's groups the dropout danger is high during this stage, whereas for women we have found the dropout rate higher during the preaffiliation period. The power and control stage is the time when leaders do the most work. It is a difficult time to introduce new group members.

POWER AND CONTROL STAGE: PRACTICE GUIDELINES

Group leaders allow conflict, but they must provide boundaries, safety, and containment and let the issues sort themselves out. Members may ask to change things about the group such as meeting length, day, or location. Leaders allow for this input but make the final decision in these matters. If a group member dominates a particular meeting, it is up to the leaders to gently cut him or her off and move on to the concerns of other members. In our experience, a "check-in" period at the beginning of the group allows each member to air concerns and bring up issues he or she wishes to discuss. If a member has a crisis or particular problem that does not concern the whole group, offer some time to him or her after the meeting. If the issue appears to need more intense individual therapy, refer the group member to another qualified therapist.

Interventions in this stage are more behavioral in nature than insight-oriented. This is not an ideal time to go into family-of-origin issues. Assertiveness skills for group members are cultivated. When members confront one another, group leaders must keep this behavior appropriate, relate the issues to the group process, and help members by offering problem-solving techniques. As in the first stage, acknowledging that these reactions are normal in this stage may be helpful, but leaders must be careful to validate (not diminish) group members' feelings. When people are experiencing such intense feelings as those that arise during this stage, they may not like to be told they are "normal."

Two important examples of issues that present during the power and control stage of the group are the formation of subgroups and the phenomenon of scapegoating.

> One of our groups for men was composed of five homosexual and two heterosexual members. Over the course of several weeks, a subgroup of gay men emerged and often engaged in talk specific to gay culture. The straight men in the group did not participate in these conversations, and we wondered how they were affected. Did they feel left out, uncomfortable, or possibly offended? As if to answer our concerns, the gay men in the group brought up these very questions for discussion. Two of the straight men in this group professed that this cultural talk "went right over" their heads.

Although in this case concerns arising when a subgroup forms were addressed by the subgroup itself, if this does not happen, the group leaders should bring up the issue. A potential risk of not discussing these issues is that people in the less dominant subgroup may drop out. Discussions of these issues pave the way to address other differences, which may prepare the group for the next stage, intimacy.

Another and potentially harmful phenomenon is that of scapegoating. A scapegoat may be someone in the group who does not follow the rules. In the preaffiliation stage, it may be appropriate for a member to miss a group meeting and/or arrive late to one or two meetings. However, in the power and control stage, this same behavior leaves the member open to becoming a target of the group's anger. If power and control issues block the group from addressing the real issues and feelings members are experiencing, the scapegoat may be the person who will exhibit these emotions by reacting excessively angry or depressed. If a group member is obviously different from the majority of the membership by virtue of his or her physical appearance, mental deterioration, or level of illness, this member can also become the scapegoat.

George, a member of one of our gay men's groups, developed Kaposi's sarcoma with large, raised purple lesions over most of his body, particularly his face. Returning to the group after a few weeks' absence due to his illness, he appeared to have markedly deteriorated. As he began to share his experiences, other group members were not listening to him. Others started separate conversations while he was speaking. He was angry and hurt. Group leaders gently silenced the extraneous conversations, redirected the group to George's concerns, and identified for the others where their discomfort may have come from. Leaders concentrated on George's concerns and then spoke in a general way about how scary it might be to deal with becoming more ill.

In this instance the scapegoat needed protection by group leaders, but the other group members did not need to be chastised. Their reactions were very normal. If a group member's mental condition renders him or her unable to participate appropriately in the group, the leaders (in a separate meeting with this member) may need to ask him or her to leave the group. Fortunately, we have never had to confront such an unpleasant situation.

Although the death of a group member may occur at any stage of a support group for HIV-infected individuals, it is during the power and control stage that such a loss is most difficult for other group members. Because there is not yet an open expression of feelings at this stage, the loss of a member may be very frightening. With this death, members may wonder, "Will this group fall apart?" This loss, at any stage of the group, moves people back to the approach-avoidance phenomenon of the preaffiliation stage. If group leaders understand this, are consistent in their support, but do not probe too deeply for feelings, group members may begin to deal with their greatest fear—death.

INTIMACY

Garland, Jones, and Kolodny (1978) describe the power and control stage as the group's attempt to defend against intimacy. What does intimacy mean to members of an HIV group? The main task of the intimacy stage is intensification of personal involvement. This movement toward increased closeness carries with it many benefits, but it also has consequences. One major consequence is that members risk losing members to whom they have grown close. Another consequence is moving close to facing one's own mortality. These consequences are obviously more pronounced in HIV groups in which the death of members is common. Despite this and other consequences, the group as a whole moves more strongly toward affiliation, and the power and control struggles decrease.

Members in this stage begin to disclose more about their life experiences and relationships, particularly with family members. Because a degree of trust has been established, members begin to discuss both positive and negative feelings about other group members and leaders. The group begins to resemble aspects of a "family," and transference and countertransference reactions emerge. Group leaders need to pay close attention to group process as well as content discussed.

INTIMACY STAGE: PRACTICE GUIDELINES

Many family-of-origin issues emerge during this stage and can be appropriately explored within the context of the group. For example, a member who may have experienced ridicule and rejection in his or her family may expect that rejection from group members and interpret feedback as criticism. Group leaders are better able in this stage of group process to help members see the connection between past experiences and current expectations in the group. The group can then become a practice ground for reworking unfinished family business.

Some members at this stage may continue with power struggles and/or other behaviors that may distance themselves from the intimacy in the group. Group leaders can try to help members understand their distancing behaviors and also facilitate appropriate group feedback regarding the behaviors (for example, frustration at chronic lateness to group, domination of group discussion, hurtful sarcasm).

Group leaders also are likely to experience more countertransference at this stage. As leaders become more connected to the group and its members, fear of loss can also emerge, particularly if leaders have experienced much loss in their own lives. These fears may be expressed in various ways. Group leaders may disclose more about their own lives at this stage as a means of identifying with clients. Leaders may also become bored or distant in the group or feel avoidant before the group begins. Group leaders are at risk for many of the same behaviors as group members when faced with intimacy and the threat of death. This is why supervision is essential when running these groups.

Another aspect of group process that occurs at the intimacy stage is that group members may have more contact with each other outside of the group and friendship dyads develop. These friendships were encouraged by us as they provided additional support for group members. Possible consequences of this contact, however, are that some members may feel left out and conflict outside of the group may lead to tension inside the group. Members at the beginning of the group agree to bring in and discuss outside conflict, and it is up to the leaders to reinforce this rule. Group leaders may also need to confront the group if members are being alienated.

Another possible consequence is that members may become sexually involved. Again, many groups have as a rule no sexual contact between members. At the intimacy stage, the group adopts a family quality. In one group in which sexual contact occurred between two members, several group members talked about feeling uncomfortable and left out. Some members did mention the sexual involvement as feeling incestuous. Other members felt okay about it. This lead to a very interesting conversation about boundaries, family-of-origin issues, and even the leaders' role as watchful authority. In the end, the group made the decision to reinforce the rule. Such a conversation would have been unlikely at an earlier stage of group development.

Because there is more trust and a greater ability to share intimate feeling at this stage, the group is now better able to cope with the death of a group member. During the intimacy stage, rituals emerge concerning the death of a member. In one group we led (the group that met in the church library), the meeting following the death of a member was of particular importance. Each person spoke about the deceased member, and at the end of the group, we would move into the chapel and each light a candle for him or her. Even after this group ended, the ritual was carried out. Upon the death of a former group member, one of the leaders and another former group member returned to the church and lit candles. This private ritual addresses the complex issues raised by a most public ritual, that of the wake and funeral. The following example will describe this complexity.

> Tim had been a core member of the group since its inception. He was also the first member to die. Tim attended group meetings regularly for about a year until he became too ill to attend. Some group members would visit him at home while others would openly discuss how it was too difficult for them to do so. Members allowed for and understood these differences in coping. Group leaders also made home visits, knowing that to do this meant making the same commitment to other group members if they became ill. Members appeared comforted by this commitment and genuine caring by the leaders.

When Tim died, many of the group members and the two leaders attended his wake. The group sat together. Some members held hands to comfort each other, and one group member reached over and held hands with the group leader as everyone sat looking at the former group member, now dead.

A true sign that this group had entered the intimacy stage was the fact that they could sit and tolerate this experience without fleeing. The courage of these men was tremendous. Issues that emerged for the leaders included how strong and/or how vulnerable should leaders allow themselves to be in such a situation. Is it okay to cry or hold hands with a client? Boundaries in this type of work are constantly challenged.

Although this experience was extremely painful, the group became more solid. After Tim's death some members avoided group for one or two sessions (back to approach-avoidance), but the group soon returned to a more intimate status quo.

The decision to attend or not attend the wake or funeral of a group member brings up many issues for group leaders as well as members. In one of our groups, leaders made the decision to attend all funerals if they were held in town. We felt this to be part of our commitment to the membership. Attendance by group members was always clearly stated as voluntary. In the beginning stages, the funeral of the first member was attended by only two other group members, sitting in the back of the church, not together. By the last stages, the group went as a group, sitting together and with the group leaders. All of the rituals, private or public, answer for the group membership the following questions: What will happen when I die? What will the group do? What will the leaders do? How will I be remembered? If group leaders and members can survive the intense experiences of the intimacy stage, the next stage, differentiation, will follow more easily.

DIFFERENTIATION

Garland, Jones, and Kolodny (1978) describe the differentiation stage of group process as one in which members accept each other as distinct individuals, accept the differences between them, and at the same time, understand their common ground. The attendant cohesion is based on mutual identification and understanding. Movement into the differentiation stage is easier if the group has surpassed the power and control struggles and has moved into the intimacy stage. The intimacy stage provides the climate for group members to accept individual needs and gives them the ability and the freedom to differentiate and "to evaluate relationships and events in the group on a reality basis" (Garland, Jones, and Kolodny, 1978, p. 52). Group members experience closeness in a more genuine way. They also discover the nature and meaning of the group itself and how it might compare with other groups or social situations known to them.

DIFFERENTIATION STAGE: PRACTICE GUIDELINES

In the differentiation stage, group leaders can step back a little. Transference and projection may decrease among members and toward leaders. Group members may feel comfortable enough to risk telling others they are going to stop all medications or never tell their children about their illness—two issues that would not have been accepted earlier. A level of closeness and a feeling that "this group can handle anything" emerge. The death of a member will not threaten the group, and new members may be admitted when appropriate.

When to allow new persons to join a support group after the death of a member brings up several issues, and our experience in this area is varied. How many weeks should leaders wait? If a new member comes in directly after the death, does that mean to the others that he or she is readily replaceable, not important to the group? What burdens are placed on the new member? Are other group members angry with the new member because he or she is not the lost member and does not know what others have experienced? In one of our groups, the tradition was to wait at least two weeks and then confer with the group as to their wishes. If the deceased member was particularly important to the others, they usually wanted to "wait a little longer" before allowing a new member into the group. At this point in the group process, group leaders probably understand the dynamics enough to, with consent of group members, make decisions about new members. The group will also be autonomous enough to make their own decisions. How do leaders help a new member through the stages of an already advanced group? In the first meeting, leaders provide the history and goals for the group, restate ground rules, and introduce themselves to the new member. They then ask other members to introduce themselves to the new member and tell him or her what the group means to them. Often as this process occurs, the individual telling the story will describe his or her progress through the early group stages, thus providing a model for the new member. The new member is then asked to introduce him- or herself with the reassurance that he or she may say as much or as little as he or she wishes. Throughout the assimilation process of a new group member (which may take several meetings) leaders need to focusing on normalizing the different stages the new member may be going through and protect the new member from being scapegoated.

Two examples will highlight the increased autonomy that is present in the differentiation stage. In one of our men's groups that ran from June 1987 through April 1990, this autonomy emerged when several group members formed another organization with a separate purpose. These men formed a local chapter of the Persons with AIDS Coalition and began to run open informational forums and support sessions for any and all persons in the community affected by HIV. This local PWA Coalition joined the national organization and provided information and service to the community long after the original support group disbanded.

Another example of the ability of an established group to act as a unit and interact with others in the community was demonstrated by one of our women's groups. The group made a decision to attend a Women and AIDS conference in another state. Some members chose not to attend, a decision accepted by the whole group. Members arranged for shared accommodations and transportation.

As indicated earlier, the differentiation stage allows group members to mutually support each other's individuality. For persons with HIV this may take the form of having AIDS in one's "own way," for example, choosing to take or not take antiretroviral medications or engaging in "alternative" treatments such as acupuncture or holistic healing. At this stage, the group is ready to hear and support these individual decisions without feeling threatened. Leadership continues to support individual experiential differences.

Another facet of the differentiation stage is that group members may feel secure enough to engage in life-review work. This is a salient component of any group composed of persons dealing with HIV and important in helping individuals come to terms with mortality. During this time, efforts may also be made to finish "unfinished business" with family members, using the group both as a family "model" to practice on and to return to for support after attempts to resolve family-of-origin issues. Part of this life-review work may include group members examining more closely their own deaths. Members may begin to plan their funerals, incorporating aspects of their lives that they have identified as meaningful. Discussions about spirituality and the afterlife are common.

SEPARATION

Tasks outlined by Garland, Jones, and Kolodny (1978) in this stage of group process fail to adequately mirror those experienced by a group of persons with HIV or AIDS. Garland's tasks are related more to a time-limited group, and our experience has never included setting a limit to the running time of our support groups. Issues that do relate to our experiences include separation anxiety, recapitulation and evaluation of group experience, and learning to take the group as a "frame of reference for approaching new social, group and familial situations" (Garland, Jones, and Kolodny, 1978, p. 57).

SEPARATION STAGE: PRACTICE GUIDELINES

Terminating a support group for people facing HIV/AIDS is full of complex issues having to do with attachment, loss, grief, and death for group members and leaders alike. Death may have decimated the number of members, and referrals may not be forthcoming. In our experience group leaders have trouble ending groups, possibly because the anxiety of telling people facing terminal illness that the group needs to end is too great. Group members who wish to leave the group for any number of reasons also have difficulty, and it is the leader's responsibility to allow them "off the hook." One way to facilitate a group member's voluntary departure is to establish a group rule at the beginning asking him or her to give a two-session warning to the group and to use those sessions to explain why he or she is leaving the group. Thus, the members can process the issues of loss that will inevitably arise. Separating from the group can also offer a member an opportunity to address issues of separation and loss within his or her family.

> Richard, a man with full-blown AIDS, had been struggling for several months with the idea of moving with his lover to another state. A major consequence of this was moving further away from his mother, with whom he was very close. His mother had expressed a desire to care for him as his illness progressed. Richard also feared losing the group's support. As he talked about feelings associated with separation from his mother and the group, he gained clarity and strength regarding his decision to move.

During the separation stage, members express their individual ways of saying good-bye—to the group, to family members, and to themselves.

Issues of separation for the social worker are always part of the reasons for ending a long-running support group that suffers loss after loss. Honesty on the part of the leadership is essential to forestall any personal responsibility that group members might feel. The session during which the ending of The Thursday Night Group was brought up will punctuate this point.

> During the preceding three months, the group had dwindled from ten to six members due to the deaths of several longtime members. No new referrals had been forthcoming and after several soul-searching sessions with our supervisor, we agreed the group needed to end. This was more for our mental health than anything else, but both of us were unwilling to admit this to ourselves or our supervisor. The night came to begin termination and with some trepidation I, as the social work leader, began the list of reasons why the group ought to end. At the end of the list, Paul looked me straight in the eye and said quietly, "You're lying. Tell us really why you're ending this group!" I began to cry and said "Because I can't watch you all die, one by one." He was right, and I told him the truth. Other members came to comfort me, and another group member (a social worker) defended me by saying how difficult it was to keep an open-ended group of this intensity running for three years. The group was able to deal with the leader's grief (as was the leader), and the last several sessions of the group were a time for all of us to review and frame positively our experience. Group members stayed in touch, and leaders kept frequent contact with members until the last member was gone, about a year and a-half after the group ended.

This example, demonstrating issues that arise in the separation stage of a group, also illustrates the intense issues faced by the social worker coleading such a group. It is important to understand what the warning signs might be for a social worker experiencing what is called "secondary traumatic stress" so that he or she can obtain the necessary support to continue his or her work. Numbness, sleeplessness, agitation, anxiety, depression, and fatigue may be signals to the worker that he or she is experiencing this type of stress. Overinvolvement with and/or detachment from group members also results from the emotional stress of running these groups. When experiencing loss after loss of group members, the social worker may wonder "Can I or should I experience joy?" All of these symptoms and feelings are *normal* and *can* be ameliorated.

As stated before, good individual and dual supervision is imperative. Processing these feelings in a team with those who understand the issues from the inside can also be of great help. Individual therapy to process personal issues arising as a result of work with these groups is another way to take care of the worker. Taking "time off" between the end of one group and the beginning of another is often necessary. Extra attention to sources of physical, emotional, and spiritual nourishment are essential for the social worker engaged in this work.

CONCLUSION

In this chapter we have discussed clinical issues that arise when social workers colead a support group for people with HIV disease. We have covered general issues and have used a five-stage framework, highlighting issues that arise in each stage for both group members and group leaders. Finally, we have described possible problems that might surface for the social worker leading a group facing terminal illness. We are aware that some of what we have written may appear daunting or frightening for the social worker who is considering starting a support group for persons with HIV. Indeed this is intense, challenging, and emotional work. However, we consider the support groups that we have led to be our finest clinical social work.

RECOMMENDED READINGS

Brauer, S.B. (1994). The HIV-infected gay man: Group work as a rite of passage. In S.A. Cadwell, R.A. Burnham Jr. and M.A. Forstein (Eds.), *Therapists on the front line* (pp. 223-235). Washington, DC: American Psychiatric Press, Inc.

Carmack, B.J. (1992). Balancing engagement/detachment in AIDS-related multiple losses. *IMAGE: Journal of Nursing Scholarship, 24*(1), 9-14.

Corea, G. (1992). *The invisible epidemic.* New York: HarperCollins.

Garland, J.A., and Frey, L.A. (1976). Application of stages of group development to groups in psychiatric settings. In S. Bernstein (Ed.), *Further explorations in group work* (pp. 1-33). Boston: Charles River Books, Inc

REFERENCES

Garland, J.A., Jones, H.E., and Kolodny, R.L. (1978). A model for stages of development in social work groups. In S. Bernstein (Ed.), *Explorations in group work: Essays in theory and practice* (pp. 17-71). Hebron, CT: Practitioner's Press.

Zierler, S., Feingold, L., Laufer, D., Velentgas, P., Kantrowitz-Gordon, I., and Mayer, K. (1991). Adult survivors of childhood sexual abuse and subsequent risk of HIV infection. *American Journal of Public Health, 81*(5), 572-575.

Clinical Issues for Families

Ian Stulberg

WHY DO THIS?
STATEMENT OF THE PROBLEMS AND ISSUES

Both persons with HIV (PWHIVs) and their families are confronted with clinical issues particular to HIV, that result from the unique biopsychosocial environment of the AIDS epidemic. In addition to the clinical issues of grief and loss associated with losing a loved one to a terminal illness, the families of PWHIVs may present with a variety of other concerns, which may require mental health interventions. Among these issues are the following:

- The young age of the vast majority of PWHIVs causes a disruption of our notion of traditional developmental stages and tasks, resulting in the caretaking by families of members who would otherwise be in the most independent and productive period of their lives. This disruption may also contribute to a more complicated bereavement for parents as their children precede them in death.
- Because the vast majority of diagnosed cases of HIV in the United States occur in previously stigmatized populations (gay men and injection drug users), there is a greater likelihood that families may suffer some degree of alienation from the HIV-infected member. Thus, secrets and denial may figure more prominently in the interactions among family members.
- Perhaps most significantly, just as with PWHIVs, the stigma and accompanying discrimination that permeate the HIV environment will often result in feelings of shame and guilt for family members and a consequent isolation from sources of social support traditionally available to families with terminally ill members.

EXAMPLES OF HOW THE ISSUE MAY PRESENT

Parents or siblings of someone with HIV often seek counseling or mental health support for the first time in their lives following the disclosure by the PWHIV of his or her HIV status. The complexity of clinical issues and the intensity of the need for mental health intervention may depend on a variety of additional psychosocial factors.

What stage of the disease process the PWHIV is in may have profound implications for the family member. Clearly, a mother who first learns of her son's HIV status after he has been hospitalized in the midst of a medical crisis is liable to present with more intense needs than the mother who learns of her son's status when he is asymptomatic, with a high CD-4 count and the likelihood of years without serious illness. In addition, the bereavement experience is apt to be much more complicated for family members who learn of a member's HIV at the end stage of the illness.

If the revelation of a family member's HIV status is accompanied by the implied or explicit revelation of a lifestyle that had previously remained hidden, the "generic" clinical issues of grief and loss may be complicated by profound feelings of hurt, guilt, resentment, betrayal, and abandonment. Consider, for example, the wife who first learns that her husband of twenty years has been actively bisexual after he has been hospitalized with pneumocystis pneumonia. Consider the parents who discover, following a revelation of HIV, that their "perfect," financially successful son has been injecting heroin with his buddies for several years.

Similarly, if the PWHIV is not a member of an "official" risk group (gay men and injection drug users), the unexpected nature of the diagnosis may intensify the family member's reaction to the news. Psychological complications may rise exponentially when women and children are involved. For example, a grandmother is informed that the reason her first grandchild has failed to thrive is because he is infected with HIV, which, in turn, means that her daughter is also infected.

The degree to which family members are influenced by the societal stigmatization of HIV is yet another factor in determining how they may present for service. Individuals who feel that HIV has a pejorative connotation and implies something negative about those whom it infects are likely, as previously indicated, to be much more secretive with the information and to isolate themselves from usual sources of support. The therapy session or support group may be the only place they feel safe enough to ask for the support they need, and confidentiality may be a primary issue of concern. If the PWHIV from such families is gay or an injection drug user, family members may also have difficulty establishing and maintaining effective and supportive relationships with the PWHIV's personal support network. Conflicts may arise in hospital settings over priority of access to the PWHIV, decision making regarding medical care, legal and financial arrangements, etc.

Families may present with a myriad other clinical issues, including the following:

- Family members may need to clarify their expectations of one another and renegotiate existing familial roles, which may have been disrupted by the chronic, terminal illness of the PWHIV.
- When PWHIVs are also parents of young children, their families may present with the need to resolve guardianship issues.
- Conflicts may arise concerning how the PWHIV wants to die, the disposition of remains, who is to be designated as power of attorney for health care, or who will be executor of the PWHIV's will, etc.
- Family members often need assistance in identifying ways in which they can better take care of themselves, which may require learning how to establish boundaries and set limits with the PWHIV.

FACTS THE SOCIAL WORKER NEEDS TO KNOW BEFORE PROCEEDING

While HIV may infect one individual, the disease happens to that individual's entire family and support system, and many of the same issues that affect the PWHIV may be experienced, in a parallel manner, by family members as well. Both the PWHIV and his or her significant others share a car in the "rollercoaster ride" of AIDS. Family members' spirits can be expected to rise and fall in conjunction with the medical and psychological conditions of their infected loved one.

Recognizing the chaos that something as devastating as AIDS creates in the lives of PWHIVs and their families is important. This chaos has significant implications for the social worker's treatment plan. First of all, the worker needs to be flexible—as does the treatment plan!—and prepared for abrupt disruptions to his or her ability to provide services, whether this means frequently missed therapy sessions due to caretaking responsibilities or the necessity to reestablish therapeutic priorities based on new developments in the loved one's illness. For example, the treatment goals of supporting a mother to confront her HIV-positive son regarding long-standing interpersonal conflicts may become clinically irrelevant when the son is rushed to the hospital and placed on a respirator.

At the same time, the social worker needs to try to anticipate the potential pitfalls, problems, and psychosocial consequences of HIV/AIDS in order to lessen their impact on the family members. For example, is the client aware of resources available in the community if the loved one requires practical or financial assistance? Have legal documents—wills, powers of attorney, access to bank accounts—been completed, in the event the loved one becomes incapacitated and unable to act on his or her own behalf? If a family member is also the primary caregiver, have discharge plans been developed in consultation with this family member, who understands and is prepared for the required caretaking responsibilities?

Social workers should also keep in mind the degree to which denial plays a role in the psychological lives of people impacted by terminal illness. While it can serve an adaptive function, in terms of allowing the family member to maintain hope and provide encouragement to the PWHIV, maladaptive denial can lead to a lack of empathic support for the PWHIV, a breakdown in communication, and/or an emotional distance between the family member and the PWHIV. Even in the absence of overt denial, avoiding painful emotional discussions with a loved one is often rationalized—by both family members and PWHIVs—as a desire to "protect" the other from issues he or she "can't handle" or "isn't ready to deal with" when, in reality, the individual may simply be projecting onto the loved one his or her own ambivalence about having such a discussion. One social worker facilitated the honest communication between a PWHIV and his sister after hearing separately from both about their desire to raise the issue of funeral arrangements.

KEY QUESTIONS TO ASK THE CLIENT

The provision of clear and accurate information is often the most valuable and effective intervention a social worker can make, particularly in the early stages of working with a family member. It is, therefore, imperative that the worker ask the client not only about his or her understanding of HIV and its attendant opportunistic infections, but also what the family member knows about his or her loved one's medical status.

The worker must also know what the relationship between the family member and the PWHIV was like prior to the PWHIV's illness. Was their relationship a close and loving one or one characterized by conflict and distance? If the relationship was dysfunctional before HIV, the likelihood is that, without significant mental health intervention, the presence of HIV will significantly intensify the dysfunction.

What did the client previously know about the loved one's lifestyle? If the PWHIV is gay, was the parent aware of the child's sexual orientation prior to learning of his or her HIV status, and, if so, was the child's sexuality something that was "assumed but never discussed," or was the parent actively supportive of the child's homosexuality? What kind of relationship does the client have with the PWHIV's personal, nonfamilial support network? What is the communication like between the family member and the PWHIV? Are they able to address problems directly when they arise or do they have a history of avoiding conflict?

Finally, the development or enhancement of the client's support network is an integral aspect of working with all HIV-impacted clients; thus, it is vital to explore what emotional resources the family member has for him- or herself. Who is aware of what is happening? Who else can the client talk to? Who can be relied on for support? The more support family members have for what they are going through, the better able they will be to "be there" for their loved one with HIV.

CULTURAL COMPETENCY CONSIDERATIONS

The stigma associated with HIV may have profound implications for working with families from ethnic or cultural backgrounds other than our own. While few cultures in the world are actively supportive of homosexuality and drug use, the proscription against the two in certain cultures may be more severe than in others. Families that come from such cultures will likely have a much stronger need for secrecy and will be less willing to access traditional or established sources of support. For example, while the conventional assumption might be that individuals are more comfortable accessing support from within their own culture, the opposite may be true within the environment of HIV. For families fearful of anyone they know finding out, the last place they will go to seek support is within their own culture. For example, after spending a great deal of time tracking down a Japanese-speaking therapist for a mother of a PWHIV, a social worker was informed by the mother, in broken English, that she actually preferred an English-speaking therapist because "Japanese people gossip too much."

Another consequence of cultural difficulty with HIV may be that families will often be kept in the dark by the PWHIV as to the true nature of the illness. It was my experience when working on a hospital's immune-suppressed unit that while Latino families tended to be among the most supportive—packing the hospital room every day with extended family members—they were also the most likely not to know the real diagnosis of their loved one. Social workers must approach such situations with sensitivity, subtlety, and tact.

With family members not born in this country, it is necessary to assess their level of acculturation, as less acculturated individuals may be less aware of available services and therefore less likely to request them. Such persons are also less likely to understand the function of the social worker (although clearly this is not solely a problem for the unacculturated!). Interventions with such families may be heavily weighted toward education, case management, and advocacy.

ACTION STEPS FOR SUCCESSFUL INTERVENTION

Because social workers are traditionally more likely to assume a variety of professional hats (clinician, advocate, educator, networker, etc.), they may be uniquely qualified to respond to the variety of needs of families impacted by HIV. While the preference may be to intervene on a psychotherapeutic level with clients, the clients may have a much stronger need for information and resources—especially directly following the revelation of their loved one's diagnosis. One must remember that sometimes the provision of accurate information (whether in the form of clarifying erroneous conceptions about HIV or describing the availability of much-needed resources in the community—and how to access them) can be the most effective intervention for clients contending with the chaos of HIV. Often, assisting in this way will enhance the therapeutic bond with the client, which, in turn, will allow the social worker to intervene more effectively in a clinical capacity, if needed. I once worked with the parents of a terminally ill patient who desperately wanted to bury their son in their small, midwestern hometown, but were considering burying him in Los Angeles because they feared their community's reaction should the cause of death be known. After checking, I was able to alleviate their fears by informing them that there was no official reason that individuals handling funeral arrangements in the hometown needed to know the cause of death. The parents were so relieved by, and appreciative of, this bit of information, that I could thereafter do no wrong in their eyes, and they readily opened up to me about their feelings about losing their son.

Helping families establish or enhance a support network is another integral aspect of working with HIV. Such assistance may initially take the form of exploring the family member's own ambivalent feelings about what it means to have a loved one with HIV as this ambivalence (loving the PWHIV but feeling ashamed of the disease) is often the major factor preventing families from accessing support. Reality testing and role-playing may prove helpful in preparing family members to tell others about their loved one's illness.

These interventions commonly take place in support groups for family members and are often more effective when they come from others who have "been there" rather than from a social worker or therapist. One middle-aged couple, who were among the first participants in a "significant other" support group I was facilitating, confessed that no one outside their immediate family was aware of their son's diagnosis and that the group was the only place they felt comfortable discussing it. They expressed fearing rejection or discrimination from others if they were to be open about their son's illness. After attending the group for several months, however, and hearing differing views on this issue from others in the group, they came to realize that their son's HIV infection had nothing to do with his value as a human being, nor theirs as parents. At this point, they started telling others—at first gradually, but then quite readily. The couple eventually became spokespersons regarding HIV in their community and, for several years, were among the top fundraisers for the annual AIDS Walk in Los Angeles.

An alternative to participation in a group, for those who are reluctant or unable to do so, is to be put in individual contact with other family members of PWHIVs. Such arrangements are relatively easily achieved and often prove to be very meaningful to the parties involved.

Often the family members are not reluctant to reveal the diagnosis to others but rather the PWHIV is ("He forbids us to tell anyone about his illness!"). In such situations, it may be appropriate to explore whether it is reasonable to assume that the PWHIV's need for secrecy should supersede the client's own need for support.

This notion of the PWHIV's needs being more important than the family member's is a pervasive theme in work with HIV-impacted families. While it is understandable to want to appease the loved one with a terminal illness, such an attitude may prove to be not only condescending and infantilizing but counterproductive as well since it may lead to resentment, burnout, and emotional distance. Family members should be encouraged to be as honest as possible with their loved ones, which often means acknowledging and asserting their own needs and feelings. When all parties are amenable, it may be beneficial for the social worker to mediate family discussions of these issues. Groups for families may also be very effective in helping members assert themselves with their loved one with HIV.

Finally, education regarding the dying process may prove invaluable to family members of a loved one in the terminal stage of the disease. Anecdotal evidence suggests that the dying may have some control over when they take their leave. Sometimes, terminally ill patients may hang on beyond everyone's expectation—including their doctor's—until they reach a special day or anniversary or until the arrival of a specific loved one. Others appear to find it difficult to die as long as they are surrounded by those closest to them. These individuals may wait until everyone goes out briefly for a meal, for example, and then quickly depart. Such information may assist families in coping with the dying process and may help alleviate any feelings of guilt once the loved one has died.

POTENTIAL BARRIERS TO SUCCESSFUL INTERVENTION

As discussed, the chaos that often accompanies—and coexists—with a diagnosis of HIV can prove a major barrier to the social worker's attempts at intervening. With the multitude of practical matters that family members may need to assist with and attend to, taking time to focus on themselves and their needs may seem like a luxury. Practical matters, such as lack of transportation, may also impinge on the social worker's ability to provide clinical services. Just getting family members to attend regular sessions, therefore, may be a daunting challenge—especially when sessions with the entire family are needed. While home visits are usually considered only when clients are too ill to get to the social worker, it may be to the social worker's advantage to consider "starting where the client is" geographically because more consistent sessions may result from regular home visits.

Flexibility is one of the keys to successfully working with those impacted by HIV. Social workers who insist on clearly delineated or rigid professional settings and boundaries may have significant difficulty working comfortably with this population. In addition to a willingness to meet with clients in their homes, working effectively with families impacted by HIV may also require hospital visits, attendance at funerals and memorials, hugging and/or touching the client, etc.

Finally, as mental health professionals, we must be sensitive to any difficult countertransference issues that may result from working with both PWHIVs and their families and significant others. In addition to the feelings that may accompany working with nontraditional boundaries—as previously discussed—some social workers may also have negative or problematic reactions to the grief, hopelessness, and despair associated with death and dying as well as to the issues of homosexuality or injection drug use. Those who work with families struggling with the stigma associated with HIV may find the extent of the desire for secrecy that these families bring into the consultation room extreme and even offensive. Being aware of and monitoring these feelings are essential steps toward effective clinical work.

The social worker must also monitor his or her own reasons for working in this field, as unresolved past experiences with loss (especially losses resulting from AIDS), rescue fantasies, or personal feelings regarding the "appropriate" death process may hinder working productively with families.

INFORMATION THE CLIENT SHOULD KNOW
BEFORE TAKING ACTION

Perhaps the most commonly expressed wish of family members is to "be there" for their loved one throughout the illness. Being truly supportive to someone with HIV—or anyone with a life-threatening illness, for that matter—requires that we be sensitive to what that individual needs and wants from us. This does not imply, of course, always subjugating or denying one's own needs and feelings. However, if one wants to be helpful, it is important to know what the PWHIV would find helpful rather than to proceed based on one's personal agenda. If a family member does not know or is unsure about this, it may be incumbent upon that person to ask the following: "I want to be supportive, but I'm not sure what you need from me right now. What can I do to help?" Of course, the PWHIV's answer to this question will most likely change as the disease progresses, and the opposite of what was wanted one week may be exactly what is needed the next. For example, I have heard PWHIVs state emphatically that they do not want to be treated like sick people ("professional PWHIVs"), with loved ones always asking how they are feeling, only to have these same individuals complain subsequently that their families do not seem to care about them because no one has been asking how they are doing!

Families should also be aware that experiencing and expressing anger is often an integral part of living with HIV, and when possible, it is advantageous to avoid responding directly to the expression of anger from the PWHIV and to look for the frustration, fear, and/or hurt that may underlie it. Anger is a very effective distancing tool and may be utilized frequently by PWHIVs who are devastated by what they perceive to be the emotional consequences of their illness on their families. I once worked with a hospitalized client whose mother was visiting from Florida, where she and the client's father had recently retired. After witnessing the verbal abuse this client heaped on his mother—ultimately driving her back to Florida—I asked him what was going on. In tears, the client replied that he felt that his illness had ruined his parents' retirement, and it was too difficult for him to witness the pain in his mother's face as she hovered about, trying to help.

POLICY IMPLICATIONS AND RELATED ACTIONS

An adequate support system is vital to optimal functioning of anyone infected with HIV. Often, the larger and more substantial a PWHIV's support system is, the less he or she may need to utilize professional sources of support. Viewing the needs of those with HIV from a systems approach allows for the creation of more effective services, resulting in a better quality of life for the PWHIV. It is, therefore, incumbent upon those devising and providing services for this population to consider the needs of the families and significant others. By having counseling, HIV education, and support groups readily available, families will be more likely to successfully endure the rollercoaster ride of HIV with their loved one and be better prepared to provide the support and assistance their loved one requires.

RECOMMENDED READINGS

Bonuck, K. A. (1993). AIDS and families: Cultural, psychosocial, and functional impacts. *Social Work in Health Care, 18*(2), 75-87.

Cates, J. A., Graham, L. L., Boeglin, D., and Tielker, S. (1990). The effect of AIDS on the family system. *Families in Society: The Journal of Contemporary Human Services, 71*(4), 195-201.

Stulberg, I., and Buckingham, S. L. (1988). Parallel issues for AIDS patients, families, and others. *Social Casework, 69*(6), 355-359.

HIV Risk Assessment
in Mental Health Settings

Lee W. Ellenberg

WHY DO THIS?
STATEMENT OF THE PROBLEM AND ISSUES

Just as the HIV virus knows no barriers in terms of gender, race, class, religion, and sexual orientation, HIV enters social work offices in mental health settings in a variety of ways and must be integrated into mental health treatment. HIV has serious implications for a vast majority of mental health clients. This includes clients who:

- are currently or have recently been sexually active;
- are contemplating becoming sexually active;
- have a history of IV drug use and/or other drug and alcohol abuse;
- are currently using injection drugs; or
- use drugs and/or alcohol when sexually active.

As social workers in mental health settings, we have a responsibility and ethical obligation to help empower clients so that they do not jeopardize their health or the health of others, consciously or not. Integrating risk assessment for HIV into social work practice in mental health settings is consistent with the goal of enhancing our clients' well-being. This chapter focuses on four important considerations in conducting an HIV risk assessment in a mental health setting. They include the following:

- *Broadening the frame:* Including sexual assessment, substance use assessment, and sex education in mental health treatment
- *Psychological barriers to practicing safer sex*
- *Ethical and legal issues:* Duty to warn; assessing suicidality and homicidality
- *Countertransference*

BROADENING THE FRAME

HIV asks the therapist/social worker to step out of the nonjudgmental listener frame and become more active. The worker must provide education and proactive interventions that encourage and reinforce safe and thoughtful behavior from clients. In this context, the worker does not have the luxury of waiting for the client to bring up issues about sexual practices. Clients may have inaccurate information and unknowingly be placing themselves or others at risk for HIV infection. Clients may also deny or minimize the risks of HIV infection. The worker must intervene in a timely manner, with forethought and respect. Whether or not a client's presenting problem is related to sex, the therapist must coach and educate the client so that he or she is able to minimize his or her risk for HIV infection. This is akin to working with clients who are in acute crisis or are actively abusing substances and need active and immediate interventions.

To begin this work, it is useful to take a sexual assessment with the client. The mental health fields have been slow to acknowledge sexual functioning as an integral aspect of health and emotional well-being, but given the seriousness of AIDS, this aspect must be integrated into mental health assessments. Taking a thorough assessment of clients' sexual behavior is the first step in helping to prevent them from becoming infected with this deadly virus.

Taking a Sexual Assessment

Before you start, the worker must be familiar and comfortable with safer sex guidelines and the range of human sexual behavior.

Safer Sex Guidelines

The social worker must know the guidelines for safer sex practices and have a good understanding of the ways in which HIV is transmitted. Many AIDS service organizations and government offices of public health offer trainings and brochures that are explicit about safer sex guidelines. While there are some specific guidelines as to which behaviors are risk-free, (e.g., mutual masturbation, bodily rubbing, etc.) there are many other sexual behaviors that pose varying degrees of risk. The worker must be familiar with these gray areas—including oral sex and insertive anal sex without a condom—and the limits of the current data and its ambiguities. The worker can then help the client explore which risks he or she is willing to take, in the face of data that are neither definitive nor absolute.

Range of Human Sexual Behavior

The social worker must be familiar with the range of human sexual behavior, including specific activities and sexual orientations. How people express their sexuality varies greatly from person to person and from culture to culture. The social worker must be both familiar and comfortable with the sexual practices within a client's culture—even if these practices are different from the social worker's own experiences and beliefs about sexual activity. The worker must feel comfortable having frank and explicit discussions about sexual practices. Otherwise, crucial information will be overlooked. For example, a worker who is uncomfortable with the practice of anal intercourse may simply ask whether the client engages in anal intercourse without ascertaining whether the client has been the recipient or the insertor or both. This distinction affects the assessment significantly since the unprotected insertee is at greater risk than the insertor. The worker must be aware that sexual orientation may be fluid throughout an individual's life. The worker should not assume that the gender of one's current object choice has always been the same or that it will remain the same in the future.

The Assessment

Listed here are six suggested questions, regarding sexual behavior that a clinician might ask during an HIV risk assessment. Each clinician will need to use his or her judgment about whether these questions will overwhelm the client and create too much anxiety for the client to work on these issues. If a client is reticent to talk about sex, the clinician may begin by exploring the client's general feelings about sex and some of the messages he or she learned about sex in his or her family of origin. It is also important to give the client the option to not answer questions that may be too overwhelming. The worker can let the client know that the questions can be addressed again when the client is less anxious and more comfortable with this topic. Brochures and pamphlets about HIV risk reduction can be an effective means to communicate information and concerns about a client's risk in a more private manner. Some clients may feel more comfortable if they are given the questions in written form and are able to respond to the questions on their own, between sessions (Frost, 1994).

1. Are you currently or have you been sexually active within the past ten years? Do you anticipate sexual activity with another person in the future?
Establishing a time frame of when the client engaged in behaviors that put him or her at risk for HIV helps to ascertain the level of risk. If a client is in good health and his or her at-risk behavior occurred over ten years

ago, the likelihood of the client currently being infected is less than some-one who has engaged in higher risk behaviors more recently. Knowing if the client is sexually active currently or intends to be in the future is important so the worker can determine whether future discussion and/or education is warranted.

2. When you are sexually active, do you have sex with men, with women, or with both men and women?

Given the degree of homophobia in our culture, many people feel reluc-tant or ashamed to acknowledge being homosexual or having same-sex relations. One should also be aware of the attitudes about homosexual behavior within the client's particular culture. It is important to *not* ask whether a client is gay, straight, or bisexual, but to find out the genders of the people with whom the client has sex. Do not assume or label an individ-ual as being of one particular sexual orientation or another. Homosexual-identified people may periodically engage in heterosexual sex, just as some-one who identifies as heterosexual may periodically have sex with someone of the same gender. Assumptions and stereotypes are often incorrect.

3. Are you concerned about being HIV-infected or becoming HIV-infected? If so, please describe the circumstances that cause you to be concerned?

Help the client to be as specific as possible, including what kind of sex (i.e., fellatio, vaginal or anal intercourse, cunnilingus or analingus, mutual masturbation, SM) in which the client has engaged and which role or roles the client has taken. Try to use the same terms that the client uses. The worker must be comfortable with such terms to ensure that the client feels respected and understood. If you cannot comfortably use the same terms as the client, it is better to use terms with which you are comfortable. Getting detailed information about the client's sexual practices helps the worker assess the client's level of risk for infection and whether interven-tion is needed.

If you are not concerned about becoming infected, how do you protect yourself from HIV infection? How did you make those decisions?

People have very varied notions, which are often inaccurate, of what constitutes safer sex, and it is important that the worker knows what the client understands to be safer sex. Given the many gray areas concerning safer sex (e.g., the degree of risk associated with oral sex and unprotected insertive anal intercourse), social workers need to discuss with clients which risks they want to avoid and also help them examine how they make those decisions. It is useful to help clients look at issues of relative risk and decision-making skills using the following kinds of questions:

- Does the client generally characterize him- or herself as a risk-taking or risk-avoiding person?
- Is his or her sexual behavior consistent with his or her character?
- How does the client decide what risks are worth taking in his or her life?
- How important is sexual activity for the client in his or her life?
- Where does the client draw the line in taking risks?

4. How often do you practice safer sex? Have there been times that you have been unable to adhere to safer sex guidelines that you have set for yourself? If so, please describe the circumstances during which this has occurred?

It is important to find out if a client is able to practicing safer sex each and every time he or she engages in sexual activity. If the client is unable to do so, in spite of being aware of safer sex guidelines and having set specific guidelines for him- or herself, further explorations of the reasons why this occurs is needed. These "slips" can occur for a wide range of reasons and will be discussed later in the chapter.

5. How often do you drink alcohol or use drugs? Is drinking or using drugs ever involved when you are engaging in sex?

Drugs and alcohol impair judgment and disinhibit behavior. This is particularly true in situations that cause anxiety, such as negotiating sex. Often, people who are able to practice safer sex consistently are unable to do so when even slightly intoxicated. Drugs and alcohol are therefore a significant risk factor—even when they do not present a problem in other aspects of the client's life.

6. Do you use injection drugs? If so, do you currently or have you in the past ten years shared a needle without washing it with bleach beforehand?

If the client's drug use has not previously been discussed in the therapy, acknowledging the drug use can be difficult for the client. The therapist must be sensitive to whatever shame or embarrassment the client may feel about this issue. As concerning sex, the worker must be familiar and comfortable with communicating guidelines about safe needle use.

These questions can be used to begin a more detailed conversation about the client's practices, beliefs, and values regarding sex and drug/alcohol use. The questions set an open and direct tone for the discussion of sex and drug/alcohol use throughout the therapy and can alleviate anxieties and concerns that a client may have about introducing these topics.

PSYCHOLOGICAL BARRIERS
TO PRACTICING SAFER SEX

Sometimes clients, whether HIV negative, HIV positive, or unaware of their serostatus, may regularly or periodically engage in behaviors that increase their risk or others' risk for HIV infection. When this occurs, in spite of the clients being aware of HIV risk-reduction guidelines, the worker is challenged to think deeply about the nature of sexuality and to try to understand what role sex plays in clients' lives. The meaning of sex varies greatly in each individual's life. Sex may be an expression of closeness and attachment for one individual while for another it may serve primarily as a physical release and be a healthy means of reducing stress. For some, it may be the only means for physical contact in a life devoid of human touch. For yet others, it may be the only means to express a part of their identity that is suppressed in all other aspects of their life. Once the motivation for sexual contact is understood, the worker can better help the client get those needs met in ways that are safe and do not endanger the client's health.

For some people, underlying psychological dynamics cause them to not practice safer sex. The worker must help such clients identify the psychological underpinnings that prevent them from using safer sex practices consistently. The following case vignettes illustrate psychological barriers to consistently practicing safer sex.

Depression, Lack of Self-Esteem, Lack of Assertiveness

A young woman, who has been in therapy for five years to address intimacy problems and low self-esteem, has been dating a man for four months whom she feels she can trust and is considerate of her needs. Her boyfriend had been clean and sober for five years, but had a brief relapse, which included injection drug use, just prior to their getting together. When the therapist asks about the couple's sexual relationship, the client tells her therapist that she fears that her boyfriend is HIV positive, but has never been able to broach the topic. In addition, the couple has been having unprotected intercourse because the boyfriend does not enjoy sex with condoms. She is fearful if she brings up the issue, her boyfriend will drop her for someone better.

A client's low self-esteem and feeling unworthy of asserting his or her needs and/or wishes to others can be a barrier to practicing safer sex. Such self-defeating or self-destructive tendencies may belie an untreated depression that warrants careful evaluation, with appropriate referral for medication or ancillary services.

Survivor's Guilt

An HIV-test counselor is seeking therapy because he finds himself periodically engaging in high-risk behaviors, in spite of his vast knowledge of HIV transmission. He does not understand why he does this.

When people experience the death of another person, they may feel a sense of guilt that they survived while the other person has died. They may be acutely aware of the unfairness in life or harbor a belief that they are less deserving of survival than others. Many people who have lost friends and family members to AIDS have similar risk factors as those who have been infected and feel guilty that they have not become infected. Engaging in unsafe sexual practices may be a manifestation of guilt about surviving and an unconscious wish to join those who have died. We see this in the above case with the worker who has experienced the multiple losses of his clients. Grief work focusing on the guilt, anger, and sadness is needed. Referral for pastoral or spiritual counseling may also be useful.

AIDS Anxiety/Counterphobic Responses

Bob and Sam have been lovers for five years. Bob has known his positive serostatus for the past eight years and has been without any symptoms. Sam tested HIV negative four years ago and reports always feeling fearful about becoming infected. During a couples' therapy session, Sam blurts out that the couple has not been practicing safer sex consistently and knows he bears much of the responsibility for that. Two months later, Sam tells the therapist that he received a positive HIV test result.

Some people deal with their anxiety in counterphobic ways; their fear is so great that they dive right into it to lessen the anticipatory anxiety. Many people, particularly young gay men, are convinced that they are going to die at an early age. The anxiety of waiting for death may be so great that one may try to control this perceived inevitability by hastening it. Talking with people about their expectations for themselves and challenging their beliefs about their total powerlessness about their fate can help people resolve these feelings and find alternative ways to manage their fears and anxieties. Learning and practicing relaxation and stress management techniques can help them gain mastery over their anxiety and decrease self-destructive responses to it. Sam's case is further complicated because the closer he feels toward Bob, the more his anxiety about losing Bob is intensified. These issues need to be talked about openly in couples therapy so that Sam does not act out his fears and lose the support that he derives from the relationship. Anticipatory grief work may also be useful.

Unresolved Trauma Reenactment

> Ever since Joe has been in recovery from drugs and alcohol, he finds that he spends increasing amounts of time in gay cruising areas. He reports that he often ends up there late at night, after spending time alone in his apartment. He believes the behavior is compulsive and feels unable to stop it. While out, he often has unsafe sex. Afterward, he feels terribly guilty.

A history of trauma can deeply effect one's current sexual functioning. For some people with a sexual abuse history, sexual activity can be a frightening experience and is often avoided. For others, a sexual encounter may be an unconscious repetition of childhood sexual abuse and an attempt, albeit unsuccessful, to master the traumatizing experience. People who are sexually compulsive have a high rate of sexual abuse histories. Burnham (1994) describes how sexual contact may revive memories of earlier sexual trauma, in which the patient regresses and becomes unable to protect him- or herself. The paralysis that occurred during the abuse in childhood is reexperienced, and the adult is unable to assert him or herself against the perceived perpetrator, which is similar to what occurred during the past trauma. This is the case for Joe, who as a child was sexually abused by an uncle late at night when no one else was at home. In Joe's case, these painful feelings began to emerge when he became sober.

Trauma work with a strong psychoeducational approach that helps the client to better understand his or her behavior is very useful for clients with sexual abuse histories who are unable to protect themselves in their current sexual activity.

Denial

> At age twenty-three, Jill realized her "dream" job as a marketing agent for a local firm. She is sexually active with men and looks forward to settling down with someone in the near future. She routinely gets tested for HIV and always tests negative. When the HIV

test counselor inquires about her safer sex practices, she sheepishly admits she does not always insist that her partners use condoms as she doubts she could ever *really* become infected. "Besides," she states, "doesn't my always testing negative prove that?"

Denial or repression is a common coping mechanism. It allows us some distance from arduous emotional tasks that we are not yet ready or prepared to face. By being oblivious to a painful reality, we are able to proceed at times when the road ahead is treacherous. At the same time, denial can leave us open to taking chances that are unnecessary and foolish. Jill is young and feels invincible. She uses denial to deal with her unwanted feelings of vulnerability. In treatment, the worker must help clients such as Jill work through the feelings of helplessness and vulnerability that AIDS can cause so that their denial does not leave them without precautions against AIDS.

Substance Abuse

Dale enjoys drinking wine. She grew up in a family in which wine was plentiful and always part of the evening meal. She rarely gets drunk. She has recently become aware that when she drinks, she is more carefree about sex and is less concerned about whether her partner uses a condom. Dale tells her therapist that her best friend wondered if she had a drinking problem. Upon hearing this, Dale immediately dismissed the idea.

A tendency to abuse substances may underlie unsafe sexual practices. Under the influence of drugs and/or alcohol, judgment becomes impaired and can lead one to take unexpected and undesired risks. When a client engages in unsafe sex, a careful assessment of the client's use of substances is critical. Sometimes, the only indication of a drug and/or alcohol problem may be a client's inability to comply with the safer sex guidelines that he or she has adopted.

LEGAL AND ETHICAL ISSUES: CONFIDENTIALITY AND DUTY TO WARN

AIDS raises many complex ethical and legal issues for the social worker in the mental health setting regarding the following:

- the assessment of suicidal and homicidal behavior and mandates for hospitalization

- the limits of confidentiality
- the duty to warn others whose safety may be at risk

AIDS challenges the limits of our ethical and legal responsibilities as professionals and raises many serious questions that yield ambiguous answers with many interpretations. The following vignettes illustrate several important questions regarding HIV and mental health treatment that therapists need to consider.

Case 1

> Brian is a forty-three-year-old man who comes to therapy due to anxiety and depression. Throughout his eighteen-year marriage, he has been having sex with female prostitutes while away on business trips every two to three months. His wife is unaware of this. They continue to have unprotected vaginal intercourse on a regular basis. Brian recently got tested for HIV, but has not scheduled an appointment to receive his results.

Is Brian's behavior suicidal and/or homicidal (regarding his wife)? If so, is hospitalization warranted?

The social worker/therapist needs to know how to assess suicidality and homicidality and consider in what ways unsafe sexual practices might constitute suicidal and/or homicidal behavior. The usual psychiatric guidelines for suicidal and homicidal assessment regarding the seriousness of the intent, the lethality of the planned method, and previous history of suicidal/homicidal behavior are practical as starting points for the assessment. To make an assessment, the worker must be aware of the degree of relative risk associated with specific sexual activities. For example, performing fellatio on other people without a condom and without ingesting semen does not constitute the same risk as being the recipient of anal intercourse without a condom. The worker might consider the following questions:

- What does Brian know about HIV transmission?
- Does Brian practice safer sex when he has sex outside of his marriage? What are Brian's sexual activities when he has sex outside of his marriage? How risky are those activities?
- Does Brian intend to/wish to harm himself or his wife (consciously or unconsciously)?
- Are drugs and/or alcohol ever involved when he has sex outside of his marriage so that his judgment or control is impaired?

The challenge for the clinician is to help the client to make choices in the absence of absolute data, thereby helping the client to make informed choices about which risks he is willing to take. If the client is unable or unwilling to make decisions that do not put him or his wife at risk for HIV infection, hospitalization may be warranted until he is able to do so.

Is the therapist ethically and/or legally obligated to take action regarding the safety of Brian's wife? What actions would be appropriate?

As is true in all treatment relationships, it is important that Brian understand the limits of therapeutic confidentiality; should he be putting his wife's safety at risk, the worker may be obligated to warn her—without Brian's permission. Although there is agreement in the professions and the law that a therapist has a responsibility and duty to warn an identifiable third party of a client's alleged intent to place that person's safety in jeopardy, there are many gray areas when this law is applied to situations involving HIV. One may argue that when two people engage in consensual sexual activity, it is both persons' responsibility to make sure that the activity is safe and responsibility does not rest any more on one person than the other, particularly given the ambiguity of some of the data on HIV transmission. NASW's policy statement on HIV/AIDS states the following:

> [P]ractitioners and agencies may perceive a responsibility to warn third parties of their potential for infection if their spouses, other sexual partners, or partners in intravenous drug use are HIV-infected and the partners refuse to warn them.

Breaching a client's confidentiality may be devastating to a client and jeopardize the therapeutic alliance, seriously compromising the effectiveness of the therapy. In some cases, the trust in the therapy may be so damaged that the therapy is no longer able to continue and refering the client to another therapist becomes necessary. Laws vary from state to state and often change. "Social workers may be vulnerable to (law)suits claiming both failure to disclose confidential information to protect third parties and inappropriate or unauthorized disclosure of confidential information" (Reamer, 1991, p. 59). The social worker must become familiar with the NASW policy statement on HIV/AIDS and with state laws governing duty to warn.

Case 2

Lou is a twenty-eight-year-old gay man who comes to see a therapist because he has been "depressed his whole life" and cares very little about his health or safety. He regularly picks up men at bars and has sex with them, which usually consists of his performing fellatio without a condom. He says it is his only pleasure in life and cannot imagine giving it up or even modifying his behavior.

Does Lou's behavior warrant involuntary hospitalization for suicidal behavior?

Certainly Lou's behavior is reckless and jeopardizes his safety to some degree. Confusion exists concerning the degree of risk for HIV infection through unprotected oral sex. However, Lou is unfazed by the potential implications of his behavior. Following an educational discussion about the degree of risk that he takes with his sexual behavior, the worker should assess whether Lou is able to make an informed decision about his sexual behavior that includes valuing his safety, as well as that of others. The worker and client must then discuss the degree of risk that the client feels is reasonable to take. The worker must be careful not to impose his or her own values about the nature of risk in life and not assume this same value system is reasonable and viable for the client. At the same time, the worker needs to assess whether the client is minimizing his or her danger and acting out self-destructive wishes. The worker should assess Lou's level of depression and ascertain whether he engages in other self-destructive behaviors.

If Lou is unconcerned about his safety, hospitalization may be considered, although it is unlikely that an involuntary hospitalization could be mandated since he is not in acute and immediate danger. However, there is little doubt that Lou's behavior has elements of self-destructiveness and may be jeopardizing his health. This needs further discussion and exploration in treatment. His level of depression needs thorough assessment and treatment, including psychopharmacolgical consultation. Lou might also benefit from a psychotherapy group with other gay men in which he could learn new ways to develop relationships and how to relate to men in a variety of ways.

Is the worker mandated to report Lou's behavior to criminal authorities?

Since Lou's partners are not known to the worker, the worker is unable to warn any "identifiable party." Even if Lou's partners were known to the worker, it is unclear whether the worker is mandated by law to warn them as Lou's serostatus is unknown and he may not be posing a threat to any individual. Again, all sexual partners have equal responsibility for their sexual activity. Consultation with a lawyer who is knowledgeable about HIV, the limits of confidentiality, and duty to warn is advised.

THERAPIST ATTITUDES, VALUES,
AND COUNTERTRANSFERENCE

Finally, AIDS challenges the therapist to look at his or her own feelings and attitudes about illness, infirmity, sex, homosexuality, and injection drug use. When a worker is unaware of or has not resolved his or her own feelings about these issues, important information may be overlooked or minimized. Fear and shame about sexuality is very much woven into our culture. Each worker must confront his or her own values and beliefs about how and with whom people express their sexuality. Homophobia, regardless of the worker's own sexual orientation, must be addressed. If a worker feels too uncomfortable with this subject, it is preferable to refer the client to a worker who is more at ease discussing these issues. Nongay workers who are unaware of their own discomfort or ignorance about homosexuality and the gay community may unknowingly communicate discomfort or ignorance about homosexuality. Workers who are gay and working with gay clients may feel pressure to be a role model and minimize or disavow their own feelings regarding homophobia, thus not allowing clients to work on their own homophobia. Discomfort with sexuality and projected fears about being intrusive or creating undue discomfort lead us to minimize or completely avoid these important topics. Similarly, stereotypes abound about people who use injection drugs, as well as other drugs and/or alcohol. Some workers may deny that their clients could engage in injection drug use, as they do not fit the workers' stereotype of injection drug users. The worker needs to educate him or herself about the extent and impact of substance abuse in our society.

AIDS also challenges the clinician to deal with the limits of our ability to create a world without pain and suffering and the vulnerability we all face in the world. Not wanting to acknowledge our own risk for HIV infection, we may deny the possibility of our clients becoming infected. Supervision and peer consultation groups that focus on HIV work are enormously helpful to clinicians working on these issues.

AIDS has become woven into the fabric of our society. As social workers, we have a responsibility to help our clients understand how AIDS impacts their lives and how to protect themselves from this disease. Risk assessments for HIV infection must become an integral part of our clinical work as we help our clients reach their goal of achieving healthy and satisfying lives.

RECOMMENDED READINGS

Shernoff, Michael (1988). Integrating Safer-Sex Counseling into Social Work Practice. *Social Casework: The Journal of Contemporary Social Work,* June: 334-339.

Shernoff, Michael (1989). AIDS Prevention Counseling in Clinical Practice. In *Face to Face: A Guide to AIDS Counseling.* J. Dilley, C. Pies, and M. Helquist (Eds.). San Francisco: AIDS Health Project, pp. 76-83.

Zonana, Howard (1989). The Duty to Protect: Confidentiality and HIV in Clinical Practice. In *Face to Face: A Guide to AIDS Counseling.* J. Dilley, C. Pies, and M. Helquist (Eds.). San Francisco: AIDS Health Project, pp. 219-229.

REFERENCES

Burnham, Robert (1994). Trauma Revisited: HIV and AIDS in Gay Male Survivors of Sexual Abuse. In *Therapists on the Front Line: Psychotherapy with Gay Men in the Age of AIDS.* S. Cadwell, R. Burnham, M. Forstein (Eds.). Washington, DC: American Psychiatric Press, Inc., pp. 379-404.

Frost, Joel (1994). Taking a Sexual History with Gay Patients in Psychotherapy. In *Therapists on the Front Line: Psychotherapy with Gay Men in the Age of AIDS.* S. Cadwell, R. Burnham, and M. Forstein (Eds.). Washington, DC: American Psychiatric Press, Inc., pp. 163-184.

Reamer, Frederic (1991). AIDS, Social Work and the "Duty to Protect." *Social Work, 36*(1): 56-59.

Ethical Issues in Clinical Practice

Susan S. Patania

WHY DO THIS?
STATEMENT OF THE PROBLEMS AND ISSUES

HIV is a relatively new disease that has produced a new client population and new ethical considerations for the social work profession. People who normally would not have considered seeking social work services may find themselves in need of therapy, concrete services, or social support due to their HIV infection. Most people with HIV are from disenfranchised groups that traditionally need strong advocacy to maintain public funding for basic necessities such as medical care and to protect them from discrimination. HIV ethical issues for social workers are therefore individual, within the helping relationship, and collective, within the social work profession's advocacy for sensible and humane public policy.

This chapter will focus on ethical issues that arise within the therapeutic relationship: confidentiality, duty to protect, duty to treat, determination of capacity, and suicide. Each issue involves social work ethics that "guide, regulate, and control the behavior of social workers in their capacity, roles, and status as social workers . . . what is expected of social workers in the performance of their professional functions and in their conduct as members of the social work profession" (Levy, 1992, p. 19). Each issue also involves the worker's individual values and the law.

"Morals" or "values" are judgments of worth, standards for what is good or bad, right or wrong, just or unjust, etc. "Laws" are social values codified by elected representatives that attempt to protect constitutional rights while enforcing standards of behavior. The values of our profession are incorporated in the Code of Ethics of the National Association of Social Workers (1996), standards of conduct governing the practice of social work. The situations discussed in this chapter may involve personal,

The author gratefully acknowledges the assistance of Carol Schumaker and Ruth E. Spencer in writing this chapter.

professional, and legal values and consequences. What is right or ethical may not be legal, and legal mandates might be unethical. Fortunately, the NASW Code of Ethics, the laws of the state in which you reside, and your clinical common sense are readily available tools to help resolve ethical issues in your practice.

GENERAL PRACTICE GUIDELINES

1. Develop an adequate working knowledge of HIV transmission and prevention in order to properly educate all clients and make valid clinical judgments regarding the behavior of clients with HIV (Lamb et al., 1989; Goldberg, 1989).
2. Monitor your countertransference and be aware of your own biases, prejudices, and areas of discomfort, especially regarding sexuality, gay, lesbian, and bisexual issues, injection drug use, racism, and poverty (Lamb et al., 1989; Goldberg, 1989; Ryan and Rowe, 1988).
3. Learn the laws pertinent to HIV in your state and seek supervision and legal consultation as needed (Reamer, 1991a; Lamb et al., 1989).
4. Know the social work Code of Ethics and Policy Statement on AIDS/HIV (revised 1996) and use them to guide your practice with clients with HIV (Goldberg, 1989; Ryan and Rowe, 1988).
5. Keep careful case notes, "documenting any discussion of issues such as confidentiality, the need to protect third parties, and informed consent" (Reamer, 1991a, p. 58). In some states, "public" case notes are subject to subpoena, but "personal" case notes are not (Lamb et al., 1989, p. 42). "Any and all" case notes on the premises may be supoenaed if you practice in an agency setting, even private notes that you keep separate from the client record.

CONFIDENTIALITY

Confidentiality is a "mode of management of private information," the process of protecting information confided by a client from disclosure to others without client authorization (Levine, 1986, p. 163). In a social worker's practice, confidentiality might be demonstrated by keeping client files locked up, not discussing work situations outside of the practice setting, keeping private notes separate from the "case file," using consent forms for release of information, etc. Confidentiality is the basis for clients' belief that the practice setting is uniquely safe for their most personal and emotional disclosures. Confidentiality is a central tenet of the NASW Code of Ethics: "The social worker should respect clients' right to privacy

. . . [and] should protect the confidentiality of all information obtained in the course of professional service, except for compelling professional reasons" (p. 10).

Discrimination against people with HIV infection is common and can be damaging in the extreme. Disclosure that someone is HIV positive can lead to loss of employment, housing, insurance, health care, friendships, and family support. This ruinous potential for discrimination is what makes the privacy of people with HIV such a potent issue. In general, this privacy can be abridged only when necessary for a client's safety or when the client presents a clear and present danger to self or others (Wood, Marks, and Dilley, 1992). The standard of confidentiality in the case of HIV should be as strict as possible. In practical terms, this means that a social worker should not release information regarding a client's HIV status without the client's informed, written consent. The consent form should specify that HIV status is the information to be released. "Informed consent" requires the worker to explain the risks and benefits of the procedure (in this case disclosing the client's HIV status), ensure that the client understands the nature of the disclosure, and determine that the client has the capacity to make decisions on his or her own behalf (Wood, Marks, and Dilley, 1992). No coercion or "undue influence" can be involved, and the client has the right to refuse or revoke consent (Reamer, 1987, p. 426). The best means of documenting authorization for release of information is a form signed by the client specifying who is authorized to give and receive the information, the information to be released, the purpose of releasing the information, and the length of time the authorization is in effect (Wood, Marks, and Dilley, 1992).

Specifically discuss with the client what information will be disclosed to whom in the course of making a referral, assisting with forms for entitlements or other concrete services, or engaging in any form of networking that connects identifying information with his or her HIV status. Clients may not realize that disclosure of their HIV status is necessary or obligatory to obtain a given service, or they may not be aware that other service providers may contact them once the referral has been made. Obtaining informed consent is not just having clients sign a form. It is an ongoing process of collaboration that includes disclosing information and engaging in dialogue with the client about the work (Reamer, 1987).

Confidentiality: Practice Guidelines

1. Openly discuss the limits of confidentiality with the client early in the course of service provision, including the possibility of reporting child abuse or taking action to prevent harm to the client or third

party. Talking about the risks and benefits of receiving services is part of ensuring informed consent, and is required by the NASW Code of Ethics (p. 7-8).

2. Never release any verbal or written information that connects a client's name or other identifying information to his or her HIV status to any party without first obtaining the client's informed, written consent with "HIV status" specified.

3. A general release authorizing release of information to an insurance company, to a managed care corporation, or to another service provider does not include authorization to release a client's HIV status. If a client's HIV status is documented in his or her case file and a general release has been signed, you must still obtain separate, specific written authorization to release the record (Wood, Marks, and Dilley, 1992). Some clinicians prefer to omit any reference to a client's HIV status in the case file rather than risk unauthorized disclosure.

4. Help the client anticipate possible consequences of releasing HIV status to all third parties, including employers, insurance carriers, HIV service providers, and law enforcement officials (such as parole officers). The client may be focusing exclusively on the favorable or unfavorable aspects of disclosure and may need to consider other possibilities.

5. Do not assume that anyone, even a client's significant other(s) or family members, knows that he or she has HIV and/or is receiving social work services. Discuss with a client early in your relationship how you should make contact with him or her if the need arises. Document any constraints, such as "no phone calls" or "no mail."

6. When calling a client at home, identify yourself only by name if someone else answers. Do not leave a message containing your agency affiliation or other information that would indicate the client is ill or receiving social work services.

7. Make sure you have the client's current address if you contact him or her by mail. Use plain paper, not letterhead.

8. Faxes, cellular phone calls, and computer interactions such as e-mail are not confidential.

DUTY TO PROTECT

Is it ever appropriate for a worker to disclose a client's HIV status to prevent harm to a third party? Does the *Tarasoff* "duty to warn" apply to the therapist of a client with HIV who is regularly having unprotected sex or sharing drug injection equipment with an unknowing partner?

There is no single, simple answer to these questions. Social workers and experts from other disciplines, however, have contributed to an ongoing discussion of this issue in the literature. Though some would answer "yes," some "no," and some "maybe" to the above questions, there is a consensus that a worker doing therapy with an HIV-positive client who has not disclosed his or her status to sex or needle-sharing partner(s) has many options for intervention that do not involve violation of the client's confidentiality. The case of an HIV-positive client in therapy refusing to notify a regular sex partner after clinical intervention may be rare. In over six years of treating many people with HIV, the Ackerman Institute AIDS and Families Project team had never been unsuccessful in persuading a client to voluntarily disclose his or her HIV status to a partner in a committed relationship (Walker, 1991, p. 121). This has included discussion of the therapist's sense of moral obligation in protecting the partner.

One should keep in mind that the HIV-positive person has the primary moral and legal responsibility to protect sex or needle-sharing partners from HIV infection (Wood, Marks, and Dilley, 1992; Rabinowitz, Fletcher, and Boverman, 1989). In addition, every adult who is aware of how HIV is transmitted has the capacity to prevent infection by using appropriate precautions such as having safer sex and/or not sharing drug injection equipment. "Unless a client lies about his or her HIV infection, partners who engage in what they know to be dangerous activities assume part of the risk and contribute to the client's negligence" (Wood, Marks, and Dilley, p. 87). These assertions are valid in cases of casual or anonymous sexual encounters; they are less certain when there is a steady, identifiable sex or needle-sharing partner.

This issue becomes an ethical one for the social worker providing therapy when a client known to be HIV positive admits to having unsafe sex or sharing drug injection equipment with a partner who is unaware that he or she is at risk for HIV transmission. All social workers must therefore be prepared to (1) assess all clients' knowledge of HIV transmission and provide education on how to protect self and others from HIV infection and (2) help an HIV-positive client overcome any barriers to protecting sex and needle-sharing partners from HIV transmission.

The *Tarasoff* case was a civil lawsuit in which the parents of a murdered woman sued the murderer's therapist for wrongful death. The Supreme Court of California ruled that the therapist was negligent because he was aware that the woman was in danger from his psychotic client and failed to take the steps necessary to protect her. The standard set by the *Tarasoff* case in 1976 and by similar cases and state laws that followed is that a therapist must use "reasonable care" to protect an identified victim from a potentially dangerous client.

"Reasonable care" does not necessarily mean breaking confidentiality to warn a third party. Warning a third party is permitted, however, in the following situations: "(1) there is a genuine psychotherapist-patient relationship . . . ; (2) when the patient has communicated to the therapist a serious and imminent threat of physical violence against another; and (3) when the threat is against a reasonably identifiable victim or victims" (Wood, Marks, and Dilley, 1992, p. 35).

Depending on the nature of the "imminent threat," the duty to protect may also be discharged through clinical options such as arranging for civil commitment, medication management, or by continuing to build rapport and using the therapeutic alliance to promote client self-control. (Lamb et al., 1989, p. 39; Ryan and Rowe, 1988). State law may allow the therapist to notify the police as a means of protecting the third party.

How does this information apply to HIV? The excellent guidebook *AIDS Law for Mental Health Professionals* (1992) identifies five facts a therapist would need to have before he or she could be considered liable for not warning a third party about the possibility of becoming infected with HIV from a client:

> (1) the client is HIV infected; (2) the parties engage in unsafe behavior [unsafe sex or sharing of drug injection equipment] on a regular basis; (3) such behavior is actually unsafe; (4) the client intends to continue such behavior even after being counseled to desist by the therapist; and (5) HIV transmission will likely occur in the future. (Wood, Marks, and Dilley, 1992, p. 37)

A close examination of this list demonstrates some of the difficulties with applying the *Tarasoff* standard to a social worker and an HIV-positive client. The likelihood of HIV being transmitted during the practice of risky behavior depends on a wide variety of factors and is difficult to assess. It could be argued that a person without medical training in this situation is not qualified to assess the degree of danger involved. A social worker, for example, may not be considered qualified to judge whether or not certain sexual or needle-sharing behaviors represent an "imminent threat of physical violence." If an HIV-positive client is occasionally having unsafe sex or sharing needles with casual or anonymous partners, "imminent danger" and a "reasonably identifiable victim or victims" cannot be established.

If the five considerations listed here are met and you think that your HIV-positive client's sexual or needle-sharing behavior does represent an imminent threat to an identifiable victim or victims, you should obtain and document supervision and exhaust all alternatives before considering violating the confidentiality of your treatment relationship (Reamer, 1991a; Ryan and Rowe, 1988; Lamb et al., 1989; Goldberg, 1989; Bassford, 1991). Numerous practical and clinical reasons to exhaust alternatives before warning a third party exist. It may be illegal in your state to disclose someone's HIV status to a third party without informed, written consent. Your therapeutic alliance with the client may be disrupted. He or she may terminate, precluding any gains that might have been made, including stopping the dangerous behavior. Battering may be an unanticipated side effect of notifying the partner (North and Rothenberg, 1993), or the client may engage in self-destructive behavior or become suicidal or homicidal.

A choice to violate confidentiality must also be viewed in the context of the values of the social work profession. The Code of Ethics (1996) enjoins social workers to "respect clients' right to privacy . . . [and] protect the confidentiality of all information obtained in the course of professional service, except for compelling professional reasons" (p. 10).

The 1990 NASW Policy Statement on AIDS/HIV emphasizes the need to exhaust clinical alternatives, consult with other practitioners, consider legal counsel, and inform the client of intention to notify the partner if duty-to-warn issues arise (NASW, 1990). The 1990 NASW policy and its 1996 revision permit, but do not impose, a duty to warn:

> Social workers should use the strength of the client-worker relationship to encourage clients with HIV infection to inform their sexual or needle-sharing partners of their antibody status. Social workers should be familiar with applicable state law regarding the duty to warn. . . . Social workers have a responsibility to consult with other practitioners and to consider legal counsel if they feel they have a duty to warn. (NASW, 1996, p. 16)

Duty to Protect: Practice Guidelines

1. Make sure all therapy clients understand the limits of confidentiality at the outset of therapy, before a conflict arises. Some authors recommend using written forms to facilitate informed consent (Reamer, 1991a; Lamb et al., 1989).
2. If practicing in an organization or agency, review its written policy on confidentiality and HIV/AIDS, follow it, and document your actions. Involve your supervisor as soon as the issue arises and seek and document ongoing supervision.

3. Assess the HIV-positive client's knowledge of HIV transmission and use of safer sex and/or clean drug-injection equipment. Does the client know that partners are at risk? What is he or she willing to do to protect others? Is the client aware that unsafe sex and needle-sharing endangers his or her own health through exposure to more virus, a different strain of virus, or other diseases?

4. If the client is aware of the risks and is not willing to protect the partner, a careful and nonjudgmental exploration of his or her reasons is essential. What are the perceived barriers to disclosure? How does this issue fit with the presenting problem, the goals of therapy, and the client's history and developmental level? What consequences does the client anticipate from disclosing and/or initiating safer behaviors? How is the client rationalizing failure to protect the partner? Use this information as a starting point in your effort to empower the client to take responsibility for protecting his or her partner.

5. Focus on the fact that the client has sufficient faith in your alliance to disclose the situation to you and therefore must have some sense that help is needed (Walker, 1991; Bassford, 1991).

6. Intervene as you would with any difficult clinical problem, using your judgment of what will be effective given the client's nature and situation. Various authors have suggested using a time line, planning with the client to disclose by a certain date or the therapist will notify the partner (Walker, 1991); disclosing their own ethical discomfort with the client's choice (Goldberg, 1989); role-playing the disclosure; using the technique of "ethical listening . . . actively and selectively focusing on a person's ethical conflict" (Cameron, 1993, p. 219); and providing education about the client's duty to warn the partner (Wood, Marks, and Dilley, 1992).

7. Offer alternatives to a solo disclosure by the client. He or she may be willing to discuss the situation in a couples session (Rabinowitz, Fletcher, and Boverman, 1989); may give you, another health care provider, or other trusted third party specific informed, written consent to tell the partner; may utilize a partner notification program (if available); or may be willing to stop or modify unsafe sexual or needle-sharing behaviors.

Duty to Protect: Conclusion

In a review of the literature on confidentiality and the duty to protect, Georgianna and Johnson (1993) found the authors to be evenly divided on whether client confidentiality or protection of the third party was the counselor's primary ethical duty. Ethically, "[t]he choice is difficult because it is between two competing 'goods'" (Goldberg, 1989, p. 116). In the legal arena, social workers could be sued for not taking adequate steps to protect a third party at risk from a client and could also be sued by a client for disclosing confidential information without consent (Reamer, 1991a; Meinhardt, 1989).

Ethics experts are careful to present both sides of the "competing goods," but may emphasize one aspect or the other in order to make the discussion useful in practice. Those who emphasize that client privacy and confidentiality are paramount assert that people with HIV will avoid therapy if a risk of unauthorized disclosure of their status exists (Perry, 1989), that there are alternatives to warning a third party which preserve confidentiality (Reamer, 1991a), and that confidentiality in the case of HIV is a primary duty of the profession (NASW NYC AIDS Task Force cited in Leukefeld and Fimbres, 1987, p. x; North and Rothenberg, 1993). Others emphasize that protecting a third party who is unaware that he or she may be at risk for HIV infection should be an option for the therapist (Bayer and Toomey, 1992), that the trend in the mental health professions is away from confidentiality as an absolute (Lamb et al., 1989; Bayer, 1991), and that warning a third party is consistent with the value of promoting the general welfare of society (Zonana, 1989).

If concerted clinical intervention has failed to induce the client to notify his or her partner and adequate supervisory, medical, and legal consultation has been obtained, the decision whether or not to breach confidentiality will be based on the worker's own values and interpretation of the NASW Code of Ethics and Policy Statement on AIDS/HIV. The NASW guidelines permit, but do not require, warning the third party in this circumstance. Because no legal requirement for a social worker to warn a third party exists the decision is an ethical one with potential legal implications.

If the decision to warn the third party is made, this information should be shared with the client so he or she will have the option of disclosing first. If at all possible, the worker should utilize a health department or other public health partner notification system rather than directly contacting the partner. Partner notification programs are likely to have systematic methods of ensuring that once the partner has been notified, he or she will obtain appropriate follow-up services.

DUTY TO TREAT

Is it permissible for a social worker to refuse to work with HIV-positive clients? This question involves personal, ethical, agency, and legal considerations. It is not considered clinically advisable to work in an area in which one lacks expertise or to work with a client when countertransference is impeding appropriate service provision. This does not mean, however, that it is ethically acceptable to avoid providing services to an entire group of clients.

The NASW Code of Ethics states the following: "Social workers should provide services and represent themselves as competent only within the boundaries of their education, training, license, certification, consultation received, supervised experience, or other relevant professional experience" (p. 8). In regard to "emerging area[s] of practice, social workers should exercise careful judgment and take responsible steps (including appropriate education, research, training, consultation, and supervision) to ensure the competence of their work and to protect clients from harm" (p. 9).

Early in the epidemic, there was a lack of information about HIV except for identification of the extreme medical and psychosocial needs of infected persons. Social workers may have felt that they lacked the necessary HIV expertise to treat infected clients. They may have lived in low-prevalence areas in which they encountered few, if any, known HIV-positive clients. Many years have passed since the start of the epidemic in the United States, and currently any social worker's caseload can include people affected by HIV. No longer is it appropriate for social workers to be uninformed about HIV issues, including transmission, prevention, and psychosocial aspects.

According to the Code of Ethics "social workers continually strive to increase their professional knowledge and skills and to apply them in practice" (p. 6). To be professionally knowledgeable at this time, a social worker must obtain the information necessary to responsibly serve clients with HIV and educate clients who do not have HIV about how to protect themselves from infection.

The Code of Ethics calls upon social workers to "act to prevent and eliminate domination of, exploitation of, and discrimination against any person, group, or class on the basis of race, ethnicity, national origin, color, sex, sexual orientation, age, marital status, political belief, or mental or physical disability" (p. 27).

This does not mean that a worker is expected to be comfortable with the values and behavior of all clients. Ryan and Rowe (1988) note that values-clarification training, supervision, and peer support may be needed when clients' behaviors and practices conflict with the worker's personal system of values. The Code of Ethics makes it clear, however, that it is unethical to discriminate purely on the basis of HIV infection.

Professional codes of ethics, including antidiscrimination provisions, are incorporated into state legal standards for professional licensure. A social worker engaging in a pattern of harmful discrimination against a group of clients may be the subject of complaints filed with the NASW or the state licensing board. The Americans with Disabilities Act prohibits discrimination against HIV-positive persons. The Act does not directly impose a duty to treat every potential client with HIV, but it prohibits any policy that might limit a person's access to care (Wood, Marks, and Dilley, 1992).

Duty to Treat: Practice Guidelines

1. Explore your own feelings about working with HIV-infected clients. What are your attitudes about sexuality and drug use, and how might these play out in the treatment relationship? How has your agency, health care facility, or practice group approached HIV issues? Do you have written policies and adequate supervisory support?
2. Familiarize yourself with basic facts about HIV transmission and safer sex and needle-sharing practices. If you are HIV negative, anxiety about your own safety may periodically arise as you work with HIV-infected clients. Remind yourself of the facts and recognize this fear as countertransference. If your are HIV positive, anticipate potential disclosure situations and plan how and why you will or will not disclose to clients and colleagues. Talk to a trusted supervisor or colleague about any misgivings you may have.
3. Network with any local HIV service organizations. Share their information about local and federal services (Social Security, e.g.), and have their brochures and eligibility information available for your clients. If you are in an area with few or no HIV services, contact your regional Social Security, Food Stamp, public welfare, and private welfare organizations as well as local medical facilities. Determine where in your area people with HIV are getting help.

DETERMINATION OF CAPACITY

In this case "capacity" means the client's capacity to make decisions on his or her own behalf. The legal concept is "competence," whether or not a person has the mental capacity to make medical decisions, to care for him or herself, or to engage in activities such as driving a car or working in a position of responsibility. The determination that a person is mentally incompetent is legal, not clinical. The Superior (or Probate) Court will appoint a guardian or conservator only after "clear and convincing evidence" that the person is so mentally incompetent that he or she can not care for his or her basic needs (Wood, Marks, and Dilley, 1992, p. 81).

A social worker providing services for clients with HIV may encounter a situation in which cognitive impairment is interfering with the client's ability to safely engage in daily activities. "The therapist is placed in the unenviable position of empathizing with the patient's wish to deny his own limitations while simultaneously needing to point out to the patient where his own safety or that of others is at risk" (Beckett and Kassel, 1994, p. 153). This problem has clinical, ethical, and legal dimensions.

The first ethical duty owed by a social worker to a client with HIV who experiences a significant change in mood, cognition, or behavior is to ensure the safety of the client by thoroughly assessing the nature of the change, the client's access to medical care, and the client's degree of follow-up with medical advice. Client safety is paramount, and mental status changes can result from a variety of physical conditions, medication side effects, mental disorders, or AIDS dementia complex (Beckett and Kassel, 1994). Medical intervention is necessary for differential diagnosis and appropriate treatment. Networking with the client's primary care physician or psychiatrist can be an invaluable resource for the social worker when a client is experiencing cognitive impairment. Physicians can perform a medical evaluation to determine if a client's HIV-related impairment represents a danger in the client's work setting or operation of a motor vehicle.

A client with HIV who refuses needed medical treatment or supervision of his or her activities of daily living creates an ethical dilemma for the worker. The NASW Code of Ethics states that "Social workers respect and promote the right of all clients to self-determination and assist clients in their efforts to identify and clarify their goals" (p. 7). The issue of when to intervene against a client's wishes for his or her own protection is not a new one for practicing social workers. HIV simply adds the element of possible physical and mental impairment.

"Capacity to consent to treatment" refers to a client's mental capacity to give informed consent (or refuse consent) for medical intervention. In order to give informed consent, a client must be able to express a choice, have a factual understanding of what is to be done, be able to rationally weigh the risks and benefits, and appreciate the nature of the situation (Appelbaum and Roth, 1982). An impaired client is considered legally competent unless evidence can be substantiated otherwise and is subsequently proven in court. Mental impairment in and of itself does not mean that a person is incompetent to make medical decisions (Wood, Marks, and Dilley, 1992, p. 80).

The specific situation should be evaluated. Who believes the client needs medical attention or extra assistance? Is severe mental or physical deterioration evident to the worker? Is the client endangered by taking medications improperly, being careless when smoking or cooking, etc.? Is he or she able to pay bills and obtain food? Does he or she describe having traffic mishaps or injurious falls, or does he or she appear grossly uncoordinated? If the client is not having difficulty in these areas, the decision to avoid treatment or refuse supervision of daily activities may be a rational choice that should be respected—even though friends, family, and the social worker may not feel the choice is appropriate.

The social worker's intervention in this situation should include a careful assessment of the client's mental status, perception of the situation, fears, social supports, and sociocultural factors. Family members and friends may be responding to their own anxieties by attempting to control the client or by exaggerating his or her dependency. The client's own perspective may suggest ways of resolving the situation without disempowering him or her. A referral to adult day care, a home health agency, a volunteer care team, or a "buddy" may be appropriate. Social Security disability checks can be issued to a "representative payee" (with the client's consent) if handling finances is difficult.

If the social worker is convinced that the client has a serious need for supervision and medical attention and the client continues to refuse, the worker should attempt to meet with members of the client's support network (with the client's informed, written consent) and arrange for them to take the client for medical evaluation. As a last resort, family members or friends can petition the court to appoint a conservator or guardian to make health care decisions for the client (Wood, Marks, and Dilley, 1992).

If they are unable to do this, if there is no support system, or if the client is "gravely disabled" and continues to refuse treatment, the worker should notify Adult Protective Services or a community mental health crisis team (or equivalent authority), or they should arrange for involuntary civil commitment. Involuntary civil commitment proceedings and standards are no different for a person impaired with HIV than they are for people with mental disorders only (Wood, Marks, and Dilley, 1992).

Clients who are not severely impaired but who have some cognitive or motor problems that may interfere with their ability to perform job tasks or operate a motor vehicle safely present a different legal and ethical issue. Potential harm to others must be weighed against the client's right to work, drive, and maintain an income and sense of efficacy. If the client is not capable of performing job tasks or operating a motor vehicle safely and "harm to others is reasonably foreseeable," the therapist has a duty to take reasonable precautions to prevent the client from causing an accident (Wood, Marks, and Dilley, 1992, p. 89).

First, the worker should discuss the problem with the client, using the client's report of difficulty as a starting point. The client's physician may be able to assist the worker in making judgments regarding a cognitively impaired client's ability to work or operate a motor vehicle. If the worker thinks the client may cause an accident while working or driving, the client should be advised to avoid these activities because he or she is dangerous to others. This warning should be documented carefully. Alternatives, such as changing job duties or using the bus for transportation, should be discussed. If the client ignores these warnings, "therapists have a duty to report their concerns to higher authorities, such as the Department of Motor Vehicles" (Wood, Marks, and Dilley, 1992, p. 89).

Determination of Capacity: Practice Guidelines

1. Medical evaluation is the essential first intervention when an HIV-positive client experiences any change in cognition, mood, or behavior. Social workers are uniquely qualified to coordinate referrals and services, including networking with medical personnel.
2. In general, the fundamental issues of determination of capacity are medical in nature and should be handled by the client's physician.
3. Social work services, such as family therapy and organizing supervision and support utilizing the client's existing support system, may resolve the problem(s) once medical management is in place.
4. Familiarize yourself with local services for people with HIV. Many larger communities have a broad range of financial and social supports available.
5. When possible, use existing HIV-dedicated and "mainstream" services in your community for a client with limited capacity. Examples include Adult Protective Services, community mental health crisis teams, and police department personnel.

SUICIDE

Until recently the phrase "rational suicide" was not in use, and viewing suicide as an appropriate course of action was unthinkable. Public opinion is still divided, but the right-to-die debate is now out in the open and "Death with Dignity" initiatives have become legitimate political issues. What effect will this new, often high-profile debate have on the attitudes of social workers providing clinical services for clients with HIV?

Advocates for disabled and HIV-infected persons fear that discrimination may bias end-of-life decision making and fail to fully affirm the humanity of already disenfranchised people. Social workers' personal moral opinions about the right-to-die issue will vary greatly. As a profession, however, we must continue to think critically about social trends, our practice, and the lives of our clients. As the political debate continues and new norms evolve, we must maintain our efforts to ensure that all clients receive complete, high-quality medical treatment for mental and physical illnesses, optimal clinical social work services, and aggressive political advocacy.

"Assisted suicide," "rational suicide," and even failure to do everything medically and legally possible to postpone death from terminal illness are very controversial issues. These acts occupy a continuum of active and passive ways to hasten death. A nationwide dialogue on these issues is occurring between ethicists, religious leaders, physicians, social workers, legal experts, and organizations such as the Hemlock Society, which advocate for a person's right to die.

An important distinction exists between assisted suicide and rational suicide. Licensed physicians are the only professionals who will be affected by any changes in the legal prohibition against assisted suicide. There is currently no "specific right to commit suicide" (Wood, Marks, and Dilley, 1992). A person who helps someone with or who is present at a suicide can be "charged with assisting the suicide, manslaughter, or even murder" (Wood, Marks, and Dilley, 1992, p. 77). Moral, ethical, and legal issues for social workers with terminally ill clients will involve rational suicide as workers struggle to choose between the competing values of client autonomy and the duty to keep clients safe—even against their own wishes—and from their own self-destructive behaviors.

Mental health practitioners must take whatever reasonable steps are necessary to prevent a client from committing suicide. Many clinicians believe the desire to end one's life can be considered irrational per se, evidence that a person is in need of psychiatric treatment. Having a life-threatening illness such as HIV may call the absolute irrationality of suicide into question:

> At what point is it possible to concede that the suicidal ideation is not the result of a potentially manageable narcissistic injury or of a crisis that will pass, but a result of an honest, realistic estimation of damage that has no possibility of being healed? (Forstein, 1994, p. 123)

Therapists' actions are legally evaluated by the standard of what a mental health practitioner of "ordinary and reasonable skill" would do under the same circumstances. A therapist may be held legally liable for the wrongful death of a client who commits suicide if the therapist's care failed to meet "community standards" established by his or her profession (Wood, Marks, and Dilley, p. 66). "Social workers' primary responsibility is to promote the well-being of clients" (NASW, 1996, p. 7).

In 1993 the NASW developed a policy statement on right-to-die issues. The statement does not take a moral position on end-of life decisions and is based on client self-determination as a guiding principle. The policy affirms that, after competent clients have become informed of all options and consequences,

> choice should be intrinsic to all aspects of life and death. . . . The appropriate role for social workers is to help patients express their thoughts and feelings, to facilitate exploration of alternatives, to provide information to make an informed choice, and to deal with grief and loss issues." (NASW, 1996, p. 5)

According to the policy, social workers should remain neutral regarding any particular means of ending life, but "should be open to full discussion of issues and care options, act as liaisons with other health care professionals and help communicate concerns and attitudes to the health care team" (NASW, 1996, p. 5). The policy is geared toward clarifying the social worker's role with terminally ill clients without mandating a given course of action.

Physical pain, mental disorders, a precipitating event such as a medical setback, or any manner of temporary and/or treatable conditions can cause suicidal feelings that pass when the problem is resolved. For social workers, the ethical issue becomes how far to go in attempting to prevent the suicide of a client with HIV if the client's choice seems thoughtful and timely, and if all medical and psychiatric interventions have been exhausted. Some workers' personal values might preclude this entirely. Others, after becoming acquainted with the ethical and legal aspects of the situation, may conclude that in rare situations it is ethical to avoid taking every possible step—e.g., involuntary commitment—to prevent the rational suicide of a client.

It would be highly unethical and negligent to allow countertransference or poor therapeutic skills to result in a lack of scrutiny of the client's suicidal feelings.

> Patients deserve an aggressive and complete assessment for a potentially treatable or manageable concern. Therapists . . . have an obligation to help them access the most complete medical and psychiatric assessment possible before acceding to the purported rational nature of the suicide. (Forstein, 1994, p. 136)

The social worker might consider the following questions:

- Has the client received exhaustive medical evaluation and treatment for mental or physical illnesses that could be affecting his or her emotional state?
- Is the client's discussion of suicide thoughtful, developed over time and through interaction with important people in his or her life?
- What family, spiritual, or economic issues might be involved?
- What are the therapist's own values regarding suicide?
- What would be different to the therapist if HIV were not involved?

The continuum of options for treating suicidal ideation might include the following: scheduling extra sessions; making a contract with the client; getting informed consent to collaborate with the primary care physician; making home or hospital visits if the client is debilitated; referring for medication consultation; arranging for supervision in the home or in day treatment, voluntary hospitalization, and involuntary civil commitment. The standard of care for a suicidal client includes meticulously assessing the degree of danger that a client poses to him or herself and others, then taking steps appropriate to the client's likelihood of harming or killing him or herself.

In my experience with HIV-positive clients who expressed serious suicidal intent, consideration of whether their suicidal ideation was rational was not usually a factor. In the overwhelming majority of cases, the suicidality was obviously not a rational response to physical disability or impending death, but was a symptom of severe depression requiring immediate psychiatric treatment.

The most painful ethical dilemmas I have faced involved HIV-positive clients who clearly needed psychiatric treatment, but who had no money or health insurance. Due to limited inpatient psychiatry beds in public hospitals, only clients who have made an actual suicide attempt or who have posed a law enforcement problem may have access to emergency psychiatric hospitalization. Will attempting to get a physically debilitated, suicidal client hospitalized through an emergency department be a painful, unsuccessful ordeal? If you decide not to send the client to the hospital, are you vulnerable to accusations, however unfounded, that you failed to act responsibly to protect him or her? An unfortunate reality is that the client's socioeconomic status, rather than medical needs, might dictate treatment options. The strength of your therapeutic alliance with your client and his or her family, rather than a wide range of concrete treatment options, may be your best resource. The following practice guidelines may prove helpful.

Suicide: Practice Guidelines

1. Assess your client's potential for suicide on an ongoing basis. Make "Are you feeling so bad that you think about hurting or killing yourself or someone else?" a routine question when clients sound depressed, report stress, or verbalize "negative" affects. If the answer is affirmative, assess whether or not he or she has planned how to do it. Emphasize that you ask because you want him or her to be safe.

2. Document that the question was asked, what the client's response was, and how you intervened. Document your treatment plan if the client should need additional treatment.

3. Make discussion of the client's relationships with medical providers part of your work. Facilitate an assertive, collaborative approach to medical care. "Coach" the client through communication problems, e.g., role-play doctor/patient dialogue or help the client make a list of concerns that need to be addressed in medical encounters.

4. Thoroughly familiarize yourself with the entire range of public and private psychiatric treatment options available in your community. If you do not practice in a medical setting, try to develop a referral relationship with whomever has admitting privileges to beds at your public hospital or to psychiatry beds in private hospitals.

5. Be proactive by facilitating discussion of death and dying before a crisis arises. When the topic arises directly, ask your client questions such as "What do you imagine when you're thinking about your death?" or "When you say you're 'scared,' what are you most scared of?" If the subject arises indirectly, e.g., the client talks about the death of a grandparent, ask "How does your family deal with death?" or "What thoughts do you have about death?"

6. HIV-positive clients may anticipate a lingering death and make statements about what increment(s) of disability they will not tolerate, for example, "I'll kill myself if I can't walk any more," or "I'm not going to let myself get as sick as he did." Explore the meaning of these disabilities as they relate to control and other issues and also in terms of concrete planning, e.g., preparing a Living Will or finding out what home care services might be available.

7. Recognize and use the power of your therapeutic alliance with your client and his or her family. Acknowledge the injustice if treatment options are limited due to the client's socioeconomic status. Discuss in advance with the client and family what your limitations are regarding obtaining treatment, and engage the client's support system in problem solving.

CONCLUSION

This chapter has described how ethical issues in social work practice may manifest with HIV-infected clients and their significant others. It is intended as a practical guide, not as an exhaustive ethical or legal analysis. The most important point is the following: The social work professional's clinical skills, ethics, and ability to focus on individual and environmental factors are already equal to the task of effective work with people living with HIV. The medical, sexual, political, and existential issues that accompany HIV can be intimidating, but up-to-date knowledge, not special skill, is required for successful intervention

Social workers who (1) learn the basics of HIV transmission, prevention, and course of illness; (2) obtain, read, and understand the application of the NASW Code of Ethics; (3) insist on adequate written policy and clinical supervision within their practice settings; and (4) find out the HIV-related laws in their state and locality are prepared to skillfully handle HIV-related ethical issues. Ethical issues are first and foremost clinical issues, and need to be approached as such. Ethical and legal requirements guide, but do not replace, clinical common sense.

Though individual practice issues are most deeply felt, compelling ethical considerations for social workers exist in the area of social policy. It is there that we must publicly and forcefully uphold our ethical obligation to advocate for access to adequate health care, housing, and income for people living with HIV.

RECOMMENDED READING

Wood, G., Marks, R., and Dilley, J. (1992). *AIDS law for mental health professionals*. Berkeley: Celestial Arts.

REFERENCES

Appelbaum, P., and Roth, L. (1982). Competency to consent to research. *Archives of General Psychiatry, 39*: 951-958.

Bassford, H. (1991). Perspectives on AIDS. In *Perspectives on AIDS: Ethical and social issues*. C. Overall, and W. Zion (Eds.). Toronto: Oxford University Press.

Bayer, R. (1991). An end to HIV exceptionalism? *New England Journal of Medicine, 324*(21): 1500-1504.

Bayer, R., and Toomey, K. (1992). HIV prevention and the two faces of partner notification. *American Journal of Public Health, 82*(8): 1158-1164.

Beckett, A., and Kassel, P. (1994). Neuropsychiatric dysfunction: Impact on psychotherapy with gay men. In *Therapists on the front line: Psychotherapy with Gay men in the age of AIDS*. S. Cadwell, R. Burnham, and M. Forstein (Eds.). Washington, DC: American Psychiatric Press, Inc.

Cameron, M. (1993). *Living with AIDS: Experiencing ethical problems*. Newbury Park, CA: Sage Publications.

Forstein, M. (1994). Suicidality and HIV in gay men. In *Therapists on the front line: Psychotherapy with gay men in the age of AIDS*. S. Cadwell, R. Burnham, and M. Forstein (Eds.). Washington, DC: American Psychiatric Press, Inc.

Georgianna, C., and Johnson, M. (1993). Duty to protect: The gay community response. *Focus: A Guide to AIDS Research and Counseling, 8*(5): 104.

Goldberg, J. (1989). AIDS: Confidentiality and the social worker. *Social Thought, 15*(3/4): 116-127.

Lamb, D., Clark, C., Drumheller, P., Frizzell, K., and Surrey, L. (1989). Applying *Tarasoff* to AIDS-related psychotherapy issues. *Professional Psychology: Research and Practice, 20*(1): 37-43.

Leukefeld, C., and Fimbres, M. (Eds.). (1987). *Responding to AIDS: Psychosocial initiatives*. Silver Spring, MD: National Association of Social Workers.

Levine, R. (1986). *Ethics and regulation of clinical research*. Baltimore: Urban Schwarzenberg, Inc.

Levy, C. (1992). *Social work ethics on the line*. Binghamton, NY: The Haworth Press.

Meinhardt, R. (1989). AIDS and issues of partner notification. *FOCUS: A Guide to AIDS Research and Counseling, 4*(12): 1-2.

NASW. (1990). Social work speaks: NASW policy statement. Acquired immune deficiency syndrome/human immunodeficiency virus: A social work response.

NASW. (1996). National Association of Social Workers Code of Ethics.

NASW. (1996). NASW Policy Statement, 1996 revision. Acquired Immune Deficiency Syndrome/Human Immunodeficiency Virus: A Social Work Response. *National Association of Social Workers News,* March, 1996, p. 16.

NASW. (1996). Right to die: Guidelines, yes—Answers, no. *National Association of Social Workers News,* Social Work '95 Sessions, January, 1996, p. 5.

North, R., and Rothenberg, K. (1993). Partner notification and the threat of domestic violence against women with HIV infection. *New England Journal of Medicine, 329*(16): 1194-1196.

Perry, S. (1989). Warning third parties at risk of AIDS: APA's policy is a barrier to treatment. *Hospital and Community Psychiatry, 40*(2): 158-161.

Rabinowitz, R., Fletcher, J., and Boverman, M. (1989). Helping the HIV-infected patient disclose to others at risk: A clinical case report. *AIDS Patient Care, 3*(1): 9-11.

Reamer, F. (1987). Informed consent in social work. *Social Work, 32*: 425-429.

Reamer, F. (1991a). AIDS, social work, and the "duty to protect." *Social Work, 36*(1): 56-60.

Reamer, F. (Ed.). (1991b). *AIDS and ethics*. New York: Columbia University Press.

Ryan, C., and Rowe, M. (1988). AIDS: Legal and ethical issues. *Social Casework, June*: 324-333.

Walker, G. (1991). *In the midst of winter: Systemic therapy with families, couples, and individuals with HIV infection*. New York: W.W. Norton and Company.

Wood, G., Marks, R., and Dilley, J. (1992). *AIDS law for mental health professionals*. Berkeley: Celestial Arts.

Zonana, H. (1989). Warning third parties at risk of AIDS: APA'S policy is a reasonable approach. *Hospital and Community Psychiatry, 40*(2): 162-164.

HIV in Private Practice

Steven A. Cadwell

WHY DO THIS?
STATEMENT OF THE PROBLEM AND ISSUES

In our private practices, we need to be prepared to work with HIV because the impact of HIV is so prevalent. There have been over 500,000 reported cases of AIDS in the United States in men, women, and children. Millions are infected with HIV. Millions of others are at risk due to IV drug use, unsafe sex, and infected blood supplies. HIV is part of our lives and is bound to be part of our clinical work as we either work directly with people who are infected with HIV, their loved ones, or people who are sexually active and need to be educated about HIV prevention. AIDS is the leading cause of death for adults between ages of twenty-five and forty-four. Although HIV is primarily transmitted by male-to-male sex and needle sharing during intravenous drug use, HIV is becoming more prevalent among women who contract it through intravenous drug use or heterosexual contact.

Although skilled providers are needed, they are not always available. A recent survey of NASW members showed that only 50 percent of respondents said they were prepared to counsel clients about HIV prevention and risk-reduction practices. Less than 25 percent strongly agreed that they have sufficient knowledge to conduct a comprehensive sexual and drug-using risk assessment history. (*NASW NEWS,* October 1995) All of us need to be better prepared to deliver services, both preventative education to the uninfected and services to the infected.

Along with the enormous challenges in this work come great rewards. The most vital issues of our time converge in HIV work: sex, addiction, distribution of care and resources, cultural diversity, poverty, religious beliefs, and moral values. This work forces us all to grow intellectually. We receive gifts of knowledge and wisdom as we deal with core human experiences of hope and dread, love and loss, isolation and community, courage and anxiety, shame and pride, and life and death.

EXAMPLES OF HOW THE ISSUE MAY PRESENT

Clients may present issues related to HIV in many ways. Any sexually active client needs to know about HIV prevention. The clinician can be a

269

vital source of accurate information and provide a supportive relationship that helps the client determine what safer sex will mean to him or herself.

A client may need to talk about his or her anxiety about HIV. The anxiety may be rational or irrational. The social worker can provide a safe relationship in which all the client's concerns can be expressed, clarified, and dealt with. The client may come to the clinician because of questions he or she has about being tested for HIV. The social worker can help the client understand what it means to him or her to be tested. For example, is the client looking for a baseline for ongoing safer sex? Or is the client flooded with panic because several friends have become infected and he or she needs some reassurance that he or she is not infected? Why does the client want to be tested at this time? What risky behavior is the client worried about? Is testing a step toward changing risky behavior or is it construed as a way to hedge his or her bets and continue risky behavior?

After being tested, a client may need to talk about the emotional impact of the test results. If the client is negative, he or she may have survival guilt. He or she may be thinking, "Can I go on living and enjoying life when, but for the grace of God, I might be infected and dying?"

The client who is positive may need to talk about the meaning of his or her positive status. Is he or she feeling shame? Does he or she equate having HIV with death? (This is a frequent and damaging misconception. HIV has become a chronic disease. In contrast with the early years of the epidemic when people often died within months of diagnosis, people are living longer and longer with the disease.)

Or clients may seek you out to talk about the course of their illness with HIV. They may need a place to talk about their initial adjustment to having their first opportunistic infection. They may need to talk about their decision to go on disability. Or in the final stages of illness, they may need to have someone to talk to about their feelings concerning their life and death.

Or clients may come to you with a combination of concerns all related to the epidemic. For example, a gay man who is grieving the death of several friends to HIV may be in a state of anxiety upon learning that his T-cell count has dropped.

FACTS THE SOCIAL WORKER
NEEDS TO KNOW BEFORE PROCEEDING

Treatment of people with HIV necessitates a multidimensional assessment and also a multidimensional intervention strategy. Attention to medical, social, political, and psychological issues is critical. Because of our tradition of exploring all these dimensions, social workers are in a unique position to be able to deliver this service.

Social workers face many challenges in this work. Treatment often goes beyond the boundaries of the traditional fifty-minute office hour. The social worker must be ready to follow the client to his or her hospital room, home, or hospice bed. The therapist must be prepared to be with the client through the course of his or her illness up to death. This may be complicated by the client's inability to pay for treatment particularly if he or she stops working. Other challenging dimensions of this work include the vital importance of getting a detailed sex history and staying attuned to risks in the client's sex life; the educational-preventive role of the therapist regarding safer sex (similar to the role in substance abuse counseling); and issues of addiction, suicidality, neurological complications, confidentiality, and the duty to warn. All these issues heighten our need for vigilance about the clarity of our contract and boundaries with our clients.

Do the Client's Needs Fit Your Capability?

If you are referred a client with HIV, assess whether the two of you are a match. Consider the specifics of his or her needs. Do you think there are gender or cultural considerations that could optimize his or her work? Does your skill and experience match what you anticipate will be needed to do the work? Given the extra demands on you in doing HIV work, be careful about how many HIV-related cases you take on. Due to the roller-coaster course of the illness, the multiple losses (health, financial, psychological), and the possible multiple complications (e.g., dementia, suicidal ideation), many private practitioners keep a percentage of their practice open to HIV work and then try to balance that work with other kinds of clinical cases. Its important not to pretend you are a clinic. You alone in a private practice cannot have all the resources necessary for HIV work— either the emotional support or the concrete services. Be honest with yourself and your client about the resources you can offer and the network of resources that he or she also will need.

What About the Client's Ability to Pay?

The issue of payment in this work is often not stated, but from the outset, a social worker in private practice must realize that HIV cases are often labor intensive with fewer billable hours. The therapist may be involved in collateral calls to other members of the care team. Or he or she may need to attend team meetings, which cannot be billed. The therapist also may need to make hospital visits. In a private practice, this time can be costly and difficult to schedule. Also, the client may have a severely limited capacity to pay at some point in the treatment. How will that be negotiated? Is the social worker willing to negotiate a reduced fee? The client's dignity and autonomy may be preserved by negotiating a radically reduced rate rather than no fee, but the clinician's real need for a salary may be compromised. In some cases, the practitioner may need to be prepared to bill the estate after the client's death if a balance is due. (Although this may feel like a radical step to take, anticipating the financial realities of this work is crucial preparation.) One way to balance the social worker's willingness to take on this work and his or her need to ensure income is to keep HIV-related cases to a limited percentage of his or her caseload.

The work will require you to be willing to *extend your role* from a more limited "traditional" clinical role to include what Winiarski (1991) has described as including a *consultant's role* and a *case manager's role*—both familiar roles to social workers. The clinician should be prepared to adopt these roles and to be creative about them.

As a *consultant*, the social worker may provide information about community services or may help trouble-shoot how to deal with difficult issues, e.g., "I'm going to my dentist. Should I tell her that I am HIV positive?" As an advocate, the clinician can explain the client's needs to legal, political, and health care delivery systems. As a *case manager*, the social worker may provide counseling, act as a liaison to other service agencies, coordinate home care and financial entitlements, assess resources, develop a program of care with other resources, discuss prenatal care with a pregnant client, discuss clients' legal rights, and ensure that such issues as living wills are clarified. Other goals include the following:

- client safety
- consideration of what the client desires
- empowerment of the client
- empowerment of natural caregivers
- improvement of quality of life
- maintenance of stability
- discerning and providing structure
- use of least restrictive environment
- monitoring overmedicalization
- shoring up the situation, especially in a crisis
- anticipatory management of changing needs

- assistance with bureaucracies
- services for caregivers
- considerations of and referrals for legal documents, including wills and powers of attorney
- clarification of issues regarding "do-not-resuscitate orders and living wills. (Winiarski, 1991, pp. 102-105)

ABOUT THE CLIENT: AN ASSESSMENT GUIDE

Assess financial issues:
Chronic illness can drain personal resources. What resources does the client have? Does he or she have any insurance, savings, assets?
Assess the client's work situation:
The client may need to continue to work as long as he or she is able. Watch for job discrimination against HIV-positive clients. Will the client's job be in any jeopardy when his or her illness becomes more apparent?
Assess the level of the client's psychosocial functioning:
What is your diagnosis of the client? What is his or her mental status? Is there any character or intrapsychic conflict that predates the HIV infection?
Assess the general health status of the client:
Is coming to your practice physically possible? Would the client be better served at a comprehensive clinic where mental health and physical health services would be combined?
Assess the client's support network:
Does the client have riends or a companion who will provide case management? Will the client need you to provide case management or will you need to help him find another resource to provide this?
Assess and link the client to resources in the health care system:
Mental Health Services: Does the client need individual therapy, group therapy, a support group, psychopharmacological intervention, neuropsychological intervention? These resources are particularly vital for the private practitioner. Unlike a hospital social worker who can depend on the expertise of affiliates, a private practitioner needs to develop good collaborations with skilled professionals. AIDS organizations and HIV clinics can be sources for such networking.
Social Services: Assess the client's need for disability or welfare and then make the proper referrals.
Medical Services: Is the client seeing an HIV specialist? (Studies show that clients live longer under the care of more HIV-experienced and HIV-

skilled doctors.) Is the client part of any special protocols for treatment? Is he or she aware of the protocols?

Continue to stay linked with resources for yourself:

Network with other practitioners; do not isolate yourself! Just as clients with HIV can be isolated, so too can caregivers. Develop a support network: join a support group, develop an affiliation with an AIDS agency, hire a consultant, go to HIV conferences, develop a peer supervision group, or in rural areas develop a support group by phone conference call.

KEY QUESTIONS TO ASK THE CLIENT

First, clarify the treatment contract. Be clear as to what you and the client can expect. You will need to know the client's willingness to use the treatment relationship. Next, boundaries must be understood, i.e., if the client does anything to endanger him or herself or others, you will take measures to protect him or her or the others. Ensure that the client can expect confidentiality within the frame of state law. Spelling this out in an initial informed consent for client to read and sign is often useful.

The issue of the social worker's duty to warn should also be discussed at this time. Finally, the client should know about the therapist's availability—in case of emergency and over the course of the illness.

CULTURAL COMPETENCY CONSIDERATIONS

By competence, do not assume you have to be "the expert." In many ways, social worker needs to be open to learn *with* the client and *from* the client. Even so, it is essential to have some confidence that you are oriented within the client's culture and that you have something to offer the client within the following areas, depending on their relevance to the case:

- IV drug culture
- Gay culture
- Hemophiliac culture
- Ethnic culture

Do not presume you are an expert in every area. If you are inexperienced in an area of the client's need, it may be better to refer the client elsewhere. If no other resources are available, discuss your own limitations with the client and assure him or her in your initial treatment contract that you will learn together.

Refer to specific sections in this volume for information and suggestions concerning working with the special populations listed above.

ACTION STEPS FOR SUCCESSFUL INTERVENTION

1. Assess the needs of the HIV population in your practice area. What are the particular problems of the HIV clients you are apt to see? Are your clients gay, hemophiliacs, adolescents, college students, women, or IV drug users? Educate yourself as to their psychosocial profile.
2. Investigate resources available. Make resource lists. Go to trainings or workshops provided by local or national gay health or AIDS organizations.
3. Based on your interest and skill, offer yourself as resource.
4. Get ongoing support in a paid supervision or a peer support/supervision group.

POTENTIAL BARRIERS TO SUCCESSFUL INTERVENTION

Politics Concerning HIV Can Be Heated

Access to you may be difficult for the client. Are you an identified resource for HIV clients? Contact HIV clinics and agencies to offer your service. The shame and stigma attached to HIV are barriers for clients. How can people come to your service and not unnecessarily lose confidentiality? Is your work environment HIV-friendly or HIV-phobic? Have brochures in your waiting area that discuss HIV-related issues. On your bookshelf, include clinical literature relevant to HIV practice.

Staying Current with HIV Treatment

It is difficult to be "the expert." Trust that your client may teach you a great deal. However, you must be willing to take professional responsibility to learn and be prepared to commit to learning on your own, too.

Wonderful resources exist including the following: the newsletters such as *HIV Frontline* or *FOCUS: A Guide to AIDS Research and Counseling* from the AIDS Health Project affiliated with University of California, San Francisco; local conferences, especially given by HIV clinics or organizations; national conferences, such as International Social Work and AIDS Conference; or conferences sponsored by state and local AIDS services organizations.

Communication Breakdown

- Communicate your availability to the client as the client determines what would be useful.
- Also communicate with the client's care team. Your involvement may include participating in a range of meetings.
- You may offer family treatment at times. This is not a closed, traditional, psychodynamic psychotherapy with strict boundaries. You need to be able to flex the boundaries.
- Be available as needed.
- Be willing to be where the client is, e.g., by providing home, hospital, or hospice visits.
- Be willing to meet more of the client's support system: family, friends, and medical team.
- Communicate with the medical providers.
- Have completed release of information forms with the providers.
- Communicate to the client that this is a "team treatment."
- Good communication is vital over the course of illness.

Have the communication as part of the treatment contract in place for time when treatment does shift and become more medically intensive.

Countertransference

Countertransference is very difficult to manage in the isolation of private practice. Difficult issues are bound to trigger your feelings, for example:

- The client's suicidality versus his or her "rational" choice to die
- Your anger at his or her slips in safer sex practices
- The client's persistant denial of health risk and death
- Your wish to make the client better or have at least a "better death"
- Issues of morality; judgments of lifestyles and choices
- Loss of control—yours and hers or his
- Genuine grief at the client's death
- Your issues related to mortality, sexuality, and addiction
- Your rescue fantasies, grandiosities, and helplessness

Supervision and support for the social worker are critical.

HIV treatment should optimally include many supportive relationships extending beyond the client and therapist to therapist/supervision-support group and the larger community of HIV work. If the client dies, how does the therapist attend to his or her feelings? What is the role of the therapist at the funeral? Where can the therapist grieve his or her loss of the client and feel comforted and supported? Support groups for therapists working with people with HIV are vital for this. (Contact your local AIDS service agency to connect with existent groups or to create your own.)

Overinvolvement can lead to burnout. Dynamics to watch for include the impact of serial loss on the provider. Balance the risk of burnout with some built-in care for yourself, leaves of absence and balancing the work (see the chapter "Care for Caregiver" by Kitsy Schoen).

CARE FOR OURSELVES:
SUSTAINING OUR CAPACITY TO DO THE WORK

AIDS work delivers a range of intense and complex issues. A powerful and potentially paralyzing parallel process exists between our clients' devastation and our own in this work. In a single clinical case, we may have to deal with issues of suicidality, chronic uncertainty in health status and mental status, and economic uncertainty, as well as the usual premorbid range of possible characterological issues. There is a dangerous convergence of devastating losses—loss of careers, autonomy, economics, youth, partnerships, sanity, selfhood, life, and community. This is very difficult work indeed.

As ever, the work must include a broad understanding of ourselves. We are not immune to any of the prejudices that complicate the epidemic. Fortunately, our profession is grounded in a tradition of examining these issues within ourselves. We are also trained to see the larger picture. More important, we also have tools to address our own inner issues. The concept of countertransference must be seen as our ally in taking our own inventories to assess our own vulnerabilities. This inventory is bound to include the inevitable issues of death, illness, race, and sexuality.

We also need to take inventory of our coping styles. We may tend to overcompensate, overidentify, or detach when we are overwhelmed by the demands of our work. We need to seek prophylaxis against burnout to sustain "safer" alliances with our clients. If we are to be effective, we must closely assess our own vulnerabilities and coping styles, and we must develop tools to manage these vulnerabilites. Those tools will be as individual as our vulnerabilities. One esteemed veteran colleague recharges herself by ironing. Others may find healing and energizing reserves in meditation, music, reading, childrearing, and home improvement projects. The vital need is to take time for ourselves and ensure that our colleagues pay attention to their own needs for time for themselves.

Critical here is negotiating the fine line of empathic efficacy—not being too close nor too distant. The balance is never static. We will always be adjusting this line. Occasionally, we will move too close and get burned out. Other times, we may find ourselves at a distance that feels unnecessarily removed and uninvolved. Neither extreme position should be seen as a failure but as part of the process of learning and growing in our work. (See the chapter "Care for Caregivers" by Kitsy Schoen.)

INFORMATION THE CLIENT SHOULD KNOW BEFORE TAKING ACTION

The client should know about confidentiality in your working relationship. The client should understand the therapist's duty to warn if the client is any danger to him or herself or to others.

The client should have confidence in your level of commitment: Are you ready to see this work through from your office to his or her bedside? From his or her health to sickness? From living with HIV to dying from HIV?

The client should understand your treatment model. Do you include the consultant and caseworker model along with psychodynamic work? Clarify your own model and be able to articulate it to your client so he or she knows what to expect from you. (See the chapter "Ethical Issues in Clinical Practice" by Susan Patania.)

POLICY IMPLICATIONS AND RELATED ACTIONS

At the policy level, our interventions can help expose stigmatizing policies and develop more protective policies for people with HIV. Conferences such as the Boston College–sponsored Annual International Conference on AIDS, the continued dedication to inclusion of gay issues on AIDS care agendas, the development of special resources such as the Living Well Program at the Fenway Community Center in Boston, and the commitment to political lobbying championed by NASW are examples.

As an advocate, clinicians can explain the needs of HIV clients to political, legal, and health care delivery systems in the community so they can better understand and serve HIV-positive people. The clinician can consult to city councils, community boards, school boards, courts, and community groups.

Fundamentally, clinicians can continue to infuse hope and care to populations who may be despairing of any future.

RECOMMENDED READINGS

Cadwell, S., Burnham, R., and Forstein, M. (Eds.) (1994). *Therapists on the Front Line; Psychotherapy with Gay Men in the Age of AIDS.* Washington, DC:American Psychiatric Press.
Walt Odets and Michael Shernoff (Eds.) (1995). *The Second Decade of AIDS: A Mental Health Practice Handbook.* New York: Hatherleigh Press.
Winiarski, M. (1991). *AIDS-Related Psychotherapy.* New York: Pergamon Press.

REFERENCE

NASW News (1995). "Many found daunted by clients with HIV." September, p. 15.

Identifying and Treating
HIV-Associated Dementia

Stephan L. Buckingham

WHY DO THIS?
STATEMENT OF THE PROBLEM AND ISSUES

HIV-associated cognitive/motor complex is the most common neuropsychiatric illness in persons infected with HIV (McArthur et al., 1993). It has been estimated that approximately 66 percent of persons with symptomatic infection exhibit clear-cut cognitive and intellectual deficits on formal neuropsychological testing while approximately 20 percent have impairment sufficiently severe to warrant a diagnosis of HIV-associated dementia (Van Gorp et al., 1993). Although HIV can be recovered from the brain and cerebrospinal fluid of more than half of the persons with early stage infection, only 5 percent of those with *asymptomatic* infection demonstrate cognitive and intellectual abnormalities related to their seropositivity (McArthur et al., 1993). The likelihood of cognitive impairment increases as the individual becomes increasingly immunocompromised and symptomatic, and it has been found that at death 90 percent of seropositive individuals have evidence of brain abnormalities related to HIV infection (Navia et al., 1986) though not all will have behavioral evidence of these abnormalities.

HIV-associated cognitive/motor complex is divided into cases in which all but the most demanding aspects of work or other activities can be accomplished ("minor cognitive/motor disorder") and more severe cases in which work and activities of daily living are seriously affected ("HIV-associated dementia complex") (American Academy of Neurology AIDS Task Force, 1991).

Differential diagnosis is important because HIV-associated cognitive/motor complex can be easily confused with a major depressive disorder with quite divergent treatment implications. The risks of incorrectly informing a depressed patient that he or she is demented, or a demented patient that he or she is actually only depressed and will likely recover

281

with treatment, are obvious. Accurate differential diagnosis is crucial for appropriate psychosocial and medical management.

An abrupt change in the patient's mental status may signal a delirium or acute confusional state. Unlike an HIV-associated dementia, this condition results from an acute medical disturbance such as a metabolic abnormality or medication toxicity and will produce a rapid alteration in the patient's thinking. Differentiating a delirium from a dementia is crucial since its associated medical abnormality poses a risk of mortality and must be promptly treated. A delirium is associated with an *acute* change in the patient's mental status with a dramatic difficulty in maintaining attention. A dementia typically has a more insidious onset, and although the patient may have widespread cognitive impairment, the patient is not dramatically inattentive. When a delirium is suspected, referral for immediate medical workup is indicated. Unlike HIV-associated dementia, the mental status changes associated with a delirium will reverse once the underlying cause (e.g., medication toxicity, high fever, metabolic disturbance, etc.) is corrected.

Differentially diagnosing a patient with HIV-associated dementia versus a focal brain disturbance such as a brain tumor, stroke, or an infection producing focal brain lesions such as progressive myelo-leukoencephalopathy (PML) is crucial since each disorder has unique implications for prognosis and treatment.

EXAMPLES OF HOW THE ISSUE MAY PRESENT

Patients with HIV-associated cognitive/motor impairment will initially present in either the mental health or primary medical setting. The most prominent feature of the initial presentation is slowing—slowing of movements such as walking as well as a slowing of their thinking. They have the greatest difficulty responding quickly in situations in which *thought is tied to action*, such as driving on a busy freeway. Because the patient may also appear apathetic, social workers in mental health settings commonly encounter patients with HIV-associated cognitive/motor impairment who have been misdiagnosed as having a primary depression and who have been referred for treatment of a depressive disorder. A classic description of the presenting features of HIV-associated cognitive/motor complex was described by Navia, Jordan, and Price (1986):

> Characteristically it begins insidiously, with difficulty concentrating, impaired recent memory, and slowing of mentation and movement. Steady or, in some cases, more abrupt progression leads eventually

in many patients to severe global dementia, mutism, paraplegia, and incontinence. (p. 518)

Research has shown that patients' own assessment of their everyday cognitive difficulties is often much more related to their mood than to their actual ability to perform well on standard neuropsychological tests (Van Gorp et al., 1993). Because of this, the social worker who encounters a patient stating that he or she is having difficulty with his or her memory, attention, etc., must first determine if a primary depression is present since this could be responsible for the patient's misinterpretation of the cause of his or her cognitive problems. When in doubt, refer for structured neuropsychological testing whenever possible. These services are usually available in large medical centers or university teaching hospitals where multi-specialty services are more likely to be available. Neuropsychological consultation services are also often available by psychologists in private practice. The referral may be made by the social worker directly or in collaboration with the primary physician treating the patient.

FACTS THE SOCIAL WORKER NEEDS TO KNOW BEFORE PROCEEDING

HIV preferentially affects the deep areas of the brain (subcortical) well below the outer covering (cortex). When these deep areas are affected, patients will often exhibit poor motor coordination and precision, mood disturbances, slowed thinking and moving, and memory difficulties. These memory difficulties are characterized by a difficulty recalling what new information has been learned but with less difficulty recognizing the information when given multiple choices. This typifies the features of a "subcortical dementia." In addition to HIV-associated dementia, other subcortical dementias with which the social worker may be familiar include Parkinson's disease, Huntington's disease, and multiple sclerosis (Cummings, 1990).

Subcortical dementia stands in sharp contrast to "cortical dementia," of which Alzheimer's disease is best known. The mental health clinician should understand the contrast between cortical and subcortical dementias since cortical dementias, which more seriously impair the patient overall, are what most patients (as well as clinicians) have in mind when they hear the term "dementia." Patients with Alzheimer's disease have relatively normal speed of movements (and even seemingly normal *speed* of thinking, though indeed it is seriously impoverished), but they have serious difficulty with language. The patient with Alzheimer's disease will have "empty" speech filled with such overlearned expressions as "you know what I mean" and "the thing that they use for that, you know." The patient with Alzheimer's disease will have a severely impaired memory, which is characterized by an inability to learn new information and a consequent inability to even recognize information that was previously presented. Visuospatial difficulties are exemplified by patients being unable to locate items they have placed around the house or wandering from their home and easily becoming lost. Unlike the HIV-infected patient with a subcortical dementia who is typically painfully aware of his or her cognitive impairment, the patient with a cortical dementia is typically unaware and unconcerned regarding his or her cognitive predicament.

KEY QUESTIONS TO ASK THE CLIENT

As stated previously, HIV-infected patients who were asked to report their own appraisal of their cognitive abilities reported observations that were often unrelated to their actual neuropsychological performance and were more related to the level of depression and anxiety they exhibited. Therefore, in addition to asking the client how his or her memory is, for instance, the social worker should ask a significant other such as a partner, family member, or other caregiver if cognitive difficulties are present.

Inquiries as to recent automobile accidents or "fender benders" may elicit information useful in detecting mild impairment. The social worker should carefully inquire about *changes* in the patient's ability to function at work or school to elicit clues as to early neuropsychiatric difficulties. Inquiry into the patient's mood and affect should be made in order to rule out a primary mood or anxiety disorder, which must be differentiated from HIV-associated dementia.

ACTION STEPS FOR SUCCESSFULL INTERVENTION

Once clinicians have the necessary basic understanding of the common mental status changes involved in HIV-associated dementia, several important implications emerge for practice that can guide appropriate treatment and assist the person diagnosed.

Practical Considerations

Many patients complain that simple tasks now create the most frustration. As Table 1 indicates, several practical recommendations can greatly assist the person struggling with cognitive changes and the limitations that

TABLE 1. Practical Considerations and Recommendations for Persons with HIV-Associated Dementia

Forgetfulness

1. Use calendars and appointment books.
2. Place Post-It notes in conspicuous places as reminders.
3. Make lists (questions for your physician, groceries needed, people to call, etc.)
4. Develop list for important things to check when leaving the residence (stove, lights, etc.).
5. Use an alarm clock as a reminder for medications.
6. Keep a list of medications with dosages and times taken.
7. Ask for help if medications must be taken at different times and dosages.
8. Keep a journal detailing complex projects.
9. Use a cassette tape recorder to dictate thoughts and questions.
10. Purchase a noise-activated key chain.
11. Keep a telephone log and important numbers by the phone.

Slowed Speech

1. Allow more time to collect your thoughts and for conversations.
2. Don't hurry; give yourself permission to take your time.
3. Keep talking. Good conversation is good practice.

Visuospatial Problems

1. Do not drive if unable to do so.
2. If able to drive, plan routes in advance, allow plenty of time, and take a friend along when you can.
3. Use verbal directions instead of maps.

Depression and Social Withdrawal

1. Plan recreational activities.
2. Be an active participant.
3. Rekindle old hobbies and interests or create new ones.

Concentration Problems, Inattentiveness, or Distractibility

1. Try to limit distractions by confining your activities to a single task.
2. Meet with people one at a time.
3. Break large tasks down into more manageable jobs.
4. Turn the TV off when conversing or needing to concentrate.
5. Do not drive in heavy traffic.

Problems with Sequential Reasoning or Multistep Tasks

1. Don't take on new or unfamiliar job responsibilities.
2. Avoid tasks in which speed of performance is important.

Source: Adapted from Buckingham and van Gorp, 1988.

these changes represent. These include the conspicuous placement of a large calendar near the bedside or living space so that the individual may remain oriented to the month, date, and year. The use of frequent notes, reminders, and appointment books serve as important memory aides since research has shown that patients with HIV-associated dementia benefit from cueing and recognition approaches (Van Gorp et al., 1993).

Because many patients with HIV-associated dementia present with motor and gait disturbances, living arrangements should avoid structures with many steps because the patient may fall or have difficulty climbing steps.

The cognitive and motor slowdown that these patients experience make it difficult for them to function in situations that require quick decisions and action. For example, working in a busy office setting where the individual must act quickly may frustrate the mildly impaired patient who is in the early stages of the dementia process and may promote a sense of failure and lack of coping.

Providing structure and a familiar environment will facilitate greater independence in activities of daily living than novel and ambiguous situations. Whenever possible, demented patients should be in environments that are familiar and that have sufficient structure and support. Unfamiliar environments with no one to assist with activities of daily living may promote increased confusion in a patient with only mild dementia.

Patients with HIV-associated dementia may have sufficient *motivation* to undertake activities or tasks but may lack the necessary *initiation* to actually begin the activity. This is common to other subcortical disturbances (e.g., Parkinson's disease), and assistance with initiating desired activities and tasks by family members or loved ones may provide the crucial impetus for actually starting a desired activity.

Educational Considerations

Not surprisingly, family members or significant others are often frustrated by the physical and mental debilitation their loved one has experienced. An unconscious "need to blame" may be present, and they may unknowingly act this out by attributing a patient's forgetfulness to a willful stubbornness or intentional manipulation. This is a common occurrence, and the clinician must be vigilant to *educate* those close to the demented patient about their loved one's actual limitations. Slowing, confusion, and forgetfulness are all characteristics of HIV-associated dementia and, when present, they do not reflect intentional manipulation but rather actual brain changes that result in clinical symptomatology.

Providing information and educational resources to the patient with cognitive decline associated with HIV is another important factor in HIV care. Many patients have little or no understanding of neurological functioning or the diseases that affect cognition. Most patients, upon hearing the term "dementia," envision the most severe clinical characteristics, usually those associated with Alzheimer's disease, such as complete memory loss and vegetablelike mannerisms. Helping patients to better understand neuropsychological functioning and the nature of the changes associated with subcortical disease will greatly reduce the fears and worries of those affected.

Clinical Considerations

Assessment of clinical depression is important in any patient with HIV, but this is especially true when questions arise regarding the patient's mental functioning. When slowing, forgetfulness, and concentration problems are present, the clinician must attempt to differentiate the effects of depression from early signs of the HIV-associated dementia. This is best done by inquiring about the mood state of the individual and being alert to atypical signs of pessimism, feelings of worthlessness, and suicidality. Since most patients diagnosed with HIV-associated dementia are aware of their declining mental capabilities, they may be understandably depressed as a reaction to these changes. This, coupled with the well-established and broad range of psychosocial assaults associated with HIV, creates the potential for a high-risk situation for patients who are also experiencing cognitive impairment. If signs of depression are present, the depressive condition should be appropriately treated. Depression can further encroach upon the mental capacities of an already impaired individual. While psychiatric medications can be very effective in treating depression, their interaction with HIV-associated dementia requires that careful attention be given to this complex interplay. Consultation with a psychiatrist experienced in treating neuropsychiatric disturbances with psychopharmacology may be an important resource in your work with this population.

Assessment of suicide potential is also important in these patients in light of the increased frequency of depression in patients with subcortical disease (for instance, as is true in Parkinson's or Huntington's disease) (Dewhurst et al., 1970; Saunders and Buckingham, 1988). Crisis resources should be available to the clinician involved with this population in the event that an impaired patient experiences suicidal intent. The unique mix of psychosocial trauma with a probable biologic contribution to depression plus dementia creates fertile ground for suicidal intent and planning. The clinician must be vigilant and resourceful when signs of suicidality are present.

Psychotherapy may be an appropriate adjunctive treatment approach to help a patient cope with HIV-associated dementia, particularly in the earlier stages. Clinicians are unfortunately hesitant to utilize psychotherapeutic interventions with patients who are experiencing central nervous system compromise since for many conditions in all but their earliest stages (e.g., Alzheimer's disease), psychotherapy with the impaired individual may not be appropriate. For this disorder, however, psychotherapy provides an opportunity for patients to ventilate their frustration with declining capacities as well as other issues unique to HIV itself. Psychotherapy may assist with problem solving in a concrete fashion, educate the patient and his or her loved ones regarding the problems associated with this condition, and set limits regarding activities that may create potential problems in light of the patient's slowed thinking and motor difficulties. Appropriate planning may make the difference between success and failure and prevent further assaults on the self-concept of an individual already beset by limitations, frustration, and failure on many fronts.

In some cases, countertransference issues arise for therapists who work with patients diagnosed with HIV-associated dementia. In general, professionals who work with other cognitively impaired patients frequently experience countertransference problems. This dynamic is particularly important for clinicians who work with HIV disease because HIV is still a relatively new, lethal, and predominantly sexually transmitted disease that was first identified in socially stigmatized groups. Identification and acknowledgment of countertransference issues are crucial and require the clinician to have adequate self-awareness to respond effectively.

POTENTIAL BARRIERS TO SUCCESSFUL INTERVENTION

Psychological testing for HIV-associated dementia requires access to professional consultants with specialized training in neuropsychology. Many rural settings may not have access to professionals with expertise in neuropsychological practice and referral to a tertiary care center; thus, referral to a professional of another discipline (e.g., psychiatry or neurology) may be the only means of obtaining a consultation to assist in ruling out HIV-associated dementia.

Active collaboration by the social worker, caregivers, and loved ones to enhance the patient's level of function and achievement of the maximum degree of independence is crucial. Caregivers can provide memory aides, encouragement, and support services such as transportation and supervision of activities for a patient with dementia. As discussed, a barrier that often occurs is the desire by loved ones to minimize the patient's memory problems or to blame them on willful forgetting. "He can remember when (or what) he wants to remember" is a statement that I frequently hear from caregivers. Whether due to denial or to an unconscious anger at the situation resulting in a need to blame the patient, the belief that the patient is willfully behaving in a difficult manner poses a significant barrier to effective psychosocial intervention. This must be addressed by the social worker before effective interventions can be instituted.

Barriers to effective diagnosis also exist. The patient who is an active substance abuser will have an altered mental status and present with symptoms that can be mistaken for an HIV-associated cognitive/motor disorder. A careful history, including elicitation of all causes of altered mental function (substance use, history of learning disability, head injury or other neurological disease) represents the best means of lowering this barrier.

Medication noncompliance also represents a barrier to successful intervention. It is known that several antiretroviral medications (such as AZT) are effective in improving cognitive function in persons with an HIV-associated dementia (Schmitt et al., 1988). Intervention addressing the patient's resistance and caregiver education regarding the role of antiretroviral medication in enhancing cognitive function are the best means of addressing this potential barrier.

INFORMATION THE CLIENT SHOULD KNOW BEFORE TAKING ACTION

In addition to psychotherapy to improve the affected individual's adjustment to his or her situation, it may be helpful to inform the client that, as just noted, certain antiretroviral medications such as AZT, especially at high doses, can improve cognitive functioning in HIV-infected individuals with cognitive impairment (Schmitt et al., 1988). Medications may be helpful to the patient with HIV-associated cognitive/motor impairment, and once diagnosed, referral for medications to potentially improve cognitive functioning is important.

Patients should be informed about the importance of neuropsychological testing for this condition, as well as the details of the testing process itself. Evaluations typically last between two to eight hours and, though lengthy, are usually not otherwise painful. Experienced neuropsychologists will typically provide the patient with support and encouragement during the testing process, which involves face-to-face administration of various tests, such as memory tests, spatial tests of copying designs, and three-dimensional blocks, etc. Other neurodiagnostic tests for which the patient may be referred include brain scans such as computerized tomography (CT) or magnetic resonance imaging (MRI) or other medical studies including a spinal tap (lumbar puncture). These are important in order to rule out a focal brain lesion or secondary infectious illness affecting the central nervous system such as toxoplasmosis.

Patients should be informed that it is necessary to distinguish between HIV-associated cognitive impairment and depression. They should be told that HIV-associated dementia is relatively infrequent in the asymptomatic state and becomes more frequent as symptoms increase. Still, the majority of infected individuals will not exhibit symptoms sufficiently severe to qualify for a diagnosis of dementia though they may experience some changes in their level of cognitive functioning.

Patients should be taught compensatory techniques such as using note pads and reminders. This will assist the individual in dealing with the everyday aspects of coping with the disorder.

POLICY IMPLICATIONS AND RELATED ACTIONS

While the connection between broad social policy/health care policy and the specific complex clinical issues associated with HIV-associated dementia may be difficult to make, there is nonetheless an imperative that within the health care delivery system, standards be established which protect patients from mismanagement, promote early and accurate diagnosis, and thereby assure a more responsible and appropriate response to the problem of HIV-associated dementia.

As the evolution of health care provisions continues to be established, consideration regarding the inclusion of selective provisions that can address the unique and unexpected needs which arise in a pandemic will be an important component to any plan or policy that is developed. As social workers, we need to underscore the importance of universal provisions, comprehensive programs and services, and the inclusion of selective provisions to meet the special needs that arise in disorders such as HIV-associated dementia.

RECOMMENDED READINGS

Buckingham, S.L., and Van Gorp, W.G. (1988). Essential knowledge about AIDS dementia. *Social Work, 33*(2) (March-April): pp. 112-115.

Buckingham, S.L., and Van Gorp, W.G. AIDS dementia complex: Implications for practice. *Social Casework, 69*(6) (June): pp. 371-375.

Buckingham, S.L., and Van Gorp, W.G. (1994). HIV-associated dementia: A clinician's guide to early detection, diagnosis, and intervention. *Families in Society, 75*(6) (June): pp. 338-345.

REFERENCES

American Academy of Neurology AIDS Task Force. (1991). Nomenclature and research case definitions for neurologic manifestations of human immunodeficiency virus-type 1 (HIV-1) infection. *Neurology, 41*: 778-785.

Buckingham, S.L., and Van Gorp, W. (1988). AIDS-dementia complex: Implications for practice. *Social Casework: The Journal of Contemporary Social Work, 69*: 371-375.

Cummings, J. (1990). *Subcortical dementia.* New York: Oxford University Press.

Dewhurst, K., Oliver, J., Trick, K.L.K., and McKnight, A.L. (1970). Sociopsychiatric consequences of Huntington's Disease. *British Journal of Psychiatry, 116*: 255-258.

McArthur, J.C., Hoover, D.R., Bacellar, H., Miller, E.N., Cohen, B.A., Becker, J.T., Graham, N.M.H., McArthur, J.H., Selnes, O.A., Jacobson, L.P., Visscher, B.R., Concha, M., and Saah, A. (1993). Dementia in AIDS patients: Incidence and risk factors. *Neurology, 43*: 2245-2252.

Navia, B., Jordan, B., and Price, R. (1986). The AIDS dementia complex: I. Clinical features. *Annals of Neurology, 19*: 517-525.

Navia, B., Cho, E.S., Petito, C., and Price, R. (1986). The AIDS dementia complex: II. Neuropathology. *Annals of Neurology, 19*: 525-535.

Saunders, J.M., and Buckingham, S.L. (1988). Suicidal AIDS patient: When the depression turns deadly. *Nursing, 18*: 59-64.

Schmitt, F.A., Bigley, J.W., McKinnis, R., Logue, P.E., Evans, R.W., and Drucker, J.L. (1988). Neuropsychological outcome of Zidovudine (AZT) treatment of patients with AIDS and AIDS-related complex. *New England Journal of Medicine, 319*: 1573-1578.

Van Gorp, W., Hinkin, C., Satz, P., Miller, E., and D'Elia, L.F. (1993). Neuropsychological findings in HIV infection, encephalopathy, and dementia. In *Neurosychology of Alzheimer's disease and other dementias.* R. Parks, R. Zec, and R. Wilson (Eds.). New York: Oxford University Press, pp. 153-185.

Organizing Support Groups for People Affected by HIV

David M. Aronstein

WHY DO THIS?
STATEMENT OF THE PROBLEM AND ISSUES

Many people experience HIV as an isolating, confusing, and complex part of their lives. In addition to coping with the psychological and emotional aspects of a life-threatening illness, people with HIV must deal with a range of legal, medical treatment, and financial issues. As a result, some people with HIV who have experience dealing with a range of problems and systems often have more accurate and helpful up-to-date specific information than agency-based professionals have.

Support groups for people with HIV and their social networks can also serve a more classic function of helping people see that there are other people in similar situations. Many people with HIV are isolated from traditional sources of emotional support. Those who are gay or bisexual may be estranged from their families of origin or, at the very least, may be cautious about seeking emotional support from their families. People who have been drug-involved may have "burned out" their families after many years of substance abuse and the cycle of recovery and relapse. Those who are in recovery may find that twelve-step programs, while providing much-needed support to remaining clean and sober, are less open to support concerning HIV. Women with HIV often see themselves as isolated from their peers because of the continuing perception that there are few women with HIV or assumptions that all women with HIV are thus addicted to drugs or promiscuous.

Support groups for family members can be essential. "Family," broadly defined, can include families of origin, families of "choice," networks of close support, and care partners. The vicissitudes of HIV illness and the complexity of issues it raises for family members means that support groups, separate from the identified person with HIV, can be essential to providing perspective and practical knowledge in coping with

293

the care needs of the person with HIV. Finally they can be very helpful in the bereavement process after the death of the person with HIV (particularly for families of origin who live in more rural areas).

EXAMPLES OF HOW THE ISSUE MAY PRESENT

As a social worker, you may receive requests from other professionals and/or clients themselves for support groups for people with HIV and their networks. Thus, you are confronted with the dual tasks of determining what kind of support group should exist that would help the people who are presenting themselves and *if* a support group of any kind is the appropriate intervention for a given client.

The fact that a person who is HIV-affected does not have a strong social network may not be the only indication that he or she might benefit from a support group. Many people affected by HIV have complex social networks, but they may not be helpful or truly supportive when it comes to coping with living with HIV. High-achieving professionals may not feel comfortable discussing "personal" issues with their professional colleagues. Gay and bisexual men may not be in a position to "come out" as gay in their work setting (due to issues of stigma and discrimination) or as HIV positive (due to issues of health and disability insurance coverage). Parents may be reluctant to seek support from their friends for fear of negative repercussions on their children. Any person with HIV might benefit from the emotional and informational support that an appropriately structured support group can provide, and many feel a tremendous need to speak with others who have HIV.

FACTS THE SOCIAL WORKER
NEEDS TO KNOW BEFORE PROCEEDING

Again, it is important to understand who the "community" of potential consumers is as well as the particular needs of individuals within it. It is essential to consider the possibility of biological/neurological impairment. Often people with HIV experience mood and thinking disorders that can be successfully treated with medication and professional mental health interventions.

To organize a support group you will need to know the following:

- demographics of people with HIV (gender, race/ethnicity, ages, risk behaviors)
- health care and social service providers who can serve as sources of client referral

- convenient locations for your target group of people with HIV to meet
- other support services that are available to people with HIV in your community

Before referring an individual to a support group you need to know the following:

- the level of the client's psychosocial functioning
- the general health status of the client (Is attending a regular group meeting physically possible?)
- client's wishes about the homogeneity or heterogeneity of the group
- client's past experiences with support groups

KEY QUESTIONS TO ASK THE CLIENT

Understanding a client's expectations about how a support group might be helpful and what strengths and weaknesses he or she brings to such a group can be important in making a successful referral. Having a good sense of a client's mental status prior to referral to a support group is very useful. People often are referred for support groups when in fact they may also need psychiatric intervention to treat a mood disorder or more intensive psychotherapy for a personality or other characterological disorder. Other questions you should ask include the following:

- What does he or she hope to gain from attending a support group?
- What is important to him or her about the background and experiences of other group members?
- Is he or she in any form of psychiatric or psychotherapeutic treatment now or in the past?
- In what ways are the structure of the group important to him or her?
- What kinds of social supports does the client currently have?
- How has that changed for him or her since learning of hihe or sher HIV status?
- What logistical issues need to addressed before attending a group (child care, transportation, physical accessibility)?

CULTURAL COMPETENCY CONSIDERATIONS

Support group models must be flexible if they are going to be successful for people from different cultural and ethnic backgrounds. The following are important cultural considerations:

- *Language* is of primary importance. Most people, even if bilingual, are most comfortable dealing with highly charged and sensitive issues in their native language.
- *Location* of the group can have an important effect on the group's actual and perceived accessibility. Both the neighborhood and the actual facility (AIDS service organization, church, school, community center, etc.) will determine, to some extent, who feels comfortable attending the group.
- *Expressing emotions* in front of others is difficult for most people. In some cultures, it is thought to be inappropriate.
- *Food* can be offered as a way of "breaking the ice" and defining the group as having a more natural setting.
- In most cultures, men and women are not comfortable expressing their feelings, particularly about *sexuality and health in mixed-gender groups*. Single-gender groups can address this issue. Psychoeducational groups, in which an "expert" makes a brief presentation followed by a group discussion, can make some people more comfortable.

ACTION STEPS FOR SUCCESSFUL INTERVENTION

Starting a support group requires a certain degree of persistence and patience. In order to be successful, you need the right combination of clients, facilitators, location, and time to come together. While an ideal group has between six to ten members, it is possible to start a support group with as little as three people. You and the group members have to be willing to hang in as word of the group spreads among other potential members and local providers. Usually, it is easier to attract people to an existing group than it is to keep people interested during the formation stage. The following is a rough outline of action steps to take to form a support group:

1. *Assess the needs of your population.* What kinds of people want and need a support group in your community or agency?
2. *Recruit group facilitators for the group.* Be clear with them that this is a support group, not a psychotherapy group. Try to find people who have experience working with the specific population you are targeting (e.g., gay men, addicts, women). Make a clear contract with them about their responsibilities to the group and the sponsoring organization. Arrange for proper supervision and support for them. It is often helpful if the facilitators speak directly with potential group members prior to their joining the group. Consider cosponsoring a group with another agency

or group of organizations. This may also increase referrals to the group and produce more potential group facilitators.

3. Based on your assessment and the skills of the facilitators, *decide on the structure and format of the group.* Will it be time-limited or open-ended? Open discussion or psychoeducational? Who is it for? Is regular attendance required? What are the eligibility criteria? What kind of commitment will group members be asked to make?

4. *Identify and reserve a regular meeting spot.* If possible, the location should be convenient for potential group members, and the meetings should be at a time that potential members can attend easily (e.g., if you expect people with HIV who are employed to attend, have your group meet in the evenings). If confidentiality is an issue, try to have the group meet in a location where group members will not be afraid to be seen (this may be the local AIDS service organization and it may be a setting outside of the clients' immediate neighborhood).

5. *Prepare group members before they begin to attend the support group.* Regardless of the level of screening you do for the group, make sure that group members understand the ground rules of behavior and expectations they can have of the other group members and the facilitators.

6. *Think through how you will end the group before you start.* People with HIV experience loss all the time. Most have lost friends to HIV, and they are coping with the potential loss of functioning in many areas of their lives. What commitment do the facilitators and the sponsoring organization have to group? How will the group deal with members' deaths? For closed groups, how will the group end?

POTENTIAL BARRIERS TO SUCCESSFUL INTERVENTION

The facilitators must be flexible if the support group is to succeed. This means adjusting the structure and format of the group to meet the needs of the members of the group. For example, if after a few weeks, the regularly attending members of an "open group" want to "close" the group to new members for a while, be open to discussing this and changing the format.

In ongoing groups, members' health will fluctuate; some members may die. Obviously, this will affect the consistency of group attendance. Short-term commitments may be more conducive to group cohesion.

Creating an overly complex set of steps a person must take in order to become a member of the group can act as a disincentive to participation. Remember, for most people, beginning to attend a group is frightening and is not necessarily a high priority. Without sacrificing good care, make it as easy as possible for a person to begin attending the group as soon as possible after he or she has expressed interest.

People with HIV usually have complex lives that require them to juggle many different responsibilities in addition to their own health care. Do what you can to make it easy for people to attend a support group. Perhaps this means arranging for child care for women with HIV who are parents and scheduling the group in conjunction with a clinic visit. It may mean arranging for transportation to and from the group because the expense or exertion of travel may be too demanding on some members.

Uncomfortable furniture, an inadequately heated room, or other seemingly simple fctors can serve as barriers to success (people with HIV often need soft padded chairs and quite warm rooms, particularly if they have lost a lot of weight).

Facilitators not following through on commitments they have made to the group will also impede the group's success. Most people with HIV have a basic distrust of "the system," which has often failed them in the past. Try to create a consistent, caring, predictable environment for the group. For some it may be one of the few predictable moments in their daily lives.

INFORMATION THE CLIENT SHOULD KNOW BEFORE TAKING ACTION

Clients should clearly understand the ground rules for their own and others' behavior in the group. They should know what information divulged in the group is confidential and what information (if any) facilitators will share with other providers in the agency or elsewhere.

POLICY IMPLICATIONS AND RELATED ACTIONS

Often people with HIV are referred to support groups when a psychiatric or other intervention is more appropriate. This is due to a combination of a lack of understanding of what support groups are and a lack of availability of good mental health services for HIV-affected people.

Social workers can advocate for the creation of mental health services for people with HIV and their families in existing medical and mental health agencies.

Social workers can advocate for the inclusion of sufficient mental health coverage, including group interventions in whatever system of health care insurance is developed.

Reimbursement for support groups for family and care partners is rarely provided. If agencies had more of a financial inducement to provide family support services, people with HIV might be able to remain at home with family support for longer periods of time. This could reduce the need for hospitalization due to the lack of home support and help to lower the overall medical costs of HIV.

SECTION III:
PEOPLE IN SPECIAL CIRCUMSTANCES

Addressing HIV Risks
with Clients Who Use Drugs

Jack B. Stein

WHY DO THIS?
STATEMENT OF THE PROBLEM AND ISSUES

Drug use is considered one of our nation's most significant public health problems. Regardless of practice setting, it is likely that a social worker will encounter clients with drug-related problems. The spread of HIV among injection drug users, their sexual partners, and their offspring account for a major proportion of new HIV infections in the United States. In contrast to a decline in AIDS cases attributed to male-to-male sexual activity over the past thirteen years, cases attributed to injection drug use have steadily increased.

As of June 1995, injection drug use accounted for fully one-third of all AIDS cases reported to the Centers for Disease Control and Prevention (CDC), with women, children, and minorities disproportionately affected. For example, consider the following:

- Nearly 50 percent of all women diagnosed with AIDS have injected drugs.
- Eighteen percent of women with AIDS were sex partners of male injection drug users.
- Fifty-three percent of babies with AIDS were born to mothers who injected drugs or were sex partners of male injection drug users.
- Thirty-six percent of all male African Americans with AIDS and 38 percent of all male Hispanics with AIDS have injected drugs.

Yet the link between HIV infection and drug use goes beyond the risks associated with injection drug use. For example, alcohol and noninjected drugs are known to further the spread of HIV by impairing judgement during sexual decision making. Of growing concern is the direct link between the use of crack (a derivative of cocaine that is smoked) and risky

303

sexual activity, particularly among women who exchange sex for crack or money to buy drugs.

Among those individuals already infected with HIV, the immune-suppressing qualities of many drugs are considered a potential contributor to HIV disease progression. In addition, continued drug use after infection with HIV may also lead to increased vulnerability to opportunistic infections.

EXAMPLES OF HOW THE ISSUE MAY PRESENT

Unless you work in a practice setting that treats drug abuse, it is unlikely that drug use will be the primary problem presented by a client. There are several reasons why this may be so. Society has little tolerance for drug use and often considers such behavior as deviant and immoral. In spite of growing scientific evidence that shows drug addiction is a disease, misperceptions still prevail about its causes. As a result, clients may be hesitant to disclose information about drug-using behaviors for fear of rejection, loss of insurance coverage, or legal problems.

Denial of drug abuse is commonplace among many clients—despite all the evidence that may be presented about their actions. As a defense, denial is probably the most characteristic trademark of drug abuse. Problems associated with drug use often present themselves in a more disguised manner. For example, clients may begin to display changes in their behavior, mood, as well as their physical condition. Social and work relations often begin to falter.

Many of the changes associated with drug use can be easily mistaken for other conditions. For example, the effects of crack use can resemble those of schizophrenia. The "crash" after cocaine use can be mistaken for clinical depression. The withdrawal symptoms from heroin are similar to the signs of a stroke.

Further complicating matters is the co-occurrence of mental health problems among drug users. For example, a client might present with a myriad of symptoms—mania, depression, anxiety, paranoia, hallucinations, and incoherence. And even if the client is able and willing to report drug use, there is still the question as to whether the drug use triggered the psychological response or vice-versa. Differentiating the source of the problems is critical to developing effective treatment plans.

FACTS THE SOCIAL WORKER NEEDS TO KNOW
BEFORE PROCEEDING

Drug use is a complex and emotionally charged issue. Too often, providers take actions based on inaccurate information or their own biased attitudes. Training and field experience are probably the best means for helping caregivers understand the dynamics of addiction and to examine personal attitudes that may hinder their work with clients. At a minimum, all social workers should keep the following facts in mind when working with clients with drug-related problems:

1. The nature and extent of drug use varies.

The illegal nature of drug use makes it difficult to accurately determine the extent of drug use within a community. However, surveys conducted provide enough estimates to tell us that drug use is widespread although its use varies geographically as well as by gender, age, racial-ethnic background, and choice of drug.

2. Multiple drug use is common.

Drug users often combine drugs to enhance the effects or to counteract withdrawal symptoms of a particular drug. These days, multiple drug or "polydrug" use is considered the norm. "Speedballing," for example, is a common practice that consists of injecting heroin along with cocaine to produce a prolonged and more intense high.

3. Drug use is a spectrum.

Not only do drug use patterns differ geographically, but drug use patterns differ among individuals. However, one must remember that *frequency and level* of use are not always directly related to the *consequences* of use. Someone who uses only on weekends (often called a "weekend warrior") may experience equally devastating problems at home or at work as might a long-term user.

4. Multiple factors lead to drug problems.

The cause(s) of drug-related problems have been debated for years. Arguments have ranged from a now-discredited view that abuse is a result of "moral weakness" to it being an outcome of genetic predisposition. Today, most experts agree that there are multiple factors contributing to drug abuse and addiction. A "biopsychosocial-environmental" model is most commonly used to explain the nature of drug problems.

5. Drug use is a preventable behavior; addiction is a disease.

Not all people who use drugs become physically or psychologically dependent. Many individuals never use or simply stop after a period of experimentation. However, addiction occurs when a person becomes physically or psychologically drug-dependent and experiences withdrawal symptoms when the drug use ceases. At this point, the person is considered to have the disease of addiction, which may require treatment. However, even after treatment, the allure of drugs can be so powerful that a return to use, called relapse, is fairly common.

6. Heroin, cocaine, and crack use pose the greatest threat of HIV infection.

Although the disinhibiting effects of most drug use can lead to risky behavior, sharing of equipment to inject heroin and cocaine is the most common means of HIV transmission associated with drug use. Because the effects of cocaine do not last nearly as long as those of heroin, cocaine users tend to inject many more times a day than heroin users, thereby increasing their risks of HIV infection. Smoking crack is directly associated with increased and prolonged unprotected sexual activity, often in exchange for drugs or money to buy drugs.

7. Drug treatment works to reduce drug use and HIV transmission.

A combination of behavioral and medication-based drug treatment interventions has been shown to be effective in helping individuals with drug-related problems. Since a reduction in drug-using behaviors will result in a reduction of HIV risks, drug treatment is considered an important form of HIV prevention. In addition, drug treatment programs provide excellent opportunities to offer ongoing HIV prevention education and counseling to some of the highest risk individuals. In spite of this, treatment is still limited for the uninsured and the poor.

8. People vary in their readiness to change drug-using behaviors.

Not all individuals experiencing drug-related problems are willing or able to modify their behaviors. Even among those who do, relapse is fairly common, particularly among newly treated clients. Addiction specialists have begun to recognize the importance of assessing a client for his or her level of "change readiness" prior to determining an intervention. For example, some clients may have no interest in changing their behavior, others may have just begun to consider making a change, while other clients may be highly motivated to do so.

Assessing "where a client is" along this continuum can be helpful in determining the appropriateness of HIV prevention efforts. For example, the Gay Men's Health Crisis in New York has established a program for drug-using clients not yet ready to enter drug treatment, but clearly in need of HIV prevention counseling. The goal of the program is to lower HIV risks through the adoption of safer behaviors and to prepare a client for admission to treatment when he or she is ready to do so.

9. Harm reduction allows for greater likelihood of effective prevention.

Abstinence from drug use, although effective, is not the only option available to reduce the risk of HIV transmission. In this respect, harm-reduction efforts have become a popular (if not controversial) means to help drug users lower their HIV risks. Harm-reduction approaches emphasize that most drug users are unable or unwilling to stop drug use completely and forever, that limited drug treatment program "slots" are available, that many drug users cannot stop drug use even when they are enrolled in drug treatment programs, and that many users who do stop may relapse.

Educating clients about proper needle hygiene (such as the use of bleach as a disinfectant) has had moderate success over the past several years in modifying behavior. More recently, needle-exchange programs have gained acceptance as a means to reduce HIV risks among active injection drug users through the exchange of sterile injection equipment for used equipment, the dissemination of HIV risk-reduction information and supplies (e.g., condoms), and referral to drug treatment and other needed services.

10. Drugs users are also at risk for HIV through sexual behaviors.

Too often, prevention efforts targeting drug users focus on drug-related risks and ignore the risks incurred through sexual activity. Crack use, for example, has been intimately linked to high-risk sexual activity, particularly among women who exchange sex for drugs or money to buy drugs. Hence, it is important to screen clients for both drug and sexual risk behaviors and to incorporate discussion of HIV risk-reduction techniques into client counseling.

KEY QUESTIONS TO ASK THE CLIENT

In preparing to assist clients who may use drugs, assessing the nature of their drug use and their level of desire to address such behavior is essential. A few questions are important, particularly when drug use is not the problem with which the client presents.

1. What is the extent of the client's drug-using behavior?
2. Does he or she consider drug use to be a problem at this time?
3. Does the client believe that he or she is personally at risk for HIV infection due to drug use?
4. Is he or she willing to enter treatment for his or her drug problem?
5. What is the client's level of "change readiness" regarding drug-related risk behaviors?

CULTURAL COMPETENCY CONSIDERATIONS

Although patterns of drug use vary by gender, age, race, and ethnicity, no population is immune to drug use problems. Cultural factors, however, do contribute to the nature and extent of drug-related problems and should always be taken into account when determining a treatment plan. For example, drug (and alcohol) use may be more tolerated by some cultures than by others. In some cultures, drug use (e.g., alcohol, hallucinogenic drugs) are intimately woven into religious or spiritual rituals.

The historical mistreatment of minorities by the public health sector (exemplified by the infamous Tuskeegee Syphilis Study from 1931 to 1972, in which treatment was withheld to track the course of syphilis among African-American men) has resulted in a high degree of suspicion and skepticism regarding HIV risk-reduction efforts, like needle exchange. For many persons of color, this type of intervention is perceived as a form of racial genocide by condoning a behavior that has already taken a huge toll within minority communities (Lurie et al., 1993).

ACTION STEPS FOR SUCCESSFUL INTERVENTION

Social workers are in excellent positions to support clients affected by HIV and drug problems. This is particularly true if rapport has already been established with a client and trust has begun to develop. Some practical action steps to keep in mind include the following:

1. Screen all clients for drug use.

Screening is an initial attempt to determine whether drug use is a problem for the client. In general, questions asked are often framed in a manner that link drug use with social and employment problems. Many standardized screening tools are available to determine the extent of a client's drug problem. (The *National Clearinghouse on Alcohol and Drug Information* is a good source to access these tools; the phone number is 1-800-729-6686.) One of the more popular and easy-to-administer screening instruments is called the Drug Abuse Screening Test (DAST). Several key questions used by DAST are the following:

- What drugs other than those required for medical reasons have you used?
- Can you get through the week without using drugs?
- Have you engaged in illegal activities in order to obtain drugs?
- Have you ever experienced withdrawal symptoms (felt sick) when you stopped taking drugs?

• Have you been involved in a treatment program specifically related to drug use?

2. Assess HIV drug and sex risks.

Explore with the client his or her behaviors that may be associated with HIV transmission. What type of drugs used and how they are used provides important information concerning the nature and extent of use and HIV-related risks. Too often, not enough attention is paid to sexual risks among drug users. Asking questions about sexual practices helps formulate a better understanding of the client's level of risk and what kinds of risk-reduction plans are indicated.

3. Assess the client's level of change readiness.

Examine the degree to which the assessed HIV risks are of concern to the client. Building on the change readiness continuum model discussed earlier, attempt to determine a client's level of desire to modify those activities based on this concern. Avoid discussing these issues too generally. Be specific about what behaviors the client is willing to address at this time and to what degree is change planned.

4. Be realistic in treatment planning.

Based on the assessed needs, work with the client to develop a plan that adequately meets the client's level of change readiness. Based on this concept of harm reduction, treatment goals may vary among clients. For an injection drug user who indicates no intention to stop using, referral to a local needle-exchange program may be most indicated. For those interested in stopping their drug use, treatment options should be explored.

In using a harm-reduction model, particularly with active drug users who do not intend (or are not ready) to stop use, make sure that you understand your agency's policy regarding service delivery to active drug users. In some agencies, active drug users must be enrolled in drug treatment programs before services are provided. In other agencies, the client is encouraged to participate in a "recovery readiness" program designed to prepare him or her to eventually seek drug treatment.

5. Determine needed community referral sources.

Rarely can one agency address the multiple problems associated with HIV- and drug-related risks. Hence, it is critical to have access to community services that are capable and willing to accept client referrals. It is a good idea to establish these linkages prior to needing them, thereby expediting the referring process. Determine the kinds of services available to such clients and what policies they may have in serving such a population.

Such referral services include AIDS service organizations, medical clinics, social service programs, HIV testing and counseling centers, community outreach programs, and needle-exchange programs. Regardless of the resource, it is always important to follow up on a referral. Clients with drug abuse problems may often need help accessing these services. A case management approach has been shown to be effective in doing so.

6. Consider the likelihood of relapse.

The Alcoholics Anonymous philosophy of living "one day at a time" speaks to the challenge faced by those living a drug-free lifestyle. In an effort to better prepare the client to avoid the urge to return to drug use (or minimize the harm if they do), treatment programs now regularly incorporate relapse prevention techniques into ongoing counseling with clients. Relapse potential is probably the most convincing argument for including safer drug-injection practices into risk-reduction education and counseling with clients in recovery.

7. Be flexible.

Treatment plans are as effective as their responsiveness to client needs. Relapse, for example, can put a client's treatment in a tailspin. Treatment plans should be reviewed regularly to ensure that client goals and actions are still realistic. When necessary, treatment goals should be renegotiated and agreed upon by client and counselor.

POTENTIAL BARRIERS TO SUCCESSFUL INTERVENTION

Social workers may face several major obstacles when attending to the HIV prevention and treatment needs of injection drug users. Several important ones to be aware of are discussed in the following:

Negative Caregiver Attitudes

Unfortunately, care providers are not above stigmatizing people with HIV and/or drug-related problems. Caregivers should first "take stock" of their own personal attitudes about drug use, particularly as they might conflict with meeting the client's needs. Supervision and training are two good ways to address these issues and to ensure that the client is appropriately served.

Mental Health Problems

The issues presented by clients with HIV and drug-related concerns are further complicated by the presence of mental health problems, such as depression and personality disorders, commonly observed among individuals with drug use problems. This level of complexity requires good screening and assessment skills and a knowledge of available community resources.

Denial

As noted, denial is one of the hallmark characteristics of addiction. This can be one of the most challenging issues encountered by a provider. In spite of the tendency to do so, confronting clients about their drug use can actually have a negative impact on their willingness to change. Rather, empathy and a nonjudgemental manner in offering feedback to clients regarding their drug use has been shown to lead to positive behavioral change in clients. Interventions that involve the family and significant others have also been used successfully to help clients improve their readiness to change.

Difficult Client Behaviors

In some clients, drug use is often associated with antisocial behaviors, such as manipulation and noncompliance with treatment. Of importance is recognizing that these behaviors are merely symptoms of the underlying illness of addiction. Behavioral management techniques, such as client contracting, can be helpful, particularly when working with clients who continue to use drugs. Although a nonjudgemental attitude is always important, care must be taken to not inadvertently "reward" the drug-using behaviors.

Limited Community Resource Referrals

In an era of diminishing resources, providing adequate resources to meet clients' needs is becoming more difficult. However, some changes in our health care system may result in enhanced linkages among service providers in an effort to reduce overall costs. Becoming familiar with local drug abuse service agencies will help you meet your clients' needs. Contact your local or state drug abuse agency (often a part of the public health department) to find out what agencies are most suited to serving clients with drug use and HIV-related problems.

Client Confidentiality

In an effort to protect the confidentiality of clients in drug treatment, communication may be limited among provider agencies. However, this need not be a barrier as long as clients provide permission for such information to be disclosed and/or "qualified service organization agreements" (QSOAs) are established among agencies that commonly refer clients to each other.

Differing Agency Policy and Philosophy

Agencies involved in serving drug users affected by HIV may differ in their approach to drug-related issues. For example, a drug treatment program might view harm-reduction strategies (e.g., bleach disinfection of injection equipment) as a contradiction to the agency's drug-free philosophy. Some social service agencies may require clients with drug-related problems to be enrolled in drug treatment programs prior to services being offered. In response to these differing viewpoints and policies, many communities have established local councils consisting of representatives from various service providers to address the multitude of issues that arise in serving clients affected by HIV and drug use.

INFORMATION THE CLIENT SHOULD KNOW BEFORE TAKING ACTION

Clients should always be made aware of agency policies regarding tolerance of drug use. In particular, they should be informed of the agency's expectations for clients who are actively using as well as for those who relapse while being served. In some circumstances, enrollment in drug treatment is a prerequisite to receive services.

All clients have a right to privacy regarding such things as HIV status and drug use history. Such information can be shared only with prior approval of the client or if your agency has established a formal agreement with another referral agency. When such agreements are in place, the client should be made aware of them.

POLICY IMPLICATIONS AND RELATED ACTIONS

Social workers are in an excellent position to advocate for clients with HIV-related and drug-related problems. This is particularly important considering that many clients may not have a support system in place.

On a community level, advocating for more drug treatment services is important. At present, only a fraction of drug users can be served by available treatment programs. Nationwide, waiting lists for entry in public-funded programs are notoriously long. In addition, it is critical that drug treatment programs link with other service providers to ensure comprehensive care to clients with HIV-related and drug-related problems.

"Prescription and paraphernalia" laws impose severe restrictions on the purchase and possession of equipment used to administer drugs. In doing so, these laws are considered obstacles to HIV prevention as they discourage injection drug users from obtaining and carrying sterile equipment for fear of arrest. In response, some states, such as Connecticut and Hawaii, have begun to pass legislation that overturns these laws. In Connecticut, for example, rates of drug injection have not increased, and rates of HIV infection among injection drug users have begun to lessen. Social workers are important advocates for such legislation and should work with community groups to address these significant barriers to conducting HIV prevention.

REFERENCE

Lurie, P., Reingold, A.L., Bowser, B., Chen, D., Foley, J., Guydish, J., Kahn, J.G., Lane, S., Sorensen, J., et al. (1993). *The Public Health Impact of Needle Exchange Programs in the United States and Abroad,* Volume 1. Berkeley, A: The Regents of the University of California. Prepared for the Centers for Disease Control and Prevention.

PART A:
SERVICES FOR CHILDREN AND FAMILIES

Counseling Parents and Children with HIV

Lori S. Wiener

WHY DO THIS?
STATEMENT OF THE PROBLEM AND ISSUES

Fourteen years into the AIDS epidemic, profound psychosocial problems affecting children and families continue. Over 80 percent of families affected by HIV are from poor communities of color, many of whom are already burdened by poverty, discrimination, and limited support systems. Frequently, these families are without savings, employment, income, insurance, legal counsel, and medical or social support—all of which antedate infection with HIV. Key psychosocial issues include fears associated with disclosure of the diagnosis to family, friends, and employers due to the stigma that surrounds this disease, isolation, depression, grief, and the threat to family integrity.

A child with AIDS usually identifies a whole family at risk of infection (Wiener and Septimus, 1994). All family members are greatly affected by the impact the disease has on the family, whether or not they are HIV positive themselves. Clinical support services are essential in order to mitigate the cumulative psychological burden on both the HIV-infected child and his or her family members.

EXAMPLES OF HOW THE ISSUE MAY PRESENT

Diagnosis

The issue of disclosure initially brings most parents to seek clinical social work services. Many HIV-infected parents remain ambivalent about whether or not to inform their child about their own or the child's HIV infection. The decision to disclose one's diagnosis is very difficult. In making such a decision, several realistic concerns must be seriously considered. These include fear of abandonment by family and friends, the effect that disclosure might have on noninfected siblings, concerns about the loss of employment or housing, and worries that the child will be unable to keep this information to him or herself (Olson et al., 1989).

Once the parents disclose the diagnosis to their child, the issue of who their child can then share this information with often becomes a source of tension. Children may also begin to struggle with fears associated with a parent's progressive illness and death. Separation anxiety is not uncommon for the school-age or preadolescent child. Clingy behavior, difficulty falling asleep, refusal to go to a friends' home or engage in any peer-related activities on the weekends, and preferring only to remain with the parent at all times are symptoms parents need to watch out for. Refusal to go to school for fear of something bad happening to a loved one while they are gone is also not uncommon. Older children who fear the loss of a parent may become withdrawn, isolated, resentful, and angry, or they may begin manifesting acting-out behaviors.

FACTS THE SOCIAL WORKER NEEDS TO KNOW
BEFORE PROCEEDING

Disclosure

Parents may withhold their child's diagnosis from their children in order to protect them from painful realities (such as how they became infected and/or discussions about death) and to avoid burdening them with the knowledge of their life-threatening disease for as long as possible in an effort to preserve their happy childhoods (Tasker, 1992). However, children who observe their parents getting upset and who hear numerous discussions pertaining to medical issues often suspect that they are more seriously ill than they are being told. Families then find themselves further burdened by a lack of candor within their own home at a time when they might benefit from being able to talk openly about the situation. Both the child and family members may find themselves entangled in a web of silence. When children do learn about their own and/or their parents' diagnosis, a barrage of questions may follow. The child needs to be reassured that he or she did not cause the illness. This can be particularly difficult for a parent to assure when the infection was vertically transmitted and the parent is struggling with his or her own feelings of guilt. Simple explanations about the virus and medical procedures are important so that medical interventions are not perceived as punishment. Other questions often include how they became infected, who they can share this diagnosis with, and if they will die. Parents need to consider how they want to answer such questions in advance. Role-playing such scenarios with their social worker is often helpful.

Questions About Death

Answering a child's question about whether or not he or she will die from their disease is extremely difficult for most parents. The child's worst fears are often associated with separation, not death. They worry about how their parents and siblings will cope and the emotional pain and suffering their family might experience as a result of them being gone. Other children worry about how the family will manage financially when their own entitlement benefits are no longer available. These issues should be openly and honestly reviewed. The issue that the parent may become too sick to care for the child should also be discussed. Children need to be assured of who will care for them if that happens. When parents begin to develop symptoms of the disease, the HIV-infected child often worries about developing the same symptoms. This is especially true for the HIV-infected child who survives his or her parent's death only to become symptomatic years later. These children often keep such memories private either because they are too frightened by them or they feel no one would understand. Sharing such memories not only provides tremendous relief but also allows for misunderstandings about disease progression to be addressed and clarified.

School

Parents often are concerned about whether or not they need to inform the school of their child's diagnosis. The social worker can research the school's HIV policy and advise the family as to the process that would take place if they decided to disclose the diagnosis to the school. The social worker can also help the parent anticipate the responses of teachers and other parents while building in backup supports for the child. School-age children who have informed their classmates about their HIV infection can easily become the focus of teachers, parents, and other students. While for some HIV-infected children negative results followed disclosure, most children have returned to the classroom to find their teachers to be compassionate and the other children to be interested in remaining friends. The range of potential reactions to disclosure of the HIV diagnosis needs to be dealt with openly and honestly with the parent(s), child, teachers, and principal. Adequate education and support of the school staff is always helpful.

Adolescents

Adolescents, like children, need appropriate support, counseling, and services to help them cope with their infection. Common adolescent reactions to the diagnosis of HIV infection include disbelief ("I don't believe it . . . take it [the antibody test] again"), fear ("My life is over if anybody finds out"), panic ("I'm going to die"), as well as anger, guilt, withdrawal, and depression. Issues related to disclosure and confidentiality are expressed most frequently not only at the time of diagnosis but throughout the course of illness as well. The fear of being rejected by one's friends is often greater than the fear of dying from AIDS (Wiener and Septimus, 1994). Depending on the degree of immune compromise, the social worker can help the adolescent modify future plans while still pursuing goals. Other critical issues to be addressed are the difficulty of partner notification, "safer sex" practices, medication options, and feelings of guilt and shame. Adolescents often do not have skills in negotiating complex bureacratic systems. Social workers can also help adolescents who are in school or at work handle repeated absences. Questions about having children are common. Coming to terms with the possibility of having a baby that could be HIV-infected is difficult. Most adolescents choose not to become pregnant (or get someone pregnant), and counseling that helps the HIV-infected adolescent grieve the loss of a future family of their own is essential. As with children, an early and comprehensive psychosocial assessment of the adolescent's needs is of crucial importance. This must include an assessment of depression and suicidal risk.

As the disease progresses, the adolescent responds best to sensitive and honest discussions about what is happening. Many have preconceived ideas about dying, and these need to be explored. It is not uncommon for the HIV-infected adolescent to keep thoughts, fears, and wishes concerning their dying to themselves in an attempt to protect those who love them from further hurt and pain (*Journal of Adolescent Health,* 1993).

HIV-Affected Adolescents

Adolescents often have difficulty showing their true feelings. However, this should not minimize the many concerns, fears, and worries with which they are struggling. These include anger of having to face such a major problem and then guilt about being angry. In general, children will react in ways that are characteristic to their personality. For example, if the teenager tends to take care of others, he or she will try to become a caretaker—often making great sacrifices. Other children go to the opposite extreme and attempt any number of ways to run away from their problems. These children may try to isolate themselves from the family. Other adolescents hide their pain and fear with anger. This is particularly true for children who have a hard time expressing sad feelings. It is age-appropriate for many of these teens to appear to be more interested in their peers than in what is happening in their family. However, their struggle to balance their need for independence and autonomy with feelings of, and need for, dependency is complicated by the potential death of one or both parents. Patience and reassurance helps, as does making sure the child has at least one adult person with whom they can talk openly and honestly.

Siblings

The experience of living with a chronically or acutely ill brother or sister will severely emotionally affect the healthy siblings. The chronicity of problems within HIV-affected families are often so great that the ensuing problems of the healthy children are not a priority. As a result, the pain, fear, and confusion felt by these children can be easily dismissed. Their pain remains invisible while the suffering of their parents and ill brothers or sisters is quite apparent to all (Wiener and Septimus, 1994). Family life is strengthened when individuals are able to share information and feelings and to communicate openly a sense of hope and trust in the future. However, many families choose not to share the HIV diagnosis with the healthy children in the home, blocking healthy expressions of feelings that are needed in a time of crisis. So much energy is expended in keeping the secret of AIDS that family members lose a sense of the what the others are feeling.

In many cases, both the infected child and siblings know or suspect the presence of HIV or AIDS but are also painfully aware of the absolute need in the family to keep the secret. One nine-year-old girl illustrated this point when she and her eleven-year-old brother were watching an AIDS program on television. The nine-year-old girl responded by saying: "This is what I could die from. Please don't tell Mommy that I could die; she would be so upset." When open communications between siblings and between parents are blocked, it is detrimental to the family.

KEY QUESTIONS TO ASK THE CLIENT

Asking the parents how they feel they are coping with the disease is always helpful. For example, who provides you with the most support? Who is looking after your own medical needs? Would you be interested in meeting others in a similar situation to your own? Are you able to sleep at night? How is your appetite? How is your mood in general? What kind of community support is available to you? Do you feel you need help with disclosure issues? Would it be helpful for your own parents, extended family members, and/or close friends to have someone to talk to? Do you feel you could benefit from assistance with parenting issues or with financial issues? If you are not well, do you have anyone in mind who you trust could take care of your child(ren)? If so, have you spoken to this person yet? It is important to help parents learn not only what is within the normal range of emotions upon learning the diagnosis but also which indicators could let them know that more intensive social work intervention may be needed.

CULTURAL COMPETENCY CONSIDERATIONS

AIDS is perceived differently by different ethnic and cultural groups. One needs to have an understanding of the cultural beliefs and values of his or her clients in order to allow greater clinical sensitivity.

Using a translator to facilitate communication with a client who does not speak or understand English well is very helpful. If the client brings his or her own translator, whether it be their child or another adult, this effort should be recognized. The social worker should always maintain eye contact with and direct all questions toward the client, rather than the translator. All instructions to clients who do not speak English well should be given both orally and in writing, even if the instructions can only be provided in English. If needed, the client can then find someone to translate the instructions at the appropriate time.

People with immigration concerns may be much more hesitant to seek out help from formal care providers than those with no such concerns. If they feel they may be reported to immigration services by the care-provider, they will probably rely more on their informal support networks. Communication must be left open between the formal care providers and the client.

For many ethnic minorities with limited access to health care information, family and friendship networks are the dominant influence on health behavior and a trusted source of health information. Thus, family and friends should be included, if desired by the client, when information is being dispensed that may enhance medical compliance by raising the level of knowledge of the informal advice network (Mays and Cochran, 1987).

Latinas and African-American women are typically the care providers within their communities and may not necessarily be willing or able to take time out to meet their own needs. As a result, they may be less likely to seek out formal care for themselves. If they are raising a child who is HIV positive, they can often become overwhelmed—especially if they have already lost other family members to HIV/AIDS. They are often grieving those losses while simultaneously assuming additional burdens of caregiving (Boyd-Franklin and Aleman, 1990). Health care and support services need to be accessible to these populations. While mental health services are a preferred resource for white women, African Americans in particular are unlikely to use counseling services, frequently citing these services as contrary to their cultural experiences and insufficient to meet their needs (Bingham and Guinyard, 1982).

African Americans tend to maintain relatively close and frequent contacts with kin, receiving much support from them. Family most frequently serves as a buffer from outside assaults. However, like many HIV-infected individuals, African Americans have experienced rejection by family members. Thus, counselors and social workers should beware that the impact of such familial rejection may be more severe, given the existing cultural norms emphasizing the kinship network as the provider of both tangible and emotional social support (Mandel and Namir, 1985).

Ataque de nervios, a culturally condoned occurrence referring to a form of distress most frequently seen in Hispanic women, is triggered by an event or situation which feels overwhelming. Reported symptoms, while often brief and self-limited, include severe panic, amnesia, seizure-like movements, and/or may resemble a brief psychotic disorder. Since ataque de nervios is often seen in medical and clinical settings, it is essential that the social worker be aware of the existence and symptoms of this disorder. Such awareness will help clarify symptomatology that may indicate a coexisting disorder and promote the design of appropriate psychosocial interventions (Oquendo, 1995).

ACTION STEPS FOR SUCCESSFUL INTERVENTION

An essential component to providing psychosocial support to HIV-infected children and families is a comprehensive assessment that identifies each family's strengths and vulnerabilities. Such an assessment should be obtained as soon as the social worker meets with the family. The assessment then allows the worker to best anticipate the psychological, social, and concrete needs of the family and to plan appropriate interventions. Genograms are another useful assessment tool as they clearly demonstrate the number of family losses and potential future care providers. Once an assessment is complete, the social worker is then in a position to initiate clinical interventions and organize community agency referrals. Crisis intervention commonly begins on the first day the social worker meets the family. Obtaining emergency food or housing, identifying adequate medical care, and providing respite care are often the first interventions the social worker provides for families.

Clinical support services are often a significant resource to children with HIV and their families. These services can take on many modalities (individual, family, or group, for example) and often complement one another.

For the child, play therapy can provide a safe haven for children to work through feelings of isolation, separation, and abandonment or to learn to cope with medical procedures. Displacement activities, such as storytelling and art are other important interventions that often help school-age children begin to address their worries. For example, having the child write a story or draw a picture about what it is like for an imaginary child to live with AIDS allows them to begin to explore their own feelings within a safe modality. This most often leads to direct communication of the child's thoughts, feelings, fears, and anxieties. Adolescents also benefit tremendously from counseling. Issues related to peer relationships, secrecy, stigma, and sexual practices, and fears associated with rejection are frequently discussed in both individual counseling and support groups for HIV-infected teens.

Family counseling is often not possible until the diagnosis is revealed. Once disclosure of the diagnosis takes place, family therapy is exceptionally useful in helping families learn to communicate openly about their inner thoughts and fears as well as to plan as a family for a future in which one or both parents may be gone.

Support groups are clearly not for everyone. Even within the security of the therapeutic environment provided within support groups, many people still fear loss of confidentiality. This is unfortunate as parent support groups, support groups for children who are aware of their diagnosis, and support groups for healthy children in families with HIV are very effective in reducing emotional isolation and providing a safe haven to explore issues that cannot be discussed with peers. For those who are not comfortable talking to others face to face, telephone support groups have become a very effective modality for persons living with HIV disease (Wiener et al., 1993).

POTENTIAL BARRIERS TO SUCCESSFUL INTERVENTION

Parental refusal to openly discuss the disease will prohibit interventions that can reduce the anxiety which results from secrecy in the home. While this is frustrating for the social worker, respect for the parents' resistance is important. Working with the parent toward open communication on any level and maintaining a sense of trust between the child and parent will facilitate open communication at a later point.

Frequent changes in the home and/or care providers, lack of consistency in providing the child's medical care, and parental drug use are other factors that can potentially lead to a more unfavorable psychosocial outcome. Recognition of these high-risk indicators and ongoing interventions designed to provide consistency for the child are essential. Even with the best assessments and interventions, a child in this setting may require additional mental health services. Indicators include the following:

1. Changes in appetite or sleep patterns. This includes difficult or excessive sleeping as well as overeating or poor appetite resulting in weight loss.
2. Failing grades in school.
3. Changes in mood; appearing sad most of the time; frequent unexplained crying times, temper tantrums, or anger directed at younger or older siblings. Being elated most of the time as if ignoring completely the realities associated with the family situation can also be an indication that coping is very difficult for the child.
4. Withdrawal from activities that were once of interest to the child, for example, withdrawing from friends or resistance toward being away from the home. Other children manifest their emotional difficulties by not wanting to be at home at all, spending most of their time busy with activities outside of the family. Either extreme can be a sign that the child is having trouble dealing with the parent's illness.
5. Self-destructive behavior or acts or involvement in risky or impulsive behaviors that are new to the child. Younger children often manifest this by head banging, throwing around large toys, running into the

street, and/or excessive jumping off of high places. For adolescents, this often takes the form of drug and alcohol use and risky sexual behavior.

6. Help parents remember that they know their child better than anyone else knows their child. Encourage them to watch out for changes in behavior, mood, and temperament. Remind them that they do not have to wait until others notice changes before asking for help.

INFORMATION THE CLIENT SHOULD KNOW BEFORE TAKING ACTION

1. Timing is of great importance. Issues such as when to disclose the diagnosis, make a will, create legacies, and/or inform the school all need careful thought and consideration. For example, a parent may wish to just "spill the beans." Anticipating first the child's and then the community's response along with careful planning for backup supports will help ensure a better outcome. Such parents may need to be reminded that once the diagnosis is revealed, it can not be taken back.

2. Parents should be made aware of all supports that are available to the child and family. Lists of community agencies for emotional and financial support are useful. Providing information about local AIDS organizations and what they offer is also helpful to parents.

3. Many parents appreciate learning that they do not need to abandon their cultural beliefs because the health care system or providers are different than they are. When at all possible, the parent and child should be encouraged to seek help from their own communities, whether from a minister of their church or the less formal networks that have the respect of their particular culture. Knowing that the social worker is available to answers questions from members of their family, community, school, etc., has been of great comfort to many families.

POLICY IMPLICATIONS AND RELATED ACTIONS

1. Learn about any AIDS service agencies that are available in your immediate area. If your HIV-infected client presents with a problem that is not addressed by an AIDS organization, look into existing programs that may be willing to expand their current services. For example, a community mental health organization already servicing children and families may be comfortable providing therapy to an HIV-infected child.

2. Be aware of the confidentiality and antidiscrimination laws, and keep abreast of specific and new laws pertaining to custody, guardianship, and the rights of foster parents to make medical decisions in your state.

Remember, this work is enormously challenging and also often sad. Each loss may trigger a loss in your own life. Stay attuned to your own needs and be sure to be able to differentiate between your own sadness and possible depression.

Families greatly appreciate the support that is made available to them. It is important to remember that there is not a blueprint to working with HIV-infected children and their families. Each child and family will cope differently than the next. It is our challenge to both understand their worlds and to provide the supports they need to help buffer the catastrophic effects that the disease has on their lives. The professional skills one gains while working with these families are great. The personal rewards are even greater.

RECOMMENDED READINGS

Lynch, V., Lloyd, G., and Fimbres, M. (Eds.) (1993). *The Changing Face of AIDS.* Westport, CT: Greenwood Publishing Group.

Wiener, L.S., Halpern A., and Best, A. (1994). Children Speaking Out About HIV Infection: Learning from Their Experiences. In P.A. Pizzo, and C.M. Wilfert (Eds.), *Pediatric AIDS: The Challenge of HIV Infection in Infants, Children, and Adolescents,* second edition. Baltimore: Williams and Wilkins, pp. 937-962.

Wiener, L. Best, A., and Pizzo (1994). *Be a Friend: Children Who Live with HIV Speak.* Albert Whitman and Company.

Journal of Developmental and Behavioral Pediatrics. (1994). Supplement: Priorities in Psychosocial Research in Pediatric HIV Infection. 15(3).

REFERENCES

Bingham, R., and Guinyard, J. (1982). Counseling Black Women: Recognizing Societal Scripts. Paper presented at the 90th Meeting of the American Psychological Association, Honolulu.

Boyd-Franklin, N., and Aleman, J. (1990). Black, Inner City Females and Multigenerational Issues: The Impact of AIDS. *New Jersey Psychologist, 40*: 14-17.

Daly, D., Jennings, J., Beckett, J.O., and Leashore, B.R. (1995). Effective Coping Strategies of African Americans. *Social Work, 40*(2): 240-248.

Journal of Adolescent Health (July 1993) Supplement: Guide to Adolescent HIV/ AIDS Program Development *14*(5).

Mandel, J., and Namir, S. (1985). Overview of Treatment Issues. Presented at AIDS and Mental Health Policy, Administration, and Treatment Conference, University of California, San Francisco, September 13-14.

Mays, V.M., and Cochran, S.D. (1987). Acquired Immunodeficiency Syndrome and Black Americans: Special Psychosocial Issues. *Public Health Reports 102:*224-231

Olson, R.A., Huszti, H.C., Mason, P.J., and Seibert, J.M. (1989). Pediatric AIDS/ HIV Infection: An Emergency Challenge to Pediatric Psychology. *J Pediatric Psychology 14*: 1-21.

Oquendo, M.A. (1995). Differential Diagnosis of Ataque De Nervios. *Journal of Orthopsychiatry, 65*(1): 60-65.

Tasker, M. (1992). *How Can I Tell You?* Bethesda, MD: Association of the Care of Children's Health.

Wiener, L.S., DuPont, E., Davidson, R., Fair, C., and Steinberg, S. (1993). National Telephone Support Groups: A New Avenue Toward Psychosocial Support for HIV-Infected Children and Their Families. *Social Work with Groups, 16*(3), pp. 55-71.

Wiener, L.S., and Septimus, A. (1994). Psychosocial Support for Child and Family. In P.A. Pizzo and C.M. Wilfert (Eds.), *Pediatric AIDS: The Challenge of HIV Infection in Infants, Children, and Adolescents*, second edition. Baltimore: Williams and Wilkins, pp. 809-828.

Helping a Parent with HIV Tell His or Her Children

Lori S. Wiener

WHY DO THIS?
STATEMENT OF THE PROBLEM AND ISSUES

One of the first and most difficult questions an individual struggles with after learning that he or she is HIV positive is who to share this information with and when. This is especially true if the individual is a parent of a dependent child. For HIV-infected parents, the thought of telling their children that their parent will likely become very sick and die during their childhood is almost too painful to consider. Resistance to such disclosure is common. Years often go by before the parent feels the time has come when he or she must communicate this truthful reality.

The stigma surrounding AIDS complicates the parental decision to share information about the disease with their children. Significant public fear and ignorance regarding the nature and transmission of HIV still exists. While many communities have responded positively to persons with AIDS, too many children have been ostracized, rejected, and stigmatized when their parents' or their own illness became publicly known. In order to avoid the potential humiliation and disgrace concerning being exposed, parents with AIDS are sometimes further burdened with keeping their diagnosis a secret. Despite the legitimate reasons for keeping the HIV diagnosis a closely guarded secret, many parents yearn to leave the world of concealment and lies, a world often in conflict with their own moral values (Tasker, 1992). This decision is as personal as it is complex.

EXAMPLES OF HOW THE ISSUE MAY PRESENT

At some point, children need to be informed of important changes in their lives such as a parent's illness. Children sense when something out of the ordinary is happening. Silence and secrecy deprive children of the opportunity to share feelings and ask questions. When children are not

327

included in this process they often feel confused, alone, and abandoned. When family members do decide to share the diagnosis, they often seek help in doing so in a style appropriate to their children's age, emotional development and cognitive abilities. It is essential that all social work interventions work from a developmental understanding of children's needs.

AGE CONSIDERATIONS

Preschool Children

Children this age do not understand differences between diseases and will probably be helped best by a general description of the illness. An example might be the following: "Mommy has an infection. This means some germs have gotten into her blood that are making her sick. Mommy is doing everything the doctors are saying to get better."

The child who is under twenty-four months of age does not fully understand illness. Death is not perceived as a permanent happening. Preschoolers (children ages two to five years) need to have the parent repeat the message over time. "You know mommy is very, very sick these days and may not get well. Mommy may die. When that happens, you and your daddy and brother won't be able to see me anymore." The child may begin asking questions about death at this point. Responses should not be complicated and should be consistent with the parents' spiritual and religious beliefs.

Children Ages Five to Eight Years

Between the ages of five to seven years, the child has a better understanding of death and illness. He or she will need more detailed information, and it is important that his or her questions be answered. They will want to know the exact name of the disease, what causes it, who they can tell about it, and whether the parent will live or die. They will want to know if they can get the disease. The more facts they have the better. It is important to help the parent not to misinterpret natural curiosity as morbid or bizarre. However, the child between the ages of five and seven still lacks the ability to deal with the intensity of the feelings associated with progressive illness and/or death of a loved one. The risk at this age is that they may believe that they are responsible for bad things happening and, as a result, may feel guilty and become withdrawn. Although changing those kinds of beliefs is hard, parents must tell the child that he or she did not cause them to be sick. Children this age also fear that they will get sick and die. The child who is not HIV-infected will need reassurance that he or she is well and that death is not likely to occur any time soon. For the child who is HIV-infected, differentiating between the parent's symptoms and his or her own is important. All children need to be told that their parent is doing everything possible to get well and that this will continue. What is said is important, but how it is said will have a greater bearing on whether the child will accept the reality of the situation without having frightening fantasies. A caring, controlled tone of a parent's voice will communicate feelings more completely than any particular words. Children need to feel their parent's warmth and affection. Parents should be encouraged to provide physical comfort and to speak softly and accurately. AIDS and HIV infection comprise a stigmatizing illness, and the school-age child will need help in learning how to deal with friends. Frequently asked questions include the following: "What can I tell my friends? What if my friends ask me what is wrong with you? Should I tell them the truth? Should I lie? What exactly should I say?" These are really tough questions, and children this age benefit greatly by being able to talk openly and honestly with their parent about these concerns. Social workers can help children enormously at this point by providing them with a safe environment in which to ask questions and to begin to come to terms with the implications that HIV will have on their life. Children are also helped by participating in a support group with other children dealing with the same issues.

Children Ages Nine to Twelve Years

Children of this age may regularly ask specific questions about how their parents became ill, including questions about sexual behavior, drug use, and/or homosexuality. They want answers and need correct information though each parent must remain sensitive to how much his or her child can cope with. Children may wish to take on more responsibility in the family, but parents need to be careful not to overwhelm them with too many tasks. They need a parent emotionally, perhaps more than before learning the diagnosis, and parents should be encouraged to let their child know that he or she does not need to take over the job of providing emotional support. While children this age typically understand the finality of death, they still may have some magical thinking concerning the death of older people only (grandparents, not parents). While discussing the issues of sickness and death, many children ask to be involved in the decisions about who their future care providers will be. Such open discussions are a healthy sign that the child is beginning to cope appropriately with what the future may bring.

Adolescents

Teenagers need to know the facts about HIV, but may not be as eager to hear them as school-age children are. Children between the ages of six and eleven use concrete facts to help them deal with painful feelings. They think that if they can learn all the facts, they can change the situation. Adolescents cope differently. They see reality more accurately, and if the reality hurts, they do not want to be forced to cope with its emotional impact. Adolescents want to belong; they want the approval of friends. Thus, they want to avoid anything that makes them feel different or makes others critical of them. As with school-age children, teenagers will need help figuring out who to tell and what to say. Again, open discussion with their parent's about these concerns will be most beneficial. Teenagers will then know they can approach their parents easily, and as the illness progresses, they will often continue to do so about matters that concern them. The teenager's premorbid personality, strengths, vulnerabilities, the kinds of losses already experienced, and the quality of the parental relationship will all affect how he or she will respond to learning that his or her parent(s) is HIV-infected. For those who have a history of depression and/or impulsivity, watching carefully for suicidal ideation is of utmost importance.

FACTS THE SOCIAL WORKER NEEDS TO KNOW
BEFORE PROCEEDING

Family decision making regarding disclosure of the diagnosis must take several factors into consideration, including the psychological effects on the child and family, coping abilities, and available environmental and social support systems. Before proceeding, it is important for the disclosing parent to identify a supportive adult that will be available to help the child(ren) process and cope with the information that is given. Social workers as well as noninfected extended family members have been very helpful in this role. Support groups have been an additional resource for many children coping with parental HIV-related illness.

Discussion of a parent's HIV diagnosis often leads to other disclosures, many of which have previously remained family secrets. Some of these include a biological parent's true identity, the identity of others in the family who have AIDS or who have died of the disease, and how the disease was transmitted (Lipson, 1994). Due to fear of rejection, mothers in particular who are struggling with feelings of guilt (feeling that their behavior or choices caused the disease) are often the most resistant to disclose the diagnosis. This is an issue that can be successfully dealt with in individual and conjoint counseling sessions with the parent(s) and child.

Talking to children about a parent's HIV disease takes preparation. Parents often find it helpful to first talk to another HIV-infected parent who has told the diagnosis to his or her child(ren). Another method parents find helpful is to role-play different scenarios that could occur at the time the information is given to the child.

The issue of where the intended discussion should take place and who will be present is of importance as well. While most parents ultimately decide they want to tell their children alone in the comfort of their own home, parents appreciate a social worker's offer to be present in case they "get into trouble" (which usually means they start to cry and cannot continue).

Disclosure of diagnosis is a process that takes place over time. One cannot expect children to understand all aspects of a parent's illness after one discussion. Many parents begin by explaining first that they are ill without providing the name of the disease. Others describe a virus in their blood but again do not name the virus. In time, the parent can then build on the information already given. For example, "Remember I told you that I have a virus that affects how I fight infections? That virus, which is known as HIV, has begun causing me some new problems. . . ." The full impact of the diagnosis will take weeks or sometimes years to absorb and will depend on several factors, such as how the illness is explained. Other factors include the parent's health at the time the child learns about the diagnosis and the support systems available to the child. In an attempt to help buffer the impact of the disease, some parents focus exclusively on the fact that it is HIV they have and not AIDS. This is an issue of semantics and clearly takes away from the child's need to acknowledge the illness and the realities associated with it. Honesty is also encouraged.

KEY QUESTIONS TO ASK THE CLIENT

Fully understanding the factors associated with parents' decision to share or not to share the diagnosis with their child is essential. Are there other disclosures that need to occur prior to the issue of an HIV diagnosis? What benefits does the parent anticipate occurring following disclosure? What are the counterindications that may result from sharing this information with the child? Helping parents write down a list of pros and cons has been useful for many.

As parents move closer to actually sharing the diagnosis with their child, they frequently seek reassurance that the social worker respects and supports their decision. This is especially true when the parent feels that his or her previous desire to maintain the secrecy of the diagnosis was understood and respected. When a parent decides to share the HIV diagnosis with his or her children, there are several questions that he or she should be prepared to answer. These include the following:

- Why did this happen to you?
- Where did you get it from?
- Who else has it? (Does Daddy? Grandma?)
- Am I the reason you got sick?
- Am I going to get it too?
- Does it hurt?
- Does "so and so" know?
- Who can *I* tell?
- Are you going to die?
- What will happen to me and (siblings)?

Such preparation in anticipating the child's questions and responses is both helpful and appreciated.

CULTURAL COMPETENCY CONSIDERATIONS

Parents who are living with HIV reflect increasing diversity in terms of their age, family heritage, belief systems, economic circumstances, and geographic location (Draimin, 1995). However, regardless of their heritage, all of these parents must face the difficult issue of sharing their diagnosis with their children.

While no data are available on what role culture plays in the decision to reveal or conceal the HIV diagnosis, the way the disease is acquired will affect how it is perceived and accepted by different cultures. The decision of whether or not to discuss sensitive issues such as sexual activity (including homosexuality) and drug use varies greatly, not only between those who share a cultural heritage but between individual family members themselves. Secrecy does not rest with any one specific ethnic group. Therefore, patterns of managing other family secrets will be instrumental in understanding how a particular family might feel about sharing a parent's HIV diagnosis with the children. It is important, however, to be aware of the stigma associated with this disease in certain communities. For groups such as African Americans who have already experienced a life marked by racial discrimination, HIV threatens to add a further token of marginality or "shameful difference" (Goffman, 1962). When the illness is believed to be caused by a serious breach of widely held community values, sympathy may be diminished or nonexistent (Groce, 1995). These individuals will thus be more likely to utilize outside support services (Brancho de Carpio, Carpio-Cedrano, and Anderson, 1990).

There is no one *culturally sensitive* way to disclose the HIV diagnosis. There is a sensitive way, though, and that is for the social worker to make every effort to understand the cultural beliefs of each family. Some cultures envision the mental health needs of children differently than middle-class Anglican Americans do (Groce, 1995). A great mistrust for mental health professionals can block potentially effective social work intervention. Parents have different beliefs about how old a child should be before being "burdened" with issues concerning illness and loss. When older children are not considered mature enough to understand issues related to life and death, they may not receive any explanation if a parent becomes sick with AIDS (Groce, 1995).

The parent living with HIV disease should be the judge concerning when and how to disclose the HIV diagnosis to his or her children. When parents do decide to share the information of their disease with their children, it should be done in their own words and in their native language. Remember, no two parents are alike, even if they share the same cultural heritage or ethnic affiliation.

ACTION STEPS FOR SUCCESSFUL INTERVENTION

Assessing a parents' readiness to share the HIV diagnosis is an essential step prior to the actual disclosure. Patience on the part of the social worker is needed. In order to be successful, the parent, not the social worker, needs to be ready. When the parent is ready, he or she is frequently willing to either "practice" telling his or her child by role-playing the discussion with their social worker or with another person who is trusted. A few basic guidelines to follow in preparing a parent for this very difficult event include the following.

1. Help parents identify a place where they would like to tell their children the diagnosis and who they would like to be present.
2. Assist parents in thinking about what is the most important message they want their child to walk away with. For example, "Nothing is going to change right now," or "I will never lie to you . . ."

3. Prepare parents for their child's potential reactions—which could range from crying uncontrollably and rage to acting indifferent.
4. Provide a supportive individual to whom the parent can talk and with whom he or she can process the discussion after the disclosure.

POTENTIAL BARRIERS TO SUCCESSFUL INTERVENTION

Remember that there is often other information that needs to be shared prior to the HIV diagnosis. If the child is having a hard time coping with some of the other disclosures (such as paternity), it is contraindicated to share the HIV diagnosis at that time. Timing is essential.

Regardless of the best social work interventions, some parents will decide not to share their diagnosis with their children. This becomes quite problematic when the parent becomes ill and the child learns from someone other than their parent the true source of the illness. Ongoing supportive counseling with the children is always indicated in this case.

When a parent shares the diagnosis with his or her children, some become so angry about either not having been told earlier or for all the previous lies that they have been told (and that they then told others) that healthy communication between the children and parent becomes compromised. This can be alleviated over time by consistent support, patience, and persistence on the part of the parent.

It is usually not until days or weeks after disclosure that the child has the courage to ask more questions. However, after sharing the diagnosis with their children, some parents feel so relieved that "it is over" that they feel that they hardly ever need to talk about it again. This blocks open communication at a time when the sharing of concerns about both the disease itself and the impact it has on all family members is most important. It also provides the child with the message that one must cope with this "on his or her own" or in emotional isolation from one another. The thought of not being able to "tell a soul" places a huge burden on the child. It is essential that they are provided with at least one person to whom they can talk about their parent's disease. If not, acting-out behaviors (often manifested as running away), substance use, suicidal ideation, and/or withdrawal are often seen.

INFORMATION THE CLIENT SHOULD KNOW BEFORE TAKING ACTION

Despite having been told the best of information, children often need certain statements to be repeated frequently. Parents also benefit from having some guidelines when deciding what is most important to talk to their children about. The following "helpful hints" can be shared with clients when they are ready to talk to their children about their disease.

1. All children need constant reassurance that they did not cause the illness.
2. Assure the child that HIV is hard to get. You DO NOT get it from hugging or kissing or food or dishes or bathrooms.
3. Prepare the child that the parent may need help for a long time and that the child may need to help more around the house, more than his or her friends help in their homes.
4. The parent should also prepare the child that he or she *may* look different as the disease progresses and so not to be very frightened if this happens. The child should also be aware that the parent may need to be hospitalized from time to time and should understand what will happen and who will care for him or her during those times.
5. The parent and child should talk openly about feelings such as sadness, frustration (when the parent is too tired to play for long periods of time), anger (other parents can do things their parent is too sick to do), guilt (again assuring the child they did nothing to cause the current situation), as well as happy feelings and the future.
6. Let the child know that no matter how difficult the subject matter, he or she can always ask questions and share feelings. Some parents have found it helpful to have another person in the family, a close friend, or even a professional available on a consistent basis for the child to talk to in addition to themselves.
7. It is very tempting for parents to keep the truth from their child in an attempt to shield him or her from further pain. However, this often has the reverse effect. The child's anxiety may increase due to knowing something is wrong but not understanding what it is. Separation anxiety or other anxiety-related symptoms often appear in these children. Once the parent lies about something and the child finds out, the child frequently questions what else the parent knows and has not revealed. They also tend to keep their thoughts to themselves, in an attempt to protect their parent from their true worries and fears. Keeping communication open between the parent and child is very important. It allows for increased closeness and a feeling of togetherness during a time that is clearly difficult for everyone.
8. Encourage the family to keep life as normal as possible. Whenever possible, routines should be kept the same as before the parent became ill, for example, meal times, school-related activities, and bedtimes should remain constant.

9. Life, however, is not normal for the child. Parents often find they have higher expectations for their children now because they cannot do all the things they were able to do prior to getting sick. When the child is stressed, he or she will do less, and this can easily lead to conflict between the child and parent. Encourage the parents to take a step back and ask themselves if what they are expecting from their child is really appropriate considering their age and emotional needs.

10. Suggest that whenever feasible, the family do as many fun things together as possible. Nothing elaborate is needed. For example, a day of shopping or an afternoon at the movies is an activity they appreciate and will always remember. If the parent is feeling too ill to get out of the home, watching favorite television shows together, baking, or doing art projects can create very special times.

11. When a parent tells his or her children about the family's cultural heritage, family history, and information about their own childhood, children are provided a sense of pride, belonging, and identity. There are many different ways a parent can do this. Some choose to make memory books with their children; others choose to make one on their own. Writing letters to each child, making a videotape to leave for the family, and creating photo albums are other ways parents choose to share information with their children (see Susan Taylor-Brown's chapter on legacies).

POLICY IMPLICATIONS AND RELATED ACTIONS

When working with a child who is HIV-infected, it is important to be aware of whether or not a school policy exists for the inclusion of infected children. If it does, learning the specifics of the policy (for example, who in the school needs to be informed of the diagnosis) will help the family decide whether or not to inform the school. Generally, disclosure by medical personnel of the HIV status of a child to school officials can only be given with expressly authorized informed consent by parents or legal guardians. However, some states (such as Illinois and South Carolina) have just passed mandatory reporting of HIV status of children to school principles or superintendents (Harvey, 1995). The National Association of State Boards of Education has published a comprehensive guide to policy and procedure development for schools that examines confidentiality issues among other school-related concerns.

Social workers should also be aware of laws that could potentially affect families. These include federal antidiscrimination legislation, the Fair Housing Amendments Act of 1988, as well as HIV confidentiality statutes, which are state-specific. In addition to the protections offered by antidiscrimination laws, persons with HIV may have legal protection against unauthorized disclosure of their medical diagnosis and related information. When one reasonably expects information communicated to another to be protected against unwanted disclosure to a third party, a duty of confidentiality may be said to arise (Katz, 1994). A breach of this duty occurs when an individual under such a duty either intentionally discloses the protected information without consent or fails to reasonably ensure that the information is protected (Powers, 1991; Katz, 1994).

In addition to being familiar with the Office of Civil Rights in your own community, social workers must also be familiar with individual state regulations and local policies as they apply to issues related to HIV infection.

RECOMMENDED READINGS

Tasker, M. (1992). *How can I tell you?* Bethesda, MD: Association of the Care of Children's Health.
Wiener, L., Pizzo, P., and Best, A. (1994). *Be a friend: Children who live with HIV speak.* Morton Grove, IL: Albert Whitman and Company.

REFERENCES

Broncho de Carpio, A., Carpio-Cedrano, F., and Anderson, L. (1990). Hispanic families learning and teaching about AIDS. *Journal of Behavioral Sciences, 12*(2): 165-176.
Campos, A.A. (1988) *Puerto Rican perspective on counseling. Counselling and Treating People of Color, 1*(1): 2.
Draimin, B. (1995) A second family? Placement and custody decisions. In S. Gegalle, J. Gruendel, and W. Andiman (Eds.) *Forgotten children of the AIDS epidemic.* New Haven, CT: Yale University Press, pp. 125-139.
Goffman, E. (1962). *Stigma: Notes on the management of spoiled identity.* New York: Simon and Shuster.
Groce, N.E. (1995). Children and AIDS in a multicultural perspective. In S. Gegalle, J. Gruendel, and W. Andiman (Eds.) *Forgotten children of the AIDS epidemic.* New Haven, CT: Yale University Press, pp. 95-106.
Harvey, D.C. (1995). Confidentiality and public policy regarding children with HIV infection. *The Connection, 2*: 1-5.
Katz, D.L. (1994). Legal issues relevant to HIV-infected children in home, day care, school, and community. In P.A. Pizzo, and C.M. Wilfert (Eds.) *Pediatric AIDS: The challenge of HIV infections in infants, children, and adolescents.* Baltimore: Williams and Wilkins, pp. 907-922.

Lipson, M. (1994). Disclosure of diagnosis to children with HIV or AIDS. *Journal of Behavioral and Developmental Pediatrics, 15*(3): S61-S65.

Powers, M. (1991). Legal protections of confidential medical information and the need for antidiscrimination laws. In R. Faden, F. Geller, and M. Powers (Eds.) *AIDS, women, and the next generation: Towards a morally acceptable public policy for HIV testing of pregnant women and newborns.* New York: Oxford University Press, pp. 221-255.

Tasker, M. (1992). *How Can I Tell You?* Association of the Care of Children's Health, 42 U.S.C. SS3601-3619 (1989 Supp.).

Talking with Parents About Creating a Legacy for Their Children

Lori S. Wiener
Susan Taylor-Brown

WHY DO THIS?
STATEMENT OF THE PROBLEM AND ISSUES

One of the most difficult and painful realizations for parents with HIV to face is the possibility that they will most likely die before their children become adults (Taylor-Brown and Wiener, 1993). All parents hope to care for their children until they are ready to establish independent lives as young adults. HIV threatens a parent's ability to accomplish this developmental task and creates a painful psychosocial aspect of this illness.

This "out of season" loss is difficult for any parent to address. The stigma surrounding HIV disease complicates this task further by creating a situation in which parents are reluctant to disclose their illness for fear of rejection of themselves or their children. The stigma of HIV/AIDS may keep a parent from ever telling a child about the life-threatening illness. Even after parental death, some children are never told the reality. Caregivers frequently avoid discussing the deceased parent out of fear of upsetting the child. Others avoid talking about the parent because of their unresolved issues with the deceased parent. For children placed with nonrelatives, the new caregiver may have little if any personal information about the parent. For these reasons, helping parents to create legacies for their children has become an important social work role within the AIDS pandemic. It is a proactive approach that empowers parents by providing them with a medium to leave a legacy for their children. Parents are able to tell their children in their own words what they hope for their future and to provide ways for the children to remember them. Each form of remembrance is unique and special for the child.

Creating a legacy can lay the foundation for exploring the parent's painful reality of premature parental death. It can serve as a vehicle for addressing the need to establish guardianship for surviving children. In the context of creating a legacy for their children, you can facilitate early permanency planning by discussing this emotion-filled topic with parents while emphasizing it as a way they can positively shape their children's uncertain future. This supportive approach helps detoxify the painful possibility of a motherless/fatherless future.

The social worker can explore different legacy options including writing letters, collecting photographs, creating a family tree, and making audio or videotapes. Special jewelry, art work, clothing, or other treasured possessions are also part of preserving a parent's heritage.

EXAMPLES OF HOW THE ISSUE MAY PRESENT

Typically creating a legacy is not something that many HIV-infected parents will initiate discussion of spontaneously; usually, a social worker introduces the topic. Initial resistance is quite common. One father kept avoiding the topic by saying, "I feel too well to talk about that—it makes me too sad." Some parents will express concern about how they will be remembered by their children when they die. They *want* to be remembered. This is an opportunity to explore with them what they have done already to preserve family memories. Many families do not have a lot of family pictures and will need encouragement to systematically save things of importance. Giving a parent a disposable camera with which to take family pictures can be an inexpensive and rewarding beginning to the project. Taking a picture during an appointment can help initiate the process.

How the topic of creating a legacy is presented influences a parent's receptivity to it. Discussions related to building legacies for their children are best done within the context of future planning that emphasizes empowerment and parental creativity. A parent is simultaneously balancing hope for the future while coping with a life-threatening disease. Creating a legacy can be discussed informally in terms of taking stock of what the parent has done to preserve family memories to date. Alternately, the issue can be raised as a specific topic to address one on one or in a group addressing capturing family memories.

FACTS THE SOCIAL WORKER
NEEDS TO KNOW BEFORE PROCEEDING

In the process of healthy development, children strive on both a conscious and an unconscious level to maintain psychological access to their deceased parent (Lohnes and Kalter, 1994). They often hold on tight to whatever concrete evidence of their parent that they can find as a means of maintaining a link to him or her. Such evidence, which becomes important keepsakes, frequently includes notes, letters, jewelry, clothing, and photographs. In fact, children's memories and reminders of their deceased parents almost always become their most cherished possessions. Such memories become very important in their adjustment and their attempt to maintain an attachment to their deceased parent. Children, as well as adults who have lost someone significant in their life, frequently report that they wish they had "more" of that person by which to remember them. This is especially true for bereaved children. As a result, helping parents to leave such legacies behind is an essential component of the permanency planning process.

Legacies may take many different forms:

1. A videotape made by the parent and left for the child has proved to be extremely therapeutic and beneficial to many. It provides a parent with an opportunity to say good-bye to his or her child and to share many thoughts that either the child would be too young to understand at the time of the parent's death or that the parent had been reluctant to express face to face.

   Of the surviving children, 25 to 30 percent are also HIV-infected themselves. These infected children, while facing their own disease, may find additional solace and strength in their parents' messages. For any child old enough to appreciate such a tape, it can also provide him or her with a sense of security in being able to witness his or her parent's expression of love.

   The timing of making such tapes is of great importance. The parent should be in relatively good physical health as children want to remember their parents as "looking good." One mother had wanted to make a tape but became seriously ill before the arrangements were made. After her hospitalization, she felt that she looked too ill to make a tape. She wrote her son and daughter letters instead. The unpredictability of central nervous system involvement is another reason to tape in the earlier stages of illness rather than later.

   Parents should also be psychologically prepared to undertake such an emotionally difficult process. While emotionally draining, the process is also very rewarding. One mother described it as one of the most important things she did for her baby daughter. Tapes are best made with a social worker or mental health professional with whom the parent has worked closely.

2. For those parents who are not able or who are uncomfortable with making a videotape, other ways to create a feeling of remembrance are needed. For example, creating a memory book, or what is known as a life review book, provides extremely useful memories for children. Within such a book, parents can recall stories that they enjoyed telling their

children; stories regarding their child's first words, first steps, or first day of school; as well as stories about their family history. Actual family trees are very useful. Many parents have not told their children about their extended families; a genogram can provide this information.

Children greatly enjoy learning about their parents as well. Encourage parents to include information about themselves, for example, their childhood, education, working life, leisure activities, special memories, important friends, as well as what they want their children to remember about them. Children take great delight in hearing stories that are funny or special incidents pertaining to their childhood. "What I always want you to remember about me is that I. . . ." If at all possible, it is best if the parent can make this book with their child. The process of creating such an important document together prior to a parent's death will only add to the significance of such a book.

3. For parents who enjoy writing, creating an autobiography can be very therapeutic. The Hospice Foundation of America has produced *A Guide for Recalling and Telling Your Life Story*, which includes several books and leads a person through the process of recording his or her life. It is intended for both caregivers who may help others in the recalling and for the person who is doing the recalling. Some parents will be more comfortable creating an audiotaped version of their life stories. This is particularly effective with parents who are highly verbal but do not read or write at a comparable level. You can offer to have the audiotape transcribed so that the child will have both written and audiotape copies of the parent's message.

4. Writing a book or even a journal may not be possible for all parents. In such cases, compiling an album of photographs and stories, leaving special jewelry or clothing for the child to wear, or writing poems or letters have also been very useful. Children also enjoy listening to their parent's voice and my benefit greatly from hearing their parent read their favorite bedtime story. By recording such stories on audio- or videotapes, parents can create a valuable gift, not only for the child but also for the child's future children.

KEY QUESTIONS TO ASK THE CLIENT

The question "If only I had asked?" occurs to most adults when it becomes important to understand more about their heritage or family history. Asking parents what they would want to know from a significant person in their life who has died allows them to begin thinking about what information they want to leave for their children.

The social worker can then explore different mediums (audiotape, letters, videotapes, etc.) that the parent can use to create such legacies. All of the mediums can incorporate similar content.

Several questions can help guide the parent in this process. What do you want (or not want) your child to know about your HIV? What special accomplishments or memories do you want to share? Do you wish to share family history? Do you want to recall specific aspects of family life? Children love to hear about themselves as children. One father described his son's ability to open every safety gate that was supposed to keep him out of danger. The son loved to hear about his early adventures.

The final questions focus on how the parent hopes to be remembered. This is an opportunity to again tell the child how much he or she was loved. What coping strategies do you want your child to use during the rough times? Are there special friends and family members to turn to? How do you want to close this? Remembrance?

CULTURAL COMPETENCY CONSIDERATIONS

McGoldrick, Pearce, and Giordano (1982) have shown that health care providers must develop cultural sensitivity toward different sets of norms and beliefs held by their patients and families, and the ways in which these culturally determined attitudes aid or adversely affect the delivery of health and mental health services. HIV/AIDS in women and children is predominantly affecting African-American and Latina women. Cultural beliefs and heritage are major determinants concerning how individuals feel about death and bereavement (Dudley, 1993).

In developing a legacy project, the social worker needs to collaborate with the parent to gain an understanding of his or her personal and cultural beliefs in developing a personal remembrance. The type of legacy a parent develops will be influenced by his or her ethnicity. AIDS-related deaths are treated by many African-American families as a toxic family secret (Boyd-Franklin, 1989). Many families will think it is not appropriate to discuss this with children (Boyd-Franklin and Alemán, 1990). African-American parents may be unlikely to disclose their HIV status in their legacy activity (Daly, 1995). The important thing is to convey their love to their children, not whether they acknowledge their HIV disease or not.

ACTION STEPS FOR SUCCESSFUL INTERVENTION

HIV/AIDS work confronts all of us with our own mortality. In order to help a parent create a legacy, the social worker has to be aware of his or her own responses to confronting death. Parents may feel profound sadness when they contemplate dying before their children have grown. Social workers need the emotional reserves to listen to parents' concerns and to help them make legacies and permanency plans. In addition to self-awareness, the social worker should have ongoing supervision to examine the issues that arise and to be supported while doing this challenging work. An open acknowledgement of the inherent loss opens the door for professional caregivers to cope with their emotional responses effectively.

Many parents and children find they feel closer to each other when they have the opportunity to create a life review book together. Such a memory book will hold special importance in the years to come as it was project created side by side at a difficult time in their life together. The process of creating this book is also therapeutic for the parents as it provides an opportunity to review their life, while assuring them that once in print, it will always be remembered. Providing the parent with an opportunity to create other legacies (as described earlier in this chapter) allows family values and beliefs to be sustained in the generations to come.

Group interventions to legacy building appear promising. A psycho-educational group, Capturing Memories, is being piloted by Taylor-Brown and colleagues. This is an eight-session group that addresses the preservation of family history and creation of a family legacy. Members benefit from peer support and universalization of their concerns. Some of the pilot group members have offered to mentor parents in the next Capturing Memories session.

POTENTIAL BARRIERS TO SUCCESSFUL INTERVENTION

Some parents will find it too painful to confront their own mortality and will be unable to focus on developing a legacy for their children. Many parents have experienced a number of traumatic losses and do not have the emotional reserves to confront their impending death or to acknowledge the related losses. A parent should not be prodded into this activity if he or she is not emotionally prepared to do so. In this case, the social worker can take family notes and develop a letter for the child at a later date.

Assisting parents in recording their histories in a way that does not make them feel ashamed about their limitations is important. For example, one mother appeared disinterested in the project until she was able to share that she could not write well. This admission was surprising, given how verbal she was. She was afraid that her children would think she was stupid if she misspelled something. In order to facilitate the legacy-making process, it is recommended that the options of audiotaping, video-taping, and writing letters be offered simultaneously to parents.

Additionally, sensitivity to the clinical issues that arise during the development of the family history can provide the practitioner with an opportunity to help the parent heal. As one father prepared to make a videotape, he told about his past experiences of being sexually abused and the influence it had on his life. By openly discussing this with the social worker, he was able to gain greater insight into his life and to reconcile his experiences. In his videotape, he delivered a powerful message to his sons about not letting other people exploit them. Legacy building can help people address past difficulties and reframe them.

Sometimes parents enter care at an advanced stage of illness and are unable to create a legacy project. At the very least, they should be encouraged to create a card or an audiotape for their child. Recently, a woman was admitted to the intensive care unit from the initial clinic visit for an HIV workup. She was diagnosed with primary pulmonary hypertension, and her condition was critical. The nurse practitioner helped her make a tape of her son's favorite bedtime stories. She died the next day. While it was impossible to create an extensive legacy, her five-year-old does have a special tape of her mom telling a story and stating her love for her.

INFORMATION THE CLIENT SHOULD KNOW BEFORE TAKING ACTION

As parents begin to develop a legacy, they may experience a flood of emotions. Anticipatory guidance can help them to cope with this if it happens. Equally, this intervention may help parents reconnect with family members from whom they have become estranged. These family members may become resources for the parent's children.

Parents need reassurance that you will proceed at a pace with which they feel comfortable. In our experiences, some parents are ready immediately while others may take years to develop their legacy. Your willingness to work with them can be very reassuring, and anticipatory guidance about the range of emotions they may experience will help prepare them. Additionally, having your patients talk with a parent who has made a remembrance can help inspire them.

Encourage parents to make copies of all legacies that they create. For example, videotapes wear out; therefore, a master tape should be made. If parents make a videotape for their child to have after they die, they need to decide where the video is to be housed. They need to also consider when the video is to be seen (weeks after the parent dies for example) and who should be with the child when the video is seen for the first time. For those parents who anticipate a custody battle, it is important to clarify legally who is to have possession of the legacy they created for their children.

When creating legacies, parents should also be encouraged to think toward the future. For example, help them consider including information about not only what would be important for their child to know at this point in their development, but in the future as well. Are there key issues they want addressed? One mother spoke frankly with her daughter about abstaining from premarital sex. She felt it was essential to her daughter's sense of self. Her candor will certainly give her daughter a base upon which to build.

POLICY IMPLICATIONS AND RELATED ACTIONS

For videotaped legacies, social workers should consider where to house the master videotape. A parental release is needed, designating who can receive copies. In case the social worker who developed the tape leaves the agency in the future, the agency needs a policy regarding the family's future access to the video(s).

RECOMMENDED READINGS AND VIDEOS

Dane, B., and Levine, C. (1994). *AIDS and the new orphans.* Westport, CT: Auburn House.

Draimin, B. (1993). *Coping when a parent has AIDS.* New York: The Rosen Publishing Group. (Recommended for adolescents to read.)

Mandel, J., and Namir, S. (1985). "Overview of treatment issues." Paper presented at the AIDS and Mental Health Policy, Administration, and Treatment Conference, University of California, San Francisco, California.

Mays, V., and Cochran, S. (1987). Acquired immunodeficiency syndrome and black Americans: Special psychosocial issues. *Public Health Reports 102*: 224-231.

Taylor-Brown, S., and Wiener, L. (In Press). *If we had talked: A videotape for creating legacies.* Available from Lyn Blackburn, Community Health Network, 716-244-9000.

REFERENCES

Boyd-Franklin, N. (1989). *Black families in therapy: A multisystems approach.* New York: Guilford Press.

Boyd-Franklin, N., and Alemán, J. (1990). Black inner city females and multi-generational issues: The impact of AIDS. *New Jersey Psychologist 40*: 14-17.

Daly, A., Jennings, J., Beckett, J. and Leashore, B. (1995). Effective coping strategies of African Americans. *Social Work 40*(2): 240-248.

Dudley, R. (1993). All alike but each one is different: Orphans of the HIV epidemic. In C. Levine (Ed.), *A death in the family: Orphans of the HIV epidemic* (pp. 55-59). New York: United Hospital Fund of New York.

Lohnes, K., and Kalter, N. (1994). Preventive intervention groups for parentally bereaved children. *American Journal of Orthopsychiatry 64*(4): 594-604.

McGoldrick, M., Pearce, S., and Giordano, J. (Eds.) (1982). *Ethnicity and family therapy.* New York: Guilford Press.

Taylor-Brown, S., and Wiener, L. (October 1993). Making videotapes of HIV-infected women for their children. *Families in Society:* 468-480.

Talking with Parents
About Permanency Planning

Susan Taylor-Brown

WHY DO THIS?
STATEMENT OF THE PROBLEM AND ISSUES

As AIDS has become the leading cause of death for twenty-two- to forty-nine-year-olds, many of whom have children, there is an increasing impact that the disease is having on families. A major consequence of this pandemic is the large and growing number of AIDS orphans. It is expected that by the year 2000, there will be ten million orphans world-wide.* Extended family members and friends are trying to care for the children who have experienced parental loss. Foster care and adoption are options when the family is unable to intervene.

The social worker can explore with parents different options to pursue to ensure that their child(ren) are adequately provided for—when the parent is no longer able. An overriding concern of parents is keeping siblings together, but this desire to preserve sibling units is not always possible. Too often, siblings are separated because a relative cannot care for that many children or the foster care family is ineligible for placement of so many children. When one mother died, her five children ended up in five separate homes in three different states. These children lost not only their mother, but also each other and their lives as they had known them. Social workers are on the forefront of efforts to help the family of origin and the reconstructed family cope with parental loss.

EXAMPLES OF HOW THE ISSUE MAY PRESENT

One of the most difficult clinical issues is helping parents reach the point at which they can address future planning. Resistance is quite com-

---

*The recent report, *Families in crisis: Report of the working committee on HIV children and families* (1996), reported greater incidence rates than the original *Orphan Report.* It is now projected that by the end of 2000, in New York State alone, 58,000 children and other youths will have been orphaned since 1981 (range 40,000 to 70,000).

mon. Many HIV-infected parents will do whatever they can to care for their children while paying little attention to their own health care needs. Many others feel that if they begin to make plans for the future care of their children, this will be perceived as them being too negative or them accepting their future death. One mother stated, "I wish my case manager would stop bugging me about signing the guardianship papers. I made a deal with God when I got sober . . . If I stay clean, he'll let me see her graduate. If I sign, I'll die."

Often, not until a significant decline in a patient's immunological status or a first opportunistic infection occurs that the full implications of the disease become an emotional reality. At these stages, the need for permanency planning gains new significance. This may be the time for proactive social work intervention to be introduced and perhaps for permanency planning to initially be discussed.

The social worker can explore future childcare options with parents in order to help them avoid a situation in which custody is relinquished to the state after their death. Helping to facilitate parents' plans for their children respects their ability to make decisions for their children and increases their sense of control. Discussions related to building legacies for their children are best done within the context of future planning that emphasizes empowerment and parental creativity.

In the context of creating a legacy, a number of opportunities to introduce the long-term permanency planning arrangements will occur. Before introducing permanency planning to a parent, be sure that you know the available legal custody options for your state. Each custody option has varying degrees of parental rights and financial support (Draimin, 1995).

Social workers need to familiarize themselves with the options available to their clients. These include the following:

1. *Informal arrangements:* These are commonly made in African-American and Latino communities. The child does not have anyone monitoring him or her, and these arrangements are not legally binding.
2. *Power of attorney:* A person is designated to make decisions in the instance the parent is unable.
3. *Designation of a guardian in a will:* This clearly establishes the parent's wishes but it does not provide assurance that the person selected will become the guardian. The judge decides who will become the guardian, and the decision is made after the parent's death. Other family members can play a role in the decision, which may result in a change from the parent's wishes.
4. *Adoption:* The parent agrees to terminate parental rights permanently.

5. *Voluntary placement in foster care:* The parent requests out-of-home placement because of illness and kinship care or nonrelative care are the only options. The parent retains the right to make permanency plans.

6. *Involuntary placement in foster care:* A child is removed based upon an investigation of abuse or neglect. Kinship care or nonrelative care are the available options. The parent still retains the right to make permanency plans.

7. *Surrendering of parental rights:* The parent relinquishes his or her ability to make decisions on behalf of the child.

8. *Emergency and respite services:* The parent retains parental rights, and the family receives support services.

9. *Standby guardianship:* The parent retains parental authority, and a guardian has authority when the parent is incapacitated.

The advantages and disadvantages of each option should be explained to the parent. Each option entitles the child to different services and benefits. This is complex information that changes frequently; therefore, ongoing monitoring of policy changes is very important.

Standby guardianship, which allows parents to retain parental authority, is currently available in only a few states. Other states are reviewing similar legislation; thus, having accurate information for the parents with whom you are working is crucial. Different benefits are available with each guardianship option. For many families, successfully becoming a guardian as designated by a permanency plan is often contingent upon adequate financial support. For example, in New York a relative who becomes a standby guardian is ineligible to become a foster care parent to an orphaned child. The foster care parent is eligible for remuneration while the standby guardian is not. For a poor family, the addition of one, two, or more children without some financial assistance may be financially prohibitive. Since keeping siblings together is an overriding parental desire and is also developmentally desirable, all efforts should maximize the viability of siblings being placed together.

Custody planning forces a parent to address complex and emotionally charged issues. Some parents find it impossible to go through the planning process. It is not unusual for a parent to wait until end-stage disease or to never be able to make guardianship arrangements. Careful monitoring of a parent's emotional state and supportive counseling may help prepare him or her make the necessary arrangements. Clinicians must respect the parent's ability or inability to do this and plan accordingly for the children. The social worker who works closely with parents should be prepared to intervene when the parent requests it or when the parent dies.

Some parents are never able to designate a guardian because the task is simply too emotionally challenging. One must respect their level of readiness and support their emotional connection with their children. Equally important is being prepared to intervene on the child's behalf at any point in the disease course. It is too easy for these children to fall between the cracks because no tracking system is in place. Very little information is available regarding whether children who are orphaned are cared for by the guardians designated by their parents. No tracking system exists for children whose parents die of AIDS-related causes, and permanency planning programs focus on developing a guardianship plan without including an assessment of the viability of that plan at the same time of parental incapacity or death. To date, Gamble's (1992) unpublished report is the only known follow-up study.

"An unpublished, independent 1992 study by Ivy Gamble, MSW, on 43 Division of Aids Services (DAS) cases in the Bronx, noted that 84% of parents who had died of AIDS were between 20 and 50 years of age at death, more than 90% were people of color, and nearly two-thirds had more than one child (42% with two or three children)" (Gamble, 1996, pp. 19-20). "The legitimacy of this fear is affirmed by data from the Gamble study, which included the disheartening statistic that 57% of siblings were separated after the parent's death" (Gamble, 1996, p. 20).

Grandparents and aunts are by far the most likely new caregivers. Gamble (1992) reported that of fifteen families who had made permanency plans, not one was still with the designated caregiver after one year.

If possible, children should be allowed to have as much interaction as possible during the terminal phase of their parent's illness. If the dying parent cannot have visitors, ways to maintain the closeness between the parent and children become important. Telephone contact, handmade cards and presents, and other concrete items help the child feel connected and assists in processing the death and his or her loss (Dubik-Unruh, 1989). While most children say little during this phase, they are acutely aware of what is going on. Listen patiently to what the child is saying and what the child is asking. Respect that he or she may need some distance. The old social work proverb is of key importance here: *Be where the child is.* Answer questions, but do not give more information than is asked for.

Parental death is often a symbolic ending of the child's life as he or she has known it. The reconstituted family will benefit from clinical services addressing the losses experienced and the adjustments needed as the new family begins to function as a unit. Such losses include parental loss, loss of the family as the child knew it, and often the loss of sibling relationships when children are placed in separate homes. Bereaved children may act out their feelings of loss. The new guardians may feel uncomfortable about the child's response and uncertain about how to help the child grieve. They will benefit from education and guidance about the process of grieving and assistance in being supportive to the child who is trying to make sense of all that has happened.

KEY QUESTIONS TO ASK THE CLIENT

There are several questions that help guide the parent in this process. These include the following:

- Who would care for your children if you were hospitalized?
- Have you begun to think about an alternative guardian for your child(ren)? If so, who would this be?
- Is there anyone you know who would oppose your guardian decision?
- Have you thought about involving your children in choosing a guardian?
- Have you considered legal help?
- Would you like assistance finding legal counsel?
- If you cannot be here to raise you children, what do you want them to always remember about you and your family?
- What about any special times you spent together?
- Would you want to share with your children the goals and hopes you have for their future?
- Do any of your children have specific needs that you would like to see addressed?
- Would you like my [social worker's] assistance in helping you make permanency plans?

Encourage early permanency planning and normalize it by saying, "All parents should have backup guardianship arrangements for dependent children." Explain to parents how children frequently become caught in a custody battle between relatives once their biological parent dies. Sometimes a parent who has not been involved in rearing the child(ren) tries to assert his or her right to have custody, disregarding designated extended family members. For example, a mother had left her daughter in the care of her partner; however, she did not make legal arrangements. In the month following her death, the maternal grandmother took the child from the woman's partner. She has refused to let him have any contact with the little girl since then. She also rejected all of the mother's friends, whom the mother had worked with to provide support and guidance to her daughter. Despite the mother's clearly stated wishes, her daughter is not receiving the care or comfort she had desired because formal arrangements were not made. It is impossible to enforce informal requests such as this. They rely on the goodwill of all involved. The negative impact this has on children is clear to see.

CULTURAL COMPETENCY CONSIDERATIONS

For families with HIV, psychosocial support requires meaningful, ongoing communication with their social worker. The most basic element of this communication is through the sharing of the same language. A parent's basic understanding of the English language may be inadequate for the profound knowledge needed for dealing with such in-depth issues as medical care, confidentiality, and family beliefs (Wise, 1994).

Beyond language, social workers must possess some basic understanding of the meaning of illness, traditions, cultural beliefs, values, and family structure in the communities in which they work. Cultural beliefs and heritage are major determinants of how the family will make custody and placement decisions, as well as how its members feel about death and bereavement (Dudley, 1993). Therefore, it is essential that the social worker fully understand each family's personal and cultural beliefs, values, and family structure prior to discussing placement.

Each family defines family members differently. For some, it includes only immediate biological family members. For others, nonbiologically related kin may have more rights and responsibilities than the biological ones. Therefore, the social worker should not assume the child will be raised by biological family members until custody arrangements have been legalized through the court system.

Within many African-American families, the family is conceptualized beyond the nuclear family and may encompass distant relatives and "fictive kin" or members of the family who are not blood relatives (Daly et al., 1995). Within Latino families, *hijo de crianza* ("reared child") refers to a child who is raised by another family but whose parents have terminated their custodial rights. While such informal adoptions are common in many Latino communities, they are not legal custody plans. Some bicultural families avoid family court proceedings, which are seen as government interference in what should be a private matter. However, parents' wishes will be more binding when stated legally.

There are subtle differences among Southeast Asians and profound differences among Koreans, Chinese, and Japanese. It is essential that the social worker not make "culture-specific" generalizations but rather ask each parent what his or her personal wishes are for his or her children.

It is also very helpful for the social worker to be aware of distinctive cultural rituals for death, including how extended family members grieve. For example, in some cultures, expressions of grief are found in forms of dress, the color of clothes worn, the styling of hair, or the use of body paint or makeup. Feasts, wakes, rituals of light with candles or torches, offerings of flowers, incense, food, music and dance, poems, stories, or masses all comprise various grief rituals to which children are exposed (Hersh, 1995). Social workers must also specifically assess and differentiate between acculturated family members (those who have taken on the values and belief system of the dominant culture) and those who are bicultural (those who have learned to function in the dominant culture while retaining their original cultural identification, values, and belief system). It is important that the rituals reflect the parent's cultural stance. Knowledge of the client's immigration status is also essential because services are linked to immigration status. One woman from Zimbabwe has been refused services for the past six months while the Immigration Service is determining her status. As a result, her medical care is being donated, but her psychosocial services were terminated because she no longer has Medicaid.

ACTION STEPS FOR SUCCESSFUL INTERVENTION

A relationship based on trust is of utmost importance prior to discussing the issue of permanency planning. Patience, respect for the parent's timing, and knowledge of the legal system concerning wills, guardianship, and custody are crucial elements for success. Future guardianship plans must be discussed with the child and, if possible, the child, parent, and future guardian should spend time together discussing this matter as well.

Parents and practitioners alike, wonder, "Who will care for the children?" The reality is that no one will care for the child as the parent did. In many instances, we do not have adequate supports in place for surviving children and their caregivers. The social worker must do his or her best with limited resources at times.

Many parents and children find they feel closer to each other when they have the opportunity to create a life review book together. Such a memory book will hold special importance in the years to come as it was a project created side by side at a difficult time in their life together. The process of creating this book is also therapeutic for the parents as it provides an opportunity to review their life and assures them that they will always be remembered. Providing the parent with an opportunity to create other legacies (as described in the previous chapter) allows family values and beliefs to be sustained in the generations to come.

POTENTIAL BARRIERS TO SUCCESSFUL INTERVENTION

Permanency planning is a complex issue both emotionally and legally. Some parents find it too painful to confront their own mortality and make the appropriate plans for surviving children. Equally, the complex legal requirements may prevent the successful completion of permanency planning.

Due to an inability to care for their children, a minority of parents decide to relinquish their children prior to their death. However, in most cases, the child stays with the parent until the time of death. Many community AIDS organizations offer free legal services, and parents should be encouraged to make a will. Who should have possession of whatever legacy the parent leaves should also be specifically described in the will. Without such legal authorization, many personal legacies will not reach the child.

Frequently, the guardians selected may be unable to care for children either due to their own health or changing family circumstances. For some children, permanency planning involves a series of plans of limited duration. For example, one child was left with his mother's sister who subsequently died. His next guardian was his grandmother who become too frail to care for him. Permanency planning can be temporary for stressed family systems.

Despite parental desires to keep siblings together, they are often separated (Draimin, 1995). Regulations limit the number of children who can be placed in a foster home. The number of children allowed is based on the number of bedrooms. If the prospective guardian does not have adequate living space, a new residence may need to be located. Because this may be too costly for the guardian, the social worker may need to help secure housing funding. Siblings may be separated when one of them displays disruptive behavior. For example, one young man was placed in emergency foster care when he had aggressive outbursts. In this placement, he was hostile and withdrawn. The foster parents decided that he was a risk to their children, and he was placed subsequently in a group home.

INFORMATION THE CLIENT SHOULD KNOW
BEFORE TAKING ACTION

As parents make permanency plans, they should be encouraged to realistically assess potential guardians and to consider alternative guardians in the case that their first choice is unable to assume the responsibility. Parents need to talk to the prospective guardian. Parents whose children are already in foster care can participate in their child's permanency plan. They have a right to state their wishes regarding the type of guardian and to participate in the process of identifying a guardian. This can help parents and children to connect meaningfully although living separately.

Encourage parents to make copies of all legacies that they create. For example, videotapes wear out; therefore, a master tape should be made. If parents make a videotape for their child to have after they die, they need to decide where the video is to be housed. They need to also consider when the video is to be seen (for example, soon after the parent dies) and who should be with the child when the video is seen for the first time. For those parents who anticipate a custody battle, clarifying legally who is to have possession of the legacy they created is important.

When creating legacies, parents should also be encouraged to think toward the future. For example, help them consider including information about not only what would be important for their child to know at this point in their development, but in the future as well.

POLICY IMPLICATIONS AND RELATED ACTIONS

Most HIV-infected parents will describe the legal system as insensitive to their unique family needs. The law assumes that once a parent is ill or dies, the other parent is able and willing to provide care, a false assumption if the other parent is absent or has already become ill or died from AIDS (Geballe, 1995). In most states, the current law does not provide legal mechanisms for shifting responsibility for care of children during periods of temporary parental incapacity (Geballe, 1995). In a few states, such as New York, a standby guardian is a new option for terminally ill parents. This law allows parents who believe that they are at risk of dying within two years either to petition for a court appointment or to execute a designation of a standby guardian to become effective at a future date (Herb, 1993). The parent names the guardian of his or her choice. Once the standby guardianship goes into effect, the standby guardian fulfills the same functions as a traditional guardian (Herb, 1993). Guardianship does not terminate parental rights. The parent is still the decision maker for the child.

Advocacy efforts should focus on developing standby guardianship options in all states. The ability of parents to preserve their relationship and authority with their children while coping with a life-threatening illness should be paramount.

It is easy for practitioners' focus to remain primarily on those sick and in emergent need. However, in the midst of this disease, our attention must also focus on the needs of those children who are not infected. These children have lost so many of their family members to AIDS. Their needs must be addressed swiftly and with compassion, for they are the survivors of tomorrow (Fanos and Wiener, 1994).

RECOMMENDED READINGS

Bingham, R. and Guinyard, J. (1982). "Counseling black women: Recognizing societal scripts." Paper presented at the 90th Meeting of the American Psychological Association, Honolulu, Hawaii.

Boyd-Franklin, N. and Alemán, J. (1990). Black inner city females and multigenerational issues: The impact of AIDS. *New Jersey Psychologist 40*: 14-17.

Dane, B. and Levine, C. (1994). *AIDS and the new orphans.* Westport, CT: Auburn House.

Draimin, B. (1993). *Coping when a parent has AIDS.* New York: The Rosen Publishing Group. (Recommended for adolescents to read.)

Geballe, S., Gruendel, J., and Andiman, W. (Eds.) (1995). *Forgotten children of the AIDS epidemic.* New Haven, CT: Yale University Press.

Levine, C. (1993). *A death in the family: Orphans of the HIV epidemic.* New York: United Hospital Fund of New York.

Lipson, M. (1994). Disclosure of diagnosis to children with Human Immunodeficiency Virus or Acquired Immunodeficiency Syndrome. *Journal of Developmental and Behavioral Pediatrics 15*(3): S61-S65.

Lohnes, K. and Kalter, N. (1994). Preventive intervention groups for parentally bereaved children. *American Journal of Orthopsychiatry 64*(4): 594-604.

Mandel, J. and Namir, S. (1985). "Overview of treatment issues." Paper presented at the AIDS and Mental Health Policy, Administration, and Treatment Conference, University of California, San Francisco, California.

Mays, V. and Cochran, S. (1987). Acquired Immunodeficiency Syndrome and black Americans: Special psychosocial issues. *Public Health Reports 102:* 224-231.

REFERENCES

Committee on HIV, Children, and Families (1996). *Families in Crisis.* Report of the working on HIV, children, and families. Federation of Protestant Welfare Agencies, New York.

Daly, A. Jennings, J., Beckett, J., and Leashore, B. (1995). Effective coping strategies of African Americans. *Social Work 40*(2): 240-248.

Draimin, B. (1995). A Second Family?: Placement and Custody Decisions. In S. Geballe, J. Gruendel, and W. Andiman (Eds.), *Forgotten children of the AIDS epidemic*, (pp. 125-139). New Haven, CT: Yale University Press.

Dubik-Unruh, S. (1989). Children of chaos: Planning for the emotional survival of dying children of dying families. *Palliative Care 5*: 10-15.

Dudley, R. (1993). All alike but each one is different: Orphans of the HIV epidemic. In C. Levine (Ed.), *A death in the family: Orphans of the HIV epidemic* (pp. 55-59). New York: United Hospital Fund of New York.

Fanos, J. and Wiener, L. (1994). Tomorrow's survivors: Siblings of Human Immunodeficiency Virus-infected children. *Journal of Developmental and Behavioral Pediatrics 15*(3): S43-S48.

Gamble, I. (1992), as cited in *Families in Crisis,* pp. 19-20.

Gamble, I. (1993). In whose care and custody: New York: New York City Human Resources Administratio of AIDS Services.

Geballe, S. (1995). Toward a child-responsible legal system. In S. Geballe, J. Gruendel, and W. Andiman (Eds.) *Forgotten children of the AIDS epidemic* (pp. 140-164). New Haven, CT: Yale University Press.

Herb, A. (1993). The New York State Standby Guardianship Law: A new option for terminally ill parents. In C. Levine (Ed.), *A death in the family: Orphans of the HIV epidemic* (pp. 87-93). New York: United Hospital Fund of New York.

Hersh, S. (1995). The gentle psychiatrist. *Journeys Children's Issue.* Hospice Foundation of America Newsletter.

Wise, P. (1994). Expanding access to health care for infants, children, and adolescents. In P. Pizzo and C. Wilfert (Eds.), *Pediatric AIDS: The challenge of HIV infections in infants, children and adolescents* (pp. 975-984). Baltimore: Williams and Wilkins.

Working with Children with HIV in Day Care, Elementary, and Secondary Schools

Susan Taylor-Brown

WHY DO THIS?
STATEMENT OF THE PROBLEM AND ISSUES

The inclusion of a child with HIV (CWHIV) in day care or school settings has been controversial since the onset of the HIV/AIDS pandemic. The controversy reflects a blend of conflicting responses including the following: the fear of contagion versus the reality that casual transmission does not occur; the fears of some communities versus the courage of many individual parents, students, schools, and health officials; and the perception that schools are intent on excluding HIV-infected children versus the reality that most school systems have policies to protect the right to education for these students (Santelli, Birn, and Linde, 1992). These controversies have been very public, and as a result, many parents of CWHIV are reluctant to disclose their child's status.

As medical treatment has improved, more CWHIV are reaching the age to attend day care or school. Also, some CWHIV who were congenitally infected are being diagnosed during latency and early adolescence when they are already enrolled in school. A child's ability to function in the classroom depends on his or her health. Seventy-eight to 93 percent of children with symptomatic infection experience some developmental abnormality, which may affect classroom functioning (Task Force on Pediatric AIDS, 1991). Many of these children will need specialized placements to function in a school setting.

As the disease progresses, neuropsychological changes may occur, necessitating adaptations in the child's educational program. When children become more ill, medical appointments and hospitalizations increase, adversely affecting school performance. The child's functioning needs to be monitored on an ongoing basis and modified as warranted. Some children will need home tutoring or may be in school for only part of the day. Others

361

elect to be home-tutored because they cannot tolerate the questions from their peers about why they are sick so often or why they look different. Many children report that they are teased for being small-statured, which is a side effect of HIV medications. CWHIV report that this teasing about being small is more disruptive to their school experience than having HIV. Some schools promote home tutoring to avoid addressing the fears of teachers and/or other parents who oppose having a CWHIV in the classroom.

Parents respond uniquely to the educational needs of their children. Some adopt the stance that everything is the same as it has always been. These parents pressure their children to "keep up" their level of academic performance. Others perceive school as providing a needed opportunity for the child to socialize and continue life as if it were normal. Other parents are too ill themselves, or too busy caregiving other infected family members, to be interested in the child's educational experience.

Families may or may not feel comfortable telling the day care or school about their child's infection. As a result, many CWHIV may enter the school setting without parents sharing the diagnosis with the school. CWHIV want to be a part of their peer group and to blend in.

Families experience isolation as they hide the diagnosis from the teachers, school nurse, and other personnel. With each illness, the child and family worry about their secret being discovered. Parents are concerned about the child becoming sick while in school, and their reluctance to disclose their child's diagnosis stems from the early, widely publicized traumatic experiences of families. The media focused on children who were excluded or ostracized, including Ryan White and the Ray brothers. These media portrayals created anxiety for families with CWHIV and families whose children attended school with them. Both groups worry about how their respective children will be affected.

CWHIV strive to be "normal" in school and to maintain an appearance of "everything is fine." They struggle to keep up with the classroom expectations while knowing that their life expectancy is limited. For example, as a child focuses on her math assignment, she is simultaneously thinking that the next day she will be in the hospital for treatment or she may be worried about the health of other family members. Many of these children are grieving the loss of one or both of their parents. Their grief is often unacknowledged because the disease and its related losses are a family secret.

Creating a supportive school environment can enhance a CWHIV's coping. Developmentally, children thrive on being with their peers and interacting with others. The peer group assumes increasing importance for the maturing child. Each family and school responds uniquely to this challenge. Both the Centers for Disease Control (CDC) (1985) and the American Academy of Pediatrics (AAP) (Task Force on Pediatric AIDS, 1993b; 1988) released guidelines regarding the placement of children with HIV in the classroom. These guidelines provide a framework for making placement decisions based upon available knowledge while countering the fear expressed in communities. Each child's placement should reflect an individualized assessment of the child's medical, educational, and psychosocial needs. The guidelines have become progressively less restrictive, reflecting the continuing epidemiologic evidence that HIV is not casually transmitted (Santelli, Birn, and Linde, 1992). Many school districts have developed their own policies that incorporate these guidelines. Additionally, the development of local guidelines allows for community input.

EXAMPLES OF HOW THE ISSUE MAY PRESENT

One of the most challenging issues is helping parents decide whether or not to disclose their child's diagnosis to school personnel. Many parents are afraid that their children will be rejected or stigmatized if the diagnosis is revealed. Some may be reluctant to share the diagnosis with others because their son or daughter has not been told the diagnosis yet. The more people who know the diagnosis, the greater the likelihood that the child will find out from someone other than the parents. Although children may not know the exact diagnosis, they are painfully aware of their illness. They know what it is like to endure multiple medical procedures and to see health care providers regularly. Frequently, the child pressures the parents to disclose what is occurring.

When a CWHIV is ready to enter day care or school, parents are apt to ask you for assistance regarding whether or not to notify the school about the infection. Many will defer the decision until their child's illness becomes more apparent. Functionally, during its early stages, HIV may not be interfering with the child's performance. The first hospitalization often stimulates parents to examine school-related issues.

The social worker can explore possible reactions to the disclosure in order to help parents consider their options. Careful consideration of the advantages and disadvantages of disclosure should be explored. Unfortunately, some schools may respond negatively to a CWHIV, and anticipatory guidance can prepare parents for this possibility. (For further discussion, see Action Steps for Successful Intervention in this chapter.) By engaging parents in this process, you strengthen their sense of control as a parent. A cooperative school can be a source of tremendous support for parents. Frequently, parents who do receive support from the school wish that they had disclosed earlier. They describe a tremendous sense of relief.

When the school is uninformed, the possibility for supplemental services does not exist. Once the diagnosis is known, a child may be eligible for specialized services, such as peer support groups or specialized educational services. For example, the child may be placed in a group for children coping with loss, where he can learn a number of techniques for coping with his frustrations about being sick. This relieves some of his parents' burden. Those children with HIV/AIDS who do not require special education are protected by Section 504 of the Rehabilitation Act of 1973 (Smith, 1990). Section 504, also known as the *Rehabilitation Act of 1973,* prohibits discrimination in any federally funded program against a qualified handicapped person solely on the basis of his or her handicap.

Taking medication during the school day is often the foremost issue for CWHIV. Some try to sneak their medications without a school authority or other students knowing. In fear of being "caught," they frequently alter their medication schedule, which places them at risk for developing a serious illness. The child's medication schedule should be modified to maximize the child feeling comfortable about taking the medicine.

FACTS THE SOCIAL WORKER
NEEDS TO KNOW BEFORE PROCEEDING

Every child with a chronic illness strives to maintain as normal a lifestyle as possible. Attending day care or school is a key source of social interaction. A child's entry into a program sets the tone for his or her subsequent experiences in that setting. As a result, checking with the day care center about its HIV policy and prior experiences dealing with CWHIV is imperative. You can do this on behalf of the family without acknowledging who they are. Hopefully, the center has a policy that is supportive of CWHIV. In reviewing the policy, it is helpful to ask the following:

- Has anyone experienced the policy before?
- How many people have, and what was (were) the outcome(s)?
- Who needs to know the child's serostatus?
- How long before a decision will be made about the child's educational plan?

In instances in which a policy does not exist, national policies can be used to develop a local policy. Santelli, Birn, and Linde (1992) describe how Baltimore adopted the CDC and AAP guidelines. Each placement decision should be made on a case-by-case basis. You can serve as a resource in the policy development. Developing a general HIV/AIDS policy is preferable to formulating a child-specific one. So, timing is a key factor. The social worker can explore this issue in anticipation of the child's future needs. Early initiation of this effort will create an opportunity to address negative responses without the family being involved. Understandably families often perceive and experience the negative reactions as a personal rejection.

Since HIV is not casually transmitted, school attendance is favored over isolation of the child with HIV/AIDS. Universal precautions for group settings ensure that all children and staff are protected. For CWHIV who have neurological impairments, open lesions, or behavior problems, a more restrictive placement may be necessary (Task Force on Pediatric AIDS, 1993a,b; 1991; 1998; CDC, 1985). The CWHIV's medical treatment team may need to consult with the day care center/school to appropriately place a child and to provide guidance as medical concerns arise. It is very reassuring for school personnel to have medical backup.

Confidentiality laws vary from state to state. The child's right to privacy is weighed against the broader community's need for protection from infection. Since it is difficult to transmit HIV, the child's rights typically take precedence. In most states, the "need to know" principle guides who is told the child's diagnosis. The "need to know" principle refers to the concept of who needs medical information in order to care for a child. Typically, very few—if any—people need to know a child's serostatus. Disclosure is frequently left to the parents, who are encouraged to notify the school principal or nurse. Parents must sign a written release for their child's status to be disclosed to anyone else. Unless there is a compelling reason to tell, such as a child is needing to take medication, parents frequently withhold the diagnosis. They may tell the school that their child is sick or has cancer instead of HIV. School personnel may learn the diagnosis inadvertently by noticing that the child takes medications specific to HIV treatment.

Confidentiality can adversely affect the CWHIV. While school officials should notify all parents of infectious disease outbreaks, this may not always happen in a timely manner. The CWHIV is more vulnerable to infection and may be needlessly exposed to devastating illness. Parents need to consider this as they weigh the pros and cons of disclosure.

Parents and teachers often want to know who is infected. There is not a compelling reason for them to have access to this information. Instead, they should be well versed in universal precautions.

Public Law 94-142, Education for All Handicapped Children Act of 1975; Section 504, Rehabilitation Act of 1973; and the American Disabilities Act (ADA) are used to protect access to education (Jones, 1986; Klindworth et al., 1989). If efforts to work collaboratively to develop an educational placement are unsuccessful, legal assistance is warranted.

KEY QUESTIONS TO ASK THE CLIENT

As a parent considers sharing the diagnosis with the school, a thorough understanding of his or her expectations of the disclosure process is central. The following questions should be considered:

- Does the child need to be told before the school?
- What will be the benefits of telling?
- Who are the people in the school who you feel comfortable talking with?
- Has the school had a CWHIV before?
- Does you child know his or her diagnosis?
- Do any of his or her friends know the diagnosis?
- Do any other parents know?
- How helpful is it for the CWHIV to have at least one person in the school who is aware of the diagnosis to turn to if the child is feeling ill, upset, or worried?

As parents prepare to share the diagnosis with the school, they frequently seek guidance from the social worker that their decision is the "right" one. Since there are no guarantees how the day care or school staff will respond, they should be prepared for all possible outcomes. Schools accepting federal funding have to accept an HIV-infected child, and schools without this funding may reject an HIV-infected child. Your earlier contact with the school should give an indication of the school's readiness to respond. Parents also need to consider how they will react if other parents find out and are upset. Will they participate in parent meetings to help allay fears?

CULTURAL COMPETENCY CONSIDERATIONS

Frequently, African-American and Latino parents have experienced stressful relationships with community care providers (Billingsley and Giovannoni, 1972; National Commission on AIDS, 1992). As a result, such agencies are frequently viewed ambivalently. Assessing how a family has related to schools or health care providers can help you identify possible barriers to a successful integration of a CWHIV. Efforts should be directed toward maximizing a productive relationship.

ACTION STEPS FOR SUCCESSFUL INTERVENTION

CWHIV are most often living with one or more infected family members. The majority of these families are from traditionally disenfranchised racial and ethnic groups (Pozen, 1995). The family's past negative experiences may create a barrier to your work with them. You will need to establish a working relationship and explore their relationships with the school professionals. You cannot assume that you will be perceived positively. By talking openly about this, you can help parents begin to trust you and to model interactions that may be useful in their dealings with the school. Also, providing guidance to the families about how to negotiate with the school system can be beneficial.

The social worker can enhance the responsiveness of the day care center to the child's needs. By first contacting the center regarding its generic approach to CWHIV, you can identify barriers to the child's successful integration.

Schools have a twofold responsibility to CWHIV. First, appropriate education for CWHIV must be provided; second, HIV/AIDS prevention curriculum designed to prevent the spread of HIV should be provided (Pozen, 1995). These responsibilities have been met with varying degrees of success around the country.

Before you have a case with a CWHIV, contacting your local schools to determine what educational efforts for students and staff are underway is helpful. It is preferable for a school to be AIDS-educated prior to a CWHIV attending. The more time teachers and staff have to become educated and to explore their reactions to AIDS, the more beneficial it is for everyone involved.

The quality (or lack of quality) of the HIV/AIDS curricula is an important indicator of the school's receptivity to CWHIV. Risk-reduction education entails specifically addressing issues regarding substance abuse and sexual behaviors. Students need clear and explicit messages. If your examination of the curriculum reveals a superficial review of these issues, you can advocate for a better-informed presentation of the material.

Contacting a school prior to having a case may appear to be putting the cart before the horse; however, in practice, it is just the opposite. This intervention opens the door for a collaborative approach to delivering services to all CWHIV and their affected siblings. For the family, the benefit of this approach is that the family does not have to carry the burden of educating an ill-prepared day care center or school. Then, you can help parents with their decision making regarding disclosure. The decision is theirs to make, and they may need a substantial time period to explore this issue. Being respectful of parental decision making and the process of developing a plan for working with the school will reinforce parental functioning.

As a social worker doing HIV/AIDS work in the community, you may be positioned to arrange supplemental HIV/AIDS education to the day care center or school to address misconceptions regarding HIV. Fears about catching the virus casually continue to persist and can adversely affect the child's integration into the classroom situation. Your efforts can help many children.

You can assist in the plan development and create backup plans to respond to possible reactions. For example, one mother decided to not tell the school. Despite her wishes and extensive discussions with her daughter about keeping the "secret," her daughter "accidentally" told her class the first week of school. By anticipating the possibility of accidental disclosure with the mother, the social worker had explored this possibility prior to its occurrence. This anticipatory guidance of the "worst case" scenario helped the mother to respond effectively to the teacher's questions. It also helped the mother to not overreact to her daughter's need to tell others.

For children entering school at the day care, school or high school levels, key features of each are highlighted in the following.

DAY CARE

A primary concern for infants and toddlers is the exposure of the CWHIV to infectious diseases from the other children. It will be important to know if a communicable disease such as chicken pox is being transmitted. Chicken pox can be a life-threatening illness for a CWHIV. Immediate medical attention is needed. For other non-life-threatening illness, early parental notification of illness can minimize the CWHIV's exposure. Parents may elect to keep the child home during such outbreaks.

In day care settings, infants and toddlers have limited control over their bodily functions. Staff deal with bodily fluids including nasal secretions, blood, vomit, urine, and feces, making universal precautions essential (Osterholm, 1994). Education and ongoing consultation can help staff members respond effectively to the child and maintain an environment that minimizes disease transmission.

Parents may be unwilling to disclose their child's diagnosis. They can withhold the diagnosis and still communicate to the center that their child's immune system is compromised, thus increasing vulnerability to illness. This allows them to be notified about illnesses within the center.

SCHOOL CHILDREN

Parents with school-age children face a different challenge. Many have not told their children the diagnosis. Some fear that their children will be unable to share the information discriminately, and others fear how their child will react to the diagnosis. Clearly, children are aware that something is happening to their bodies. For CWHIV, the repeated hospital visits to infectious disease or immunology clinics and other specialists let them know that something is happening with their bodies. Most children do not undergo these experiences; thus, at the very least, the child will be aware that something is awry. Parents need to consider the burden placed on their children when they are asked to keep the HIV secret. It is very challenging emotionally for the CWHIV to worry about being "found out." You can help parents examine how much their child knows and then whether or not to tell the school personnel.

Medications may need to be given during school hours, which forces the disclosure issue. Sometimes medication schedules can be changed to avoid this.

HIGH SCHOOL

Adolescents with HIV want to be like their peers and may opt to withhold the diagnosis. They have less of a need to notify school personnel since they can function more independently than younger children. It is not difficult for a teen to take his or her medication without supervision. But the stress of hiding in the bathroom to take it is often so great that stress reactions occur and compliance problems ensue.

Disclosure may follow the adolescent's experience of a major illness. As the disease progresses, it becomes more difficult to hide it.

The social worker can help the adolescent consider whether or not to disclose. If supportive people are available in the school, the adolescent may find it helpful to share his or her experience. While other kids are preparing for jobs, careers, or college, it is important to help the HIV-infected teenager maintain hope and plan appropriately. It is a balancing act between being optimistic and while being realistic.

POTENTIAL BARRIERS
TO SUCCESSFUL INTERVENTION

While many day care centers and schools successfully integrate CWHIV, some are not as receptive. Fears of staff and other parents need to be addressed. Staff and students need education regarding HIV disease and universal precautions. Most important, they need an opportunity to examine their fears and to become more educated. The social worker is ideally situated to facilitate a more successful school response. Parents need to be educated about their rights to obtain an education for their child while the school may need to be reminded about its responsibility to provide this care. You may facilitate meetings between the parents and school to develop a viable plan for the child. There may be a need for additional meetings as the child's illness progresses.

Many parents of CWHIV have had difficult relationships with the school and other human service agencies before HIV became an issue. It may not be possible for parents to establish a trusting relationship with staff whom the parents do not perceive as supportive.

Social workers working with HIV-affected families may experience a stigma similar to that experienced by the families. This can limit your effectiveness. There will be limits to what you are able to accomplish with an unreceptive school. Persistence and ongoing efforts to productively engage the school system are part of the professional role in working in this arena. You can model for parents how to work with a hostile partner and when to seek legal assistance if efforts fail.

INFORMATION THE CLIENT SHOULD KNOW
BEFORE TAKING ACTION

A child's entry in day care or school may be the first time a parent has relied on others for care for the child. Assessing the parent's level of comfort in entrusting the child's care to others is an important area to explore. It is natural for a parent to feel that no one will care for his or her child as effectively. Validating these feelings can open the door to discussion of whether or not the parent is ready to let the school know about the child's HIV. Role-playing can help a parent rehearse the information he or she wants to share with the school.

Some parents will be empowered by the legal safeguards for their children's education while others will be frightened by them. Frequently, the legal safeguards are misunderstood. Many fear that the authorities will remove their children. Many parents are unaware of these safeguards and will benefit from learning about them. For a parent, knowing that established ways to counter negative responses by the school exist can buffer the pain of a nonsupportive response.

Disclosure decreases secrecy. Children may not know who in their family is struggling with HIV. One little girl was sent to a camp for affected children. When she came home, she asked her mother, "Who has HIV?" Her mother had never told her daughter her own diagnosis. Hudis (1995) reported that only 61 percent of the youths reported that they knew the HIV status of their HIV-infected parent; almost all of them had been specifically instructed not to speak about it with anyone outside the family. Equally, the school is in the dark regarding the family secret. A natural outcome of the secrecy is limited access to either informal or formal support networks. Parents will benefit from establishing connections with outside support networks that can help their children cope with the multiple related losses.

School-age children and older children may benefit from counseling and play therapy, which can provide a safe setting to explore their fears. For example, many CWHIV are small in stature and are teased by their peers. Feeling different than peers is a very important dynamic for CWHIV to examine. By sharing their concerns, they can develop more effective coping skills. Peer groups can provide an opportunity to universalize feelings of isolation, secrecy, and being different as well as the realities of HIV.

POLICY IMPLICATIONS AND RELATED ACTIONS

All programs serving children should have policies regarding the process for inclusion of CWHIV. The national guidelines discussed earlier can be used to develop local policies. Ideally, the policy should be in place before a CWHIV enters the school setting. As an advocate, you can assist day care centers and schools in the development of an HIV/AIDS policy. You should anticipate some resistance from either staff or parents. The fear of AIDS continues despite extensive evidence that it is not casually transmitted. Legal safeguards ensure that children have access to education in the least-restrictive environment possible. Social workers need to familiarize themselves with these safeguards and assist families in accessing legal counsel when warranted.

HIV is a family disease. An infected child is often the entry point for a family with multiple infected members. Affected and infected children remain largely invisible in our school districts. They need supportive services that emphasize normative development and coping. There also needs to be greater efforts to help children adjust to and survive the family illness.

Previously, schools have not considered this their responsibility. While schools do not perceive this as their responsibility, they are dealing with its impact on students daily.

Hudis (1995) found a wide range of children's responses to living with a parent with HIV/AIDS. Among these responses included problems in school such as truancy, disruptive behavior, or school suspension. Seventy-three percent of the children had problems in school and 58 percent had a drop in grades associated with parental illness. Additionally, these children also had a tendency to be more likely to engage in high-risk behaviors than their counterparts.

Schools may play a crucial role in helping children adjust to the major changes and challenges they are facing with HIV disease. If school staff are made aware of the issues facing these children, they would be in a position to better provide a critically needed support structure for these students. It is also important that the staff not place judgment on such students and their families. Given this consideration, school staff and personnel need to be provided a better understanding of HIV/AIDS facts, myths, and related issues. In doing so, the school staff will be better equipped to help support these children instead of placing judgment on them and their families.

Schools also have a key role to play in prevention efforts. While schools are mandated to provide HIV/AIDS education, they too are compromised in their efforts to provide sexuality and AIDS education. Frequently, AIDS curriculums are ambiguous, and condom distribution has been blocked.

To effectively stop HIV transmission, our youth need the skills to remain uninfected. They need specific information about transmission and how to decrease its likelihood. Just as we teach children to be safe when crossing the street, we need to teach them to decrease the possibility of HIV transmission. For the sexually active adolescent who is unwilling to abstain, he or she can reduce the risk of transmission by using latex condoms or the female condom. Equally, the drug-using teen needs to know how to clean "works" and about needle exchange to minimize the likelihood of transmission. Drug treatment should also be offered. You can help your schools implement more effective prevention programs.

RECOMMENDED READINGS

Baker, L. (1991). *You and HIV: A day at a time*. New York: Sauder and Company.
Bauman, L. and Wiener, L. (June 1994). Priorities in psychosocial research in pediatric HIV infection. (supplemental issues). *Journal of Developmental and Behavioral Pediatrics 15*(3).

Billingsley, A. and Giovannoni, J. (1972). Children of the storm.
Boyd-Franklin, N., Steiner, G., and Boland, M. (Eds.) (1995). *Children, families, and HIV/AIDS: Psychosocial and therapeutic issues.* New York: Guilford Press.
Girard, L. (1993). *Alex the kid with AIDS.* Morton Grove, IL: Albert Whitman and Company.
Wiener, L., Best, A., and Pizzo, P. (1994). *Be a friend: Children who live with HIV speak.* Morton Grove, IL: Albert Whitman and Company.

REFERENCES

Centers for Disease Control (1985). Guidelines for education and foster care of adenopathy-associated with human T-lymphotrophic virus type II/lymphadenopathy-associated virus. *MMWR 34*: 517-520.
Centers for Disease Control (1988, Jan. 29). Guidelines for effective school health education to prevent the spread of AIDS. *MMWR*, 1-14.
Draimin, B. (1995). A second family? Placement and custody decisions. In S. Geballe, J. Gruendel, and W. Andiman (Eds.), *Forgotten children of the AIDS epidemic* (pp. 125-139). New Haven, CT: Yale University Press.
Geballe, S., Gruendel, J., and Andiman, W. (Eds.) (1995). *Forgotten children of the AIDS epidemic.* New Haven, CT: Yale University Press.
Heagarty, M. (1993). Day care for the child with Acquired Immunodeficiency Syndrome and the child of the drug-abusing mother. *Pediatrics* suppl.:199-201.
Hudis, J. (1995). Adolescents living in families with AIDS. In S. Geballe, J. Gruendel, and W. Andiman (Eds.), *Forgotten children of the AIDS epidemic* (pp. 83-94). New Haven, CT: Yale University Press.
Jones, N. (1986). The education of all handicapped children act: Coverage of children with Acquired Immune Deficiency Syndrome (AIDS). *Journal of Law Education 15*: 195-206.
Klindworth, L., Dokeski, P., Baumeister, A., and Kupstas, F. (1989). Pediatric AIDS, developmental disabilities, and education. *AIDS Education Press 1*: 291-301.
Morrow, A., Benton, M., Reves, R., and Pickering, L. (June 1991). Knowledge and attitudes of day care center parents and care providers regarding children infected with Human Immunodeficiency Virus. *Pediatrics 87*(6): 876-883.
National Commission on AIDS (December 1992). *The challenge of HIV/AIDS in communities of color.* Washington, DC: Author.
Osterholm, M. (December 1994). Infectious disease in child day care: An overview. *Pediatrics 94*(6): 987-990.
Pozen, A. (1995). HIV/AIDS in the Schools. In N. Boyd-Franklin, G. Steiner, and M. Boland (Eds.), *Children, families and HIV/AIDS: Psychosocial and therapeutic issues* (pp. 233-55). New York: Guilford Press.
Santelli, J., Birn, A., and Linde, J. (May 1992). School placement for Human Immunodeficiency Virus-infected children: The Baltimore City Experience. *Pediatrics 89*(5): 843-848.

Schonfeld, D., O'Hare, L., Perrin, E., Quackenbush, M., Showalter, D., and Cicchetti, D. (1995, April). A randomized, controlled trial of a school-based, multi-faceted AIDS education program in the elementary grades: The impact on comprehension, knowledge, and fears. *Pediatrics 95*(4): 480-486.

Smith, W. (April 5, 1990). "Guidance on application of Section 504 to children in elementary and secondary schools." Memorandum to U.S. Department of Education, Office of Civil Rights Senior Staff.

Task Force on Pediatric AIDS (1988). Pediatric guidelines for infection control of Human Immunodeficiency Virus in hospitals, medical offices, schools, and other settings. *Pediatrics 82:* 801-807.

Task Force on Pediatric AIDS (September 1991). Education of children with Human Immunodeficiency Virus. *Pediatric 88*(3): 645-647.

Task Force on Pediatric AIDS (1993a). *School health: Policy and practice,* fifth edition. Elk Grove, IL: American Academy of Pediatrics.

Task Force on Pediatric AIDS (1993b). Committee on school health and adolescents with human T-lymphotrophic virus type III/lymphadenopathy-associated virus infection. *Pediatrics 77:* 430-432.

Talking to Women with HIV About Childbearing Issues

Susan Taylor-Brown

WHY DO THIS?
STATEMENT OF THE PROBLEM AND ISSUES

Women are the fastest growing group diagnosed with HIV. The vast majority of these women are of childbearing age (twenty-two to forty-nine years old), and many have children or are considering having children. A significant proportion of these women became infected while teenagers. Frequently, women find out that they are infected during their pregnancy or when their baby is born. Psychosocially, this is one of the worst times to learn about the diagnosis.

Becoming a mother is an important part of a woman's life. For many, nurturing children is seen as the primary role of women in our society. HIV does not diminish the desire to have children. In fact, the reality of a life-threatening disease may heighten the desire to create a new life as a continuation of oneself. With other life-threatening illnesses, for example, cystic fibrosis, women and men have chosen to bear children. While it might appear inconceivable to bear a child to those who are uninfected, the promise of a new life may outweigh the risk of having a child who is infected.

The decision to have a child is complex for all potential parents. This decision is complicated for an HIV-infected woman by the possibility of transmitting the disease to her offspring (vertical transmission) and the likelihood of premature maternal death. This stark reality competes with the life-affirming desire to have children and create a family.

For some women, the decision to bear a child is not their decision. These women do not perceive themselves as having a say about whether or not to use contraception. They frequently do not have control over their sexual relationships with their partner and have no influence over the partner engaging in additional sexual relationships. Many become pregnant regardless of their wishes. All infected women need support as they cope with the decision to have children or not. Further, your support should be continued regardless of a woman's decision to bear children or to defer childbearing. Each choice is emotionally taxing and has a lasting impact for all members of the family. One woman chose to have an abortion because she felt she needed to devote herself to her three children whom she delivered prior to finding out her serostatus.

From the onset of the pandemic, controversy has surrounded an infected woman's choice to bear or not to bear a child. HIV-infected women are seen as selfish, irresponsible, or immoral if they choose to initiate or continue a pregnancy (Anastos and Martes, 1991). Central to the debate is *whose decision is it to make—the woman's or the medical provider's?* Initially, the Centers for Disease Control (CDC) recommended that women defer childbearing until more was learned about vertical transmission, which refers to a mother infecting her baby either before or during childbirth or after birth by breastfeeding her baby. Currently, between 13 percent to 30 percent of infants born to a mother with HIV will be infected themselves. Also, providers wanted to know the impact of pregnancy on the mother's survival.

Currently, the debate focuses on whether mandatory testing of all pregnant women should become law or if pregnant women should receive mandatory HIV counseling and be offered voluntary HIV testing (CDC, 1995). Advances in the management of HIV-infected pregnant women have underscored the importance of women knowing their serostatus prior to or early in pregnancy. Mandatory testing restricts a woman's civil rights regarding knowledge of her serostatus. Many are concerned that pregnant women who are afraid of learning about their serostatus may avoid prenatal care if testing becomes mandatory. The United States Public Health Service favors mandatory counseling with voluntary testing.

Another facet of this debate is the data from the HIV Survey in Childbearing Women (HSCW). HSCW is an anonymous newborn seroprevalence study that anonymously tests infants for HIV. An infant who tests HIV positive at birth indicates that the child's mother is infected and that the child may or may not be infected. This anonymous test allows public health officials to track the spread of HIV in women who may not be aware of their infection. Proposed legislation would unblind this data. The stated intent of the legislation is to get all infected children into care. This legislation would result in parents being told if their infant tested positive at birth. Many of these women are unaware of their own serostatus, and this proposal has major psychosocial implications for women. A mother, during the postpartum period, would learn of her serostatus without the benefit or pre- or posttest counseling. This is counter to the emphasis placed on the importance of patients receiving pre- and posttest counseling. It also is too late for the woman to consider her treatment options to decrease the likelihood of HIV transmission during the pregnancy.

As politicians and care providers struggle over standards of care, women's needs are frequently secondary. The CDC recently suspended the HSCW, a valuable source of information about HIV infection in women. The HCSW appears to be the latest casualty in the never-ending fight over mandatory and nonconfidential testing (Spirits, 1995).

This ongoing debate engenders strong reactions in care providers and the public alike. Practitioners frequently allow their personal biases to influence their recommendations to women. Women are frequently caught in the crossfire and are oftentimes negatively portrayed. Little concern is expressed about the medical or emotional needs of HIV-infected mothers. To call for the care of infants who test HIV positive at birth without a simultaneous call for treatment of the mother seems short-sighted. Clearly, both need care. A balanced approach to this complex issue will help clarify the issues and provide a more supportive approach to women who are considering having children. As an advocate, you can help a woman to weigh her options and then allow her to make the best decision for herself.

These transmission rates compare favorably to many genetic disease rates of transmission. For example, a mother who is a carrier of an X-linked recessively inherited disease (e.g., Duchenne's muscular dystrophy) has a 50 percent chance of transmitting if the fetus is male. HIV-infected parents, just as parents who have a genetic disorder or are a carrier, must weigh out the risks of transmitting a disease with their desire to have a family. Frequently, women living with HIV receive coercive counseling rather than counseling that helps them to make informed decisions about whether to continue a pregnancy or not. This is particularly true for women who are substance users and are perceived as less compliant with their medical care.

EXAMPLES OF HOW THE ISSUE MAY PRESENT

Childbearing is a central role for most women. For a woman living with HIV, childbearing carries a burden that most women do not have to consider "Will I give this illness to my child?" No one wants to transmit HIV to a child, but this potential reality is omnipresent for women with HIV.

Women are apt to explore this issue indirectly, if at all. Many times the issue arises when a woman thinks that she may already be pregnant. As one woman said, "I was afraid to tell you; I thought you would be mad at me for not practicing safer sex." Or it may be raised in an offhand way: "Do you think I will ever have children?" Childbearing is a frequent theme in support groups as women mourn the loss of never having a child or the loss of having a child without worrying about whether the infant will be positive or not.

As a social worker, you may receive referrals from other professionals who request that you tell the woman not to have children. Colleagues may support a woman through a pregnancy only to become very upset with a subsequent pregnancy, particularly if the first child was infected. Women sense this rejection and may leave treatment. All efforts should be directed toward helping women remain in care.

You are challenged with the simultaneous task of working with your colleagues regarding the woman's right to decide this highly personal issue while assisting women to weigh the pros and cons of having a child. Uncertainty is the reality and this can be anxiety producing for the woman and providers alike. The woman needs to consider how a child will impact her life and to explore the possibility of a motherless future for the child. Ultimately, it is her decision.

FACTS THE SOCIAL WORKER
NEEDS TO KNOW BEFORE PROCEEDING

Practitioners have an important role to play in assisting women to consider their choices. You can help a woman to weigh the options and the risks entailed in having a child. You will need updated information before meeting with the woman. Treatment recommendations for women have changed, and the knowledge base continues to grow. It is imperative to have up-to-date medical information. Appropriate medical consultation is required on a case-by-case basis. To rely on outdated information is inadequate. It is important to share the most current knowledge with her and to advise her to seek consultation regarding treatment options as necessary.

Practitioners need to be prepared to provide nondirective reproductive counseling. Such counseling entails presenting information and choices available to an HIV-infected woman and responding to those questions raised by the woman. The woman and her partner need to understand the available information and the limits of our knowledge about HIV disease. We do not have all the answers regarding whether an infant will be infected or not. It is not possible to predict whether or not a woman will give birth to an infected child. She should not be given false reassurances that her child will be seronegative. Equally, she should not be given overly pessimistic reproductive counseling. If she chooses to go ahead with the pregnancy, support will help her cope with the inherent anxiety.

Today, HIV treatment advances afford women an opportunity for a longer, more productive life coupled with the possibility of reducing the likelihood of maternal-to-infant transmission by following the Clinical Trial 076 protocol. For Trial 076, women whose T-cell count was over 200 took AZT (AZT = ZDV) and the infant was given AZT (Connor et al., 1994). A mother transmits HIV to the baby 13 to 30 percent of the time without the intervention of medication, and this rate drops to 8 to 13 percent with drug treatment (Kurth, 1995). This is a remarkable drop in transmission of HIV from mother to child. Every mother should be informed of this treatment option as she considers bearing a child. It is an exciting development in the efforts to decrease the rate of vertical transmission. Clinical Trial 076 has had very promising results, and all women need to know about this trial in order to make an informed decision.

While practitioners and women are heartened by this new advance and the possibility of having an uninfected child, the findings of clinical trial 076 have been viewed with skepticism by many. Since the study was pulled before the trial was complete, questions remain regarding what the long-term effects of AZT will be on the infant and the woman:

- Will there be adverse effects on the mother or child?
- Will a woman who takes AZT during her pregnancy not be able to use it effectively later during her illness?
- What is the impact of taking AZT for the infant who was not infected?
- Who has access to this information?
- Is there a commitment to long-term follow-up and treatment for both mother and child?

Additionally, there are questions about the efficacy if a woman has T-cell counts below 200 (Kurth, 1995). A woman with AIDS may not experience the same benefit from treatment. Further research is needed to address these concerns.

More is being learned about which factors may contribute to higher rates of vertical transmission, and new treatments are being considered. Vaginal lavage during delivery and cesarean deliveries are being studied as possible means of decreasing transmission. Vaginal lavage refers to washing the vagina during childbirth to decrease the concentration of HIV in the birth canal as the baby is being born. New clinical trials for pregnancy appear promising. For example, the ACTG 250 protocol is a phase I clinical trial evaluating the safety of and how the drug nevirapine works (Benson and Shannon, 1995). This is a good example of an alternative to AZT therapy that might be available to a wider population of childbearing women in the near future. These developments have important implications for a woman's decision to bear a child, and she needs an opportunity to consider what is known as well as what is still unknown.

The decision to have a child is linked to a number of factors that extend beyond the medical facts. This decision involves competing demands; a woman will need to consider the impact of having either an infected or uninfected infant. The woman needs to assess her relationship with her partner. Is he infected himself? If yes, will they reinfect each other trying to become pregnant? If not, does he know her status? A few sessions with the partners may help clarify these and other related issues. Many women do not feel they have an option. You can effectively help a woman explore the meaning of creating a life by examining the role of her past reproductive experiences, her religious background, her partner's expectations, and the meaning of her illness.

It will be helpful to explore the long-term realities for the child ranging from being a part of a family to coping with the reality of maternal death and needing guardianship arrangements. Careful exploration can facilitate the woman's assessment of what will be best for the infant and the parents.

The birth of a child for many symbolizes hope for the future and a continuation of the mother's family. Springer (1994) reports that a number of factors influence a woman's decision making including the following: grief and hope in the face of loss, faith in religious or medical systems, pressures from partners or society, concerns about ill effects on health for oneself or one's infant, moral beliefs about the value of life or the acceptability of abortions, and societal and personal meanings of reproduction.

Losses permeate the lives of infected women; thus, creating a life can counter a sense of depletion. A woman's reproductive history can provide valuable information about prior losses. Commonly, women with substance use histories have relinquished children or have had abortions or miscarriages. Identifying these losses and exploring the relationship of their meaning to a woman's current desire to have a child can help to clarify some of the issues. This can be an opportunity for a woman to reconnect with children who have been removed from her care and custody.

Working with women regarding childbearing also requires the clinician to understand the complexities of implementing safer sex and behavior change models. First, women need to receive education regarding contraception and reproduction. Lai (1994) reported that women living with the virus did not receive adequate counseling about reproduction and contraception. About half of the women surveyed believed that chances of vertical transmission were about 50 percent while the other half believed that the chances were 100 percent. Education can clarify the noted misperception. Women need to know the likelihood of transmission.

Yet, education alone is insufficient. A woman's ability to incorporate sexuality education will be influenced by her past sexual experiences. Frequently, infected women have experienced sexual abuse or are involved in sexual relationships in which they have limited power regarding the implementation of safer sex practices. Incest and sexual abuse within the context of poverty leave a child vulnerable to developing a chemical dependency and to tolerating sexual abuse in adulthood (Walker, 1995). These women are vulnerable to low self-esteem and may not perceive that they have any control over reproduction. You will need to take a thorough sexual history and to be prepared to help women cope with their sexual abuse disclosure. A history of abuse raises concerns regarding a woman's ability to function fully in her present sexual relationship.

Every time a couple practices safer sex, they are reminded of the underlying illness. It is unrealistic to expect a woman to implement safer sex methods in these situations without interventions that include her partners. Again, more research is needed regarding interventions in couples.

Women do not have good female-controlled contraceptive or viricide options. The female condom is a step in the right direction but is cumbersome to use, not widely available, and expensive. Also, efficacy is unknown. Birth control pills prevent contraception but not HIV transmission. Vaginal contraceptive film, a small dissolving insert, is beginning to be advertised. If effective, this is a subtle female-controlled option. Efficacy studies are pending.

Many women wish to conceive but not become HIV-infected. A viricide that kills HIV but not sperm is not yet available. The development of such a viricide is urgently needed for women who do not believe in practicing birth control but who do want protection from HIV.

A woman may seek counseling after she is told she is pregnant. A careful assessment of her reaction to the pregnancy is needed before exploring her options with her. Ambivalence is a common reaction to any pregnancy. For many women, abortion is not an option, and it is helpful to find this out before reviewing options. For these women, the mere suggestion of abortion may impede the patient relationship. Such women need support in examining their choices.

For a woman who decides to have a child, you need to provide psychosocial support throughout the pregnancy, focusing on anxiety management regarding the possibility of vertical transmission. Regular prenatal care that integrates HIV management will help her to access aggressive prophylaxis and treatment of opportunistic infections, which can adversely affect mother and child. Some areas have specialized high-risk initiatives, and in other areas, HIV care and obstetrical care are coordinated. For women in more rural or lower-incidence areas, you may have to advocate for the coordination of needed services.

The context of childbearing while coping with a life-threatening illness is not unique to HIV. Couples in which one or both partners may have a life-threatening illness choose to have children. For example, women with cancer choose to have children as do women with genetic illnesses or other life-threatening diseases. The desire to have a child is powerful for all of us. We do not know when a cure for HIV will be found. It may be next year or in the next decade. HIV care has been transformed in the past decade, and the future holds promise. Your job is to help women make an informed decision.

KEY QUESTIONS TO ASK THE CLIENT

You can help a woman clarify the issues regarding having a child. Careful questioning offered in a supportive manner can facilitate a woman's decision making. Many questions will need to be explored repeatedly. As a woman considers her options, a myriad of emotions will surface including frustration about having a life-threatening disease, uncertainty regarding how long she will be able to care for her children, and pain about the inherent losses. Some useful questions include the following:

- What does having a baby mean to you?
- Are you being pressured to have a child?
- What are your hopes for the baby? Fears?
- How will bearing a child affect your health? Your ability to care for your other family members?
- Who are your supports?
- What is your understanding of the possibility of your baby becoming infected from you?
- Are there things you do not understand about transmission?
- How will you feel if your child is negative? Positive?
- Who will love and care for your child when you are not able? Will this person care for your child until he or she grows up?

CULTURAL COMPETENCY CONSIDERATIONS

African-American and Hispanic/Latina women account for 21 percent of all United States women, yet they represent 75 percent of the cumulative AIDS cases reported among women. Further, African-American women have rates twenty-eight times higher than white women (National Minority AIDS Council, 1995). HIV in women is primarily about HIV in women of color. Not only are women of color being infected, but they are also the caregivers of family members who are are infected.

Women of color value their role as mothers, and they receive validation from family members by becoming mothers. Extended family members frequently take an active role in parenting children. As a result, the woman may see her family as a future resource in the event she succumbs to HIV.

Historically, women of color have experienced difficulty in accessing needed medical services; thus, mistrust of medical services is pervasive. Historical barriers include the Tuskeegee syphilis study, a governmental study that failed to offer treatment to African-American men who had syphilis (National Commission on AIDS, 1992). The demands of urban poverty create adversarial relationships between poor families and the larger institutions with which they must interact (Walker, 1995).

The current legislative initiatives to require mandatory testing of pregnant women or to unblind seroprevalence studies of infants perpetuate the conflictual relationship between women and providers. These initiatives may discourage women from seeking care. As the CDC (1995) concluded, all pregnant women should receive counseling regarding the risks and benefits of HIV antibody testing coupled with voluntary testing. It is believed that this approach will help women establish trusting relationships with their providers.

ACTION STEPS FOR SUCCESSFUL INTERVENTION

The decision to bear children is complex, and you can help a woman clarify the issues for herself. All clinicians are ethically bound to present the contraceptive and reproductive information in a nonjudgmental manner (Kurth, 1995). Frequently, clinicians fail to be nonjudgmental when discussing these issues. Case consultation with colleagues can facilitate examination of their biases.

You can strive to deliver the material to the woman in a nonjudgmental fashion that will help her make an informed decision. You can help your client interpret the scientific data and protocol requirements. By responding to your client's questions and concerns, you can assist her decision making regarding an intervention that may lead to adverse effects for mother, infant, or both. There are a few guidelines to follow in preparing a parent for this very difficult decision:

1. Help the woman to identify what the motivating factors are for having a child.

2. Assist her in weighing the possible outcomes of the pregnancy and evaluating the child's future.
3. Prepare her for potential reactions from her family and the medical team.
4. Provide a supportive relationship for her to explore the impact of this decision. (Kurth, 1995)

Support groups can provide a safe place for HIV-infected women to explore these complex issues. By sharing their experiences, group members can help another member to decide what is best for her. Also, she may benefit from learning about available community services from other consumers.

It is not helpful to approach a pregnant woman by focusing exclusively on her infant. Her needs must also be taken into consideration or else her commitment to treatment may be minimal. Women are more than vessels of infection; they are patients in their own right. The success of your intervention will rest on your ability to respect a woman's decision making and to not impose your own values.

POTENTIAL BARRIERS TO SUCCESSFUL INTERVENTION

Unintended pregnancies are common, regardless of a woman's HIV status. The decision to have children is highly personal and may or may not be influenced by the "facts." The decision to bear a child may be complicated by the high degree of suspicion among women of color both about the medical community and the efficacy of antiretroviral treatments (Focus Group, 1995). Members of the focus group on clinical trial 076 expressed a pervasive mistrust of health care providers both within the research community and the health care system. Efforts to develop a trusting relationship between patient and provider will have a significant impact on their ability to work together. Unless a trusting relationship is forged, treatment recommendations may be ignored.

Some providers may be unwilling to support a woman's choice if it varies from their perspective. While a clinician is ethically bound to present the information in a nonjudgmental manner, childbearing evokes a strong provider response, which may vary from the woman's choice. At times, your colleagues may communicate their disapproval to the woman. As a result, a woman grappling with childbearing decisions may withdraw from medical care despite your efforts to assist her. Mutual recognition of the differences can be a starting point for exploring this potential problem. Ongoing outreach is essential to attempt to provide the necessary ongoing HIV care. Prenatal care is particularly important for an infected woman.

POLICY IMPLICATIONS AND RELATED ACTIONS

The combination of sexism, stigma, and racism confronting women in the HIV pandemic call for strong advocacy by social workers. In order to preserve women's rights in childbearing decisions, social workers can assist in setting national and state policies that protect a woman's right to have a child.

The proposed coercive legislative measures to test pregnant women or their infants will not advance our work in this area. Historically, it has been assumed that most mothers will act in the best interest of their children. This is clearly seen in HIV treatment, in which women typically sacrifice their own care in order to get care for their children. Mandatory testing will undermine maternal decision making. Social workers have a clear mandate to advocate on behalf of these women. Legislation in this area should not pit the needs of the mother against the child.

An infected mother needs access to quality medical care to enable her to care for herself and her children. All women should be informed of the need to know their HIV status, preferably before conceiving. Disclosure of HIV status perinatally is not desirable. Social workers must advocate for more appropriate timing of this disclosure and strive to ensure that counseling and treatment are available to mothers.

RECOMMENDED READINGS

Denenberg, R. (October/November 1993). Applying harm reduction to sexual and reproductive counseling: A health provider's guide to supporting the goals of people with HIV/AIDS. *SIECUS Report*.

Kurth, A. (1993). *Until the cure: Caregiving for women with HIV*. New Haven, CT: Yale University Press.

Lipson, M. and Berman, N. (1993). Family and reproductive issues. In *AIDS clinical care*. Boston: Massachusetts Medical Society.

REFERENCES

Anastos, K. and Marte, C. (1991). Women: The missing persons in the AIDS epidemic. In N.F. McKenzie (Ed.), *The AIDS reader: Social, political, and ethical issues* (pp. 190-199). New York: Meridian.

Benson, M. and Shannon, M. (June 1995). Nevirapine: Ethical dilemmas and care for HIV-infected mothers. *Focus: A Guide to AIDS Research and Counseling 10*(7): 5-6.

Centers for Disease Control (1994). Recommendations for the use of zidovudine to reduce perinatal transmission of Human Immunodeficiency Virus. *Morbidity and Mortality Weekly Report 43*(RR-11): 1-20.

Centers for Disease Control (February 1995). PHS guidelines for HIV counseling and voluntary testing for pregnant women [draft]. Atlanta: Centers for Disease Control.

Connor, E., Sperling, R., Gelber, R., Kiselev, P., Scott, G., O'Sullivan, M.J., VanDyke, R., Bey, M., Shearer, W., Jacobson, R. et al. (1994). Reduction of maternal-infant transmission of Human Immunodeficiency Virus type-1 with zidovudine treatment. *New England Journal of Medicine 331*(18): 1173-1180.

Focus Group on ACTG 076 Summary Report. Institute for Family-Centered Care, 7900 Wisconsin Avenue, Suite 405, Bethesda, MD, 20814.

Kurth, A. (June 1995). HIV disease and reproductive counseling. *Focus: A Guide to AIDS Research and Counseling 10*(7): 1-4.

Lai, K. (1994). Attitudes toward childbearing and changes in sexual and contraceptive practices among HIV-infected women. *Cleveland Clinic Journal of Medicine 61*(2): 132-136.

National Commission on AIDS (December 1992). *The challenge of HIV/AIDS in communities of color.* Washington, DC: Author.

National Minority AIDS Council (March 29, 1995). *Action Alert: Oppose HR. 1289, Newborn Infant HIV Notification Act.* Available from: National Minority Council (202) 544-1076.

Spirits (June/July 1995). *National Women & HIV/AIDS Project, 1*(3).

Springer, L. (1994). Reproductive decision-making in the age of AIDS. *Image: Journal of Nursing Scholarship 26*(3): 241-246.

Walker, G. (1995). Family therapy interventions with inner-city families affected by AIDS. In W. Odets, and M. Shernoff (Eds.), *The second decade of AIDS: A mental health practice handbook* (pp. 85-114). New York: Hatherleigh Press.

PART B:
SERVICES FOR SPECIAL POPULATIONS

Services to Adolescents

Mary Beth Sunenblick

WHY DO THIS?
STATEMENT OF THE PROBLEM AND ISSUES

The threat of AIDS presents an enormous challenge for adolescents. The developmental stage of adolescence is a period marked by change, confusion, and tumultuousness for many teens. Adolescents are considered to be one of the high-risk groups for AIDS. Many engage in behaviors that may put them at risk of acquiring HIV infections, other sexually transmitted infections, or infections associated with drug injections. Recent studies conducted every two years in high schools (grades 9 to 12) by the Centers for Disease Control (CDC) consistently indicate that by twelfth grade, approximately three-fourths of high school students have had sexual intercourse, less than half report use of latex condoms, and about one-fifth have had more than four sex partners. Many students report using alcohol or drugs when they have sex, and in the most recent survey, one in sixty-two high school students reported having injected an illegal drug (CDC, 1994). According to the CDC, the number of reported cases of AIDS in twenty- to twenty-nine-year-olds is increasing dramatically. Given the length of time that one can be infected with HIV and show no symptoms—an average of eight to ten years—it is reasonable to conclude that many AIDS patients are likely infected during their adolescence.

EXAMPLES OF HOW THE ISSUE MAY PRESENT

Social workers in contact with adolescents often are asked to address the issues of adolescent sexuality and sexual behavior. In exploring their sexuality, adolescents must come to terms with the reality of AIDS. The life-and-death issues of AIDS cannot be separated from an understanding of the adolescent's tendency toward experimentation and risk taking. These behaviors often include elements of denial and invulnerability—blinding the adolescent from the tragic consequences of some dangerous behaviors. Adolescents are asked to face their mortality at a time when, developmentally, feelings of immortality and invincibility are at their highest.

Consequently, social work practitioners should work toward creating environments that are safe for adolescents to talk about sex, AIDS, and mortality. Practitioners themselves must be comfortable engaging in such a dialogue. Discussions about HIV, including such topics as risk factors, safe sex, and access to good health care, can provide adolescents with the necessary information to make good and safe choices about their sexual behavior.

The social work maxim of "beginning where the client is" should be the cornerstone of the initial contact. Therefore, as part of the initial assessment, clinicians should consider the developmental level and cognitive ability of their adolescent client. Pacing of inquiries made and information given are important in this regard. The amount and intensity of information about sex and sexual practices should be measured so as to avoid flooding the adolescent with more material than is manageable. Attending to the client's spoken and unspoken language style and carefully inquiring into his or her view of sex and sexual practices are important components of a thoughtful interview. Social workers should seek clarity about how an adolescent client thinks about sex and sexual practices; for example, careful exploration of his or her relationship status, sexual history, and sexual preference are important areas to be reviewed. Attention to the client's understanding of prevalence, modes of transmission for high-risk groups, symptoms of AIDS, and safe sex practices may highlight the adolescent's misconceptions and need for clarification.

FACTS THE SOCIAL WORKER NEEDS TO KNOW
BEFORE PROCEEDING

Social workers should be well informed about all aspects of HIV and safer sexual behavior. This includes accurate, up-to-date information about HIV (including all possible modes of transmission). A solid understanding of sex, sexual practices, contraception, pregnancy, and decision making about alternatives to pregnancy is also important. Despite the benefits of an educational approach to HIV and safer sex, educational interventions alone do not necessarily result in safe sexual behavior for this age group (Sunenblick, 1988). Teaching adolescents about AIDS is especially difficult, public health officials and educators say, because teenagers often are impulsive and consider themselves "immortal."

Social workers need to keep in mind the developmental tasks of adolescence, which explain why some adolescents may continue to engage in risky sexual practices while others do not. These developmental tasks include the following: constancy of self-esteem, development of inner regulatory controls, constancy of mood, being at home in one's body, knowing where one is going, and an "inner confidence" of anticipated recognition from others who count. In their quest for identity consolidation, adolescents often experiment and take risks. For some adolescents, this includes impulsive and potentially dangerous behaviors. Impulsive behavior often reflects the notion of invulnerability or an "it can't happen to me" attitude. Adolescent invulnerability can explain why some teens do not change unsafe sexual practices in response to educational efforts alone. The vulnerable adolescent can be aided by interventions designed to teach him or her to identify and label their feelings. Helping teens use their emotional response as a form of self-signaling, rather than as a trigger for impulsivity, can also be a helpful intervention. For instance, an adolescent can benefit from recognizing that his or her pattern of substance use after fights with a boyfriend or girlfriend is a way of managing disappointment and other sad feelings about relationship problems. This can be a useful step toward identifying, then managing, distressing affect by talking about it rather than numbing the self through substance use.

TALKING WITH ADOLESCENTS
ABOUT SEX AND SEXUALITY

Discussions about sex and sexuality should be presented in a variety of ways in order to "reach" as many adolescents as possible. Social workers can create environments that allow open discussion of such topics as sex and sexual practices, using individual and group approaches. Psychodynamic, psychoeducational, behavioral, and cognitive perspectives all have something to offer. Intervention strategies that address the importance of low-risk sexual behaviors are also important to consider. Films such as *Sex, Drugs, and AIDS* and *In Our Words: Teens and AIDS* include material designed to elicit affective reactions from adolescents. This type of intervention can be conducive to small group discussion for the exchange of information on a more personal level.

Although it goes without saying that clinicians should be comfortable talking about sexual issues, many are uncomfortable discussing sexual behavior and avoid it until the client brings it up. Some are reluctant to discuss certain sexual practices, such as anal sex, and some may quickly gloss over sexual contact, leaving clients uncertain about what is risky behavior and what is recommended for safety in such situations.

Practitioners have a responsibility to help the adolescent client assess his or her risk for infection and to learn new behaviors to reduce this risk. This can be done by including a sexual history as a routine part of a psychosocial assessment. Ryan (1988), outlines a format for doing this, which includes (1) taking a sexual history as a routine part of a psychosocial assessment and (2) asking clients how AIDS has affected their lives (whether they volunteer this information or not). Additionally, one should inquirie about the adolescent's sexual practices and past efforts to alter his or her behavior to reduce risk.

Many clients avoid discussing sexual contact with their therapists. Nevertheless, they may be at high risk, be misinformed about prevention, and not know how or where to get this information. Having risk-reduction literature in the waiting room and office, in languages used by clients, is helpful so that they can continue to incorporate this information into new behavioral practices.

KEY QUESTIONS TO ASK THE CLIENT

Clinicians need to ask how adolescents make decisions concerning their sexual relationships. Questions aimed at a better understanding of the adolescent's decision-making process often can help determine his or her level of ego functioning. Ego functioning for the adolescent includes the way in which he or she regulates self-esteem, the level of identity consolidation, and the degree of autonomy. It is not uncommon to hear an adolescent girl report that she "goes along" with her boyfriend's insistence on not using a condom. Faulty self-esteem can be a contributing factor to her tendency to bypass careful decision making regarding safe sexual practices. Clinicians can be instrumental in guiding adolescents to carefully consider how they make decisions about whether to have sex. In her work with adolescent girls, Mary Pipher (1994) suggests that she and her client generate a set of criteria about what the client needs to have in place before having sex. The list can include thinking about circumstances, choice of partner, protection options, and safe sex behaviors. Role-playing with the adolescent client to counteract "ploys" that partners may use to have sex with him or her can also be a useful exercise.

In educating adolescents about safer sexual practices, it is useful to keep in mind that they need to preserve a sense of wholeness, to be in charge, and to have "total" power and control over self and environment during adolescence—a time when they experience much biological and physical change. Keeping this in mind, a skilled clinician can question and educate adolescents in a way that appeals to their interest in being in charge of their lives.

Assessment of Ego Functions

Self-Esteem Regulation

The ability to be intimate, to seek mutual sexual fulfillment, and to discuss sexuality, as well as contraceptive protection, is impeded if an adolescent has low self-esteem. Adolescents often regulate their self-esteem through external sources. In these situations it is not uncommon for the insecure adolescent to engage in a range of high-risk behaviors including reckless experimentation with drugs, alcohol, or unprotected sex. Engaging in reckless behaviors is one way adolescents protect themselves from keen feelings of vulnerability, thus denying the real-life implications of their dangerous behaviors. This is often the way an adolescent who is at risk presents. Diminished self-esteem contributes to his or her feelings of invulnerability. Clinicians should recognize that the defenses of invulnerability and denial are attempts to restore and stabilize self-esteem in an adolescent who is feeling vulnerable. For example, an adolescent male's pattern of risk-taking behavior often belies self-doubt and diminished self-esteem. His presentation of bravado can be a facade masking his insecure self. These adolescents often use sexual behavior to regulate their self-esteem and to bind their fears against regressive pulls to their parents. Consequently, in their haste to connect, they may not communicate about sexual matters with their partners or they may seek out indiscriminate sexual encounters, thus placing themselves and their partners at risk for AIDS.

Identity Consolidation

Finding new identifications, loyalties, and interests outside the nuclear family is a core feature of adolescent development. The most important and fundamental aspect of identity consolidation is the development of sexual identity. The adolescent's sense of self is partially based on the extent to which sexual impulses are successfully negotiated. In this regard, the adolescent's ability to negotiate closeness and to experience intimacy in inter-personal relationships is key. The more open an adolescent is able to be with peers, the more likely he or she can talk about intimate topics such as sexual behavior, sexual history, and contraception plans. For some adolescents, a frantic search for comfort, connection, and affirmation may be reflected in unsafe sexual behavior that places them at risk for AIDS.

The capacity for intimacy is only possible when identity formation is solidly established. Oftentimes, sexual intimacy precedes the capacity to develop true and mutual intimacy with another person. For example, an "identity crisis" often occurs upon graduation from high school and moving on into the adult world, where new relationships and behaviors challenge the adolescent's sense of self. For some adolescents, this is a vulnerable period in their development. An impressionable adolescent's experimentation with sex may include multiple partners, drug use, and other potentially dangerous behaviors. Trying out new behaviors in this way can be dangerous, even life-threatening.

Autonomy

The achievement of autonomous functioning for the adolescent involves the disengagement from family ties and engagement with the world of peers and social institutions. A fairly stable sense of identity or self resides in the autonomous person who has become emotionally emancipated from depen-dence on family and who is capable of intimate exchanges and loving relationships. As adolescents move toward autonomy and independent functioning, they search for a place where they can feel safe. Problems can arise for those who have left their families without a "firm enough" sense of their ability to function on their own. Clinicians may see adolescents who upon premature disengagement from family, turn to intense, often frantic relationships, providing the semblance of a temporary place where the ado-lescent can feel safe. The sexual component can reflect his or her attempt to flee from the regressive pulls to the family, resulting in a passionate turning to the "other" through a sexual connection. Adolescents who need others to perform self-regulating functions to make him or her feel complete often turn to impulsive sexual acting out in an effort to meet those needs.

ACTION STEPS FOR SUCCESSFUL INTERVENTION

AIDS education with adolescents works optimally when the informa-tion is presented by someone who recognizes that most behavior in adoles-cence is often psychologically motivated. Research suggests that attitudes, emotional maturity and developmental readiness for intimate relationships play a part in effective use of contraceptives and safe sexual behaviors. In working with adolescents, social workers need to consider the adolescent's ability to delay gratification, to contain impulse control, and to draw upon cognitive abilities to understand, self-soothe, and change behavior.

Social workers working with adolescent populations need to recognize that the developmental stage of adolescence involves a move toward interpersonal closeness and intimacy, which includes sexual intimacy. Feelings of a positive sense of self can be promoted with the exploration and testing of new relationships, resulting in a sense of mastery. With the AIDS epidemic, appropriate moves toward sexual intimacy may be forestalled. The negotiation of closeness and intimacy may be complicated by the frightening, fatal aspects of AIDS. For some adolescents, sexual behavior may be equated with death. In serving adolescents, social workers should consider the potential for this type of thinking and the kind of dilemma it poses for the adolescent.

One of the most important things to convey to adolescents about their sexual behaviors is that they should respect and take care of themselves and their partners. A pragmatic stance can be useful in this context. Attempts to convince teenagers that certain behaviors are "right" elicit either immediate oppositional behavior or superficial compliance. This can be managed by appealing to the inherent adolescent drive toward "making life easier," an approach that often can motivate adolescents toward getting more control over their lives. One might offer privileges contingent on responsible behavior. This is appealing and rewarding to many adolescents. Some schools and community groups offer groups for parents to learn more about adolescent development. Encouraging parents to monitor their adolescent children and especially to attend to responsible behaviors with rewards (i.e., driving privileges, extended curfews, increased allowance, offering to help pay for driver's education or car insurance) helps reinforce their appropriate behavior.

However, the more emotionally vulnerable adolescent often presents a complex challenge to the social worker. The practitioner must first work toward helping the adolescent consider that it is "worth" having a life. Adolescents who have low self-esteem, are depressed, abuse substances, or come from disorganized families may be at highest risk for acquiring HIV. These teens require careful attention and support to convince them that life is worth living. As the adolescent client moves toward a more solid sense of self, stressing safer sexual practices is then more appropriate.

Adolescents need to know that unlike most other STDs, the AIDS virus can exist inside the body for many years before any symptoms of the disease appear, and that even during the asymptomatic time, the disease can be passed on to others. Some teenagers do not believe they can become infected with HIV because they rarely see people their own age who have AIDS. Teens need to understand this discrepancy. Because the time between getting infected with HIV and developing AIDS can be ten years or more, many people with AIDS who are in their twenties (currently one of five reported with AIDS) were infected while they were teenagers (CDC, 1993). Adolescents who share needles to inject drugs (including steroids) or who have sex without a latex condom are getting infected. However, most will not show any symptoms of HIV infection or AIDS until they are in their twenties, even though they can still transmit the infection to others.

CULTURAL COMPETENCY CONSIDERATIONS

Adolescents reflect diversity in terms of socioeconomic status, cultural and ethnic heritage, belief systems, and geographic locations. Talking with adolescents about AIDS should reflect a sensitivity to cultural attitudes regarding sexual activity, including homosexuality.

Cultures have different beliefs about adolescent sexual behavior. Sexual behavior is considered more acceptable in some cultures than in others. Regardless of culture, adolescents should first and foremost be guided to practice safer sex. Assumptions, beliefs, and behaviors that appear normative across a particular group can still represent problems when manifested by individual members of that group. Montalvo and Guitierrez (1983) warn clinicians that some clients hide behind caricatures of their culture's norms to refrain from changing problematic behaviors. For example, girls and women may participate in a silent acquiescence to their male partner's casual, often promiscuous sexual practices, a position that is often unchallenged in the Latin culture. Promiscuity often involves unsafe sex practices. The cultural stereotype of the male "Latin lover" may inadvertently promote problematic behavior, especially in the age of AIDS. Regardless of clients' culture, the social worker's first and foremost charge is to guide adolescents to practice safer sex.

Sexual behavior can reflect both healthy and unhealthy psychological status for the adolescent. Psychological status often is based on the adolescent's definition of self and includes his or her "sense of future" in life (Cadwell, Burnham, and Forstein, 1994). However not all adolescents have a positive, internalized sense of self or future. As Cadwell, Burnham, and Forstein point out, a sense of future is compromised for gay/lesbian adolescents. Other adolescents may have their sense of future impeded by their socio-economic status, especially if they live in a culture of poverty with limited opportunities for the future.

A sense of future often has cultural ramifications. Different groups and subgroups offer their members a feeling of identity, an explanation for the world around them, and assumptions about what is valued. A person from one culture might define something as problematic that members of another group might see as healthy and normal. For example, in Hispanic cultures, sexual behavior often is seen as an expected pathway toward the ultimate goal of motherhood, a desired and valued identity for Hispanic women. Sexual behavior is more positively associated with a sense of future for these adolescent girls.

Dialogues about AIDS should be creative, spark interest and participation, and target "captive audiences." Such audiences might include health, science, physical education, and humanities classes; recreational and church groups; sports teams; clubs; and vocational training classes. Social workers should strive to utilize the accepted mode of gathering for various ethnic groups; for example, many African Americans have strong religious ties and listen carefully to directives from their religious and spiritual leaders.

Challenges to cultural competency include the following: (1) varying levels of comfort that organizations or institutions may have regarding the dissemination of material about sexual behavior, (2) the confusing mixed message in our culture about sex—from "just say no!" to the opposite "just do it!" axioms that adolescents so often hear, and (3) the difference between adolescents who have no sense of future and those who do—because of either cultural or psychological factors.

It is unlikely that adolescent invulnerability is represented as prominently across all cultures as it does in European-Western settings. However, cross-culturally, boys appear to engage in higher risk behaviors such as excessive alcohol or drug use, reckless behaviors (including reckless driving, and more promiscuous sexual behavior than girls. Although newly emigrating adolescents from less-developed countries in Africa, Asia, Russia, and Eastern Europe are in many respects expected to perform more serious, "adultlike" responsibilities in their families, it is unclear yet whether the cultural expectations for responsible behavior will carry over into responsible sexual behaviors.

EXPERIMENTING WITH ALCOHOL AND DRUGS

According to a survey by the National Institute on Drug Abuse, 89 percent of high school seniors reported having tried alcohol (*Sex Education in America; AIDS and Adolescents*, 1993). In survey after survey, young people admit to experimenting with and regular use of illegal drugs. Use and abuse of alcohol and drugs can lower inhibitions and impair judgment and may lead adolescents to engage in risky sexual behavior. Abandoning safer sex techniques, failing to use condoms correctly and consistently, and having sex while under the influence can lead to possible infection with HIV or other STDs. Date rape, an increasing problem, is also associated with alcohol and drug use and may present a risk for infection.

Depression and low self-esteem often lead to the use of substances for self-medication. The disinhibiting aspect of drugs and alcohol make it very hard to be careful about safe sex. Additionally, it is not uncommon to learn that the use of substances serves the function of masking worry about HIV and the importance of being careful. Some people claim that sex feels better when they are using drugs or alcohol. Others acknowledge that they do not like the way they act sexually when they have been using. In this context, social workers may be called upon to convey accurate information about how substances affect sexual pleasure and functioning. Explaining that substances often dull a person's sexual response and interfere with male erections is useful. Also, talking about how substances can interfere with the teen's ability to communicate about whether to have sex, what is pleasurable, or what to do sexually can be helpful. Adolescents who can think and talk about what is right for them are more apt to have sexual relationships that are planned and safe.

Anticipation of situations in which adolescents openly acknowledge on-going drug use forces clinicians to determine their own degree of comfort in addressing this issue. Many practitioners were trained in an era that disapproved of directive approaches that included taking value-laden stands about "what is right" for their client. However, concerning AIDS, drug and alcohol use often contribute to careless sexual behavior, and careless sexual behavior can result in death. Clinicians should consider taking straightforward approaches with clients about how substance use impairs judgment and decision making. Social workers also need to recognize that some teens will be unwilling to stop drug use altogether. Presented with this stance, practitioners will need to manage the anger, frustration, and disappointment that may erupt for them in this difficult situation. In spite of the troubling position an adolescent client may take about his or her drug use, clinicians should focus on safety by emphasizing that if the adolescent cannot stop using, at the very least, he or she should maximize protecting him or herself from AIDS by practicing safe sex.

HELPING ADOLESCENTS WITH HIV
OBTAIN GOOD HEALTH CARE

Although there is no cure for AIDS, the symptoms of AIDS can be treated. Experimental drugs alleviate some of the discomforts created by

AIDS. However, these will not reverse the immune deficiency itself or stop the disease from getting worse. One can access an expert by calling the National AIDS Hotline (1-800-342-AIDS) to find out about resources in the area. Each state has a Board of Health or a Department of Health that provides free HIV testing and treatment.

The new Americans With Disabilities Act (Public Law 101-596) helps fight discrimination against people with disabilities and can protect people who are infected with HIV or are believed to be infected with HIV. Businesses and employers have been made aware of this law. For more information, call the CDC National AIDS Hotline 1-800-342-AIDS (CDC, 1993).

Social workers should recognize that results of the HIV antibody test have the potential to be misused. Patients' rights must be clearly recognized when this test is administered. Clear guidelines have been established in administering the testing by the Centers for Disease Control, including informed counseling and follow-up referral. Because HIV-positive individuals are at risk for discrimination, which can include loss of employment, housing, health insurance, and other rights, practitioners should be especially careful that this test is conducted appropriately and that confidentiality is maintained.

Confidentiality is mandatory for AIDS testing and treatment. Health workers are forbidden, by law, to reveal a client's name. For example, if an adolescent cannot bring himself to tell his partner(s), he can report the name(s) to the Department of Health in his area, and a health worker will inform the partner(s) that he or she has been exposed to HIV and must be tested. If someone at the Department of Health or related service provider treats the adolescent harshly, this can be reported to the CDC National STD Hotline (1- 800-227-8922).

After receiving a diagnosis of HIV, many adolescents seek more information, attempting to make sense of their strange, uncontrollable, and elusive health status. Denial and acceptance alternate throughout this information-gathering process. For some, information becomes a mechanism to regulate fear and uncertainty for both patient and family. Practitioners can direct clients to appropriate journals, medical libraries, and books since mastering the medical jargon and reading about the latest treatment and research can readily enhance coping. For others in which denial operates against the painful realities of AIDS, management of their illness may occur by not wanting to know more about treatment or the status of their illness. They may show a range of behaviors including lack of cooperation regarding needed medical involvement, noncompliance with medication, problematic health or lifestyle habits, and disinterest in monitoring T-cell counts. These adolescents appear able to function psychologically only by denying the reality of their HIV status. This kind of situation is particularly challenging. Talking with adolescents about their wishes and fears, ways of managing their disease, and means of developing the semblance of a normal life can be useful. Joining their "resistance" to know about the illness can be a useful technique toward understanding adolescents' fear of knowing and their powerful defense of denial, which serves to interfere with taking precautions and behaving in healthy ways.

WORKING WITH INFECTED ADOLESCENTS

Infected adolescents will require assistance in managing the enormous social, emotional, and medical implications of their illness. A referral for individual, group, or family therapy might be warranted. Support groups for people with HIV, as well as support systems for families, friends, and caretakers can be helpful.

Clinical work with people with AIDS and HIV is not unlike traditional social casework. A clinician assesses the client's needs and develops a plan for meeting those needs. Practitioners sometimes feel inadequate or helpless when working with people with AIDS (Macks, 1988). However, social workers bring a broad range of professional and personal skills to any clinical experience. Using the practice base as a starting point, social workers can begin immediately to help clients and their support systems mobilize and respond.

Adolescents with HIV display a range of behavior in response to their HIV status. From a psychosocial perspective, these infected adolescents can present a range of behaviors including the following: (1) counterphobic stances, presenting as strong and brave, eager to reach out and teach peers about HIV and safe sex; (2) more overtly debilitated, depressed, ashamed, or hopeless; (3) angry and acting out, even sexually; (4) more psychologically healthy, presenting a mix of fear, anger, or loss, with an accompanying ability to acknowledge their feelings and access supports. The particular presentation may indicate the emotional/developmental level of the adolescent before seroconversion.

The impact of the diagnosis on the internal organization of the patient and the family system is significant. While each family is different, each must absorb and process the information about AIDS. Blame, guilt, anger, shame, anxiety, sadness, and depression must be dealt with. The diagnosis of an AIDS-related condition can be socially stigmatizing and has the potential for discrimination that can and does follow "sharing the secret." Thus, many family members and significant others are reluctant to disclose the health status of the infected individual. This can result in cutting them off from needed supports.

After receiving the diagnosis and integrating the new information, families usually pull together and provide a supportive and caring holding environment for their child. Those with more substantial emotional and material resources understandably do better. Family systems that were socially isolated, were structurally inflexible, and had poor communication and poor affectional relationships before the diagnosis will have more difficulty coping.

THERAPIST'S USE OF SELF

The therapeutic contract often requires modification in doing psychotherapy with persons with AIDS. The concrete aspects of the contract (e.g., consistent time, duration, roles, fees, seating) serve to contain anxiety and evoke a powerful transference relationship (Cole, 1992). News of the illness can be difficult for both the therapist and client. Despite the power of the therapeutic alliance, it cannot contain the client's rage at the therapist and his or her disappointment in the therapist's lack of magical protectiveness. With the HIV diagnosis, the slow, methodical thinking characteristic of the traditional treatment approach gives way to a more active, emotionally present response. In our work with relatively young, highly stigmatized clients who will be intermittently hospitalized and who become increasingly debilitated, the use of self becomes even more important to provide strength and support. This may mean reexamining one's traditional interpretation of such treatment issues as personal disclosure, the use of touch, or seeing clients in their homes, hospital rooms, or in unusual settings. Part of the task in doing therapy with this population is the willingness to reach out and to engage the client wherever he or she may be.

COUNTERTRANSFERENCE ISSUES

A frequent response to working with people with AIDS is a sense of helplessness. The feeling of being "deskilled" is a common one when confronting the complex and multiple needs of people affected by AIDS (Ryan, 1988). Feelings of professional inadequacy can reflect the underlying sense of powerlessness, helplessness, loss of control, and fears that emerge in working with these clients (Macks, 1988). The challenge to be real with clients while still preserving the working alliance is often present for the therapist. Clinicians must confront their sadness and anger while managing their sense of futility about their clinical work as they see their clients dying. For example, to finally confront the death of a client who grew tremendously through the therapeutic relationship can be difficult.

Social workers find themselves in positions of not knowing what to do or say or how to make decisions. Going into a hospital or home, if this is a new procedure, creates anxiety for the therapist. The issue of how sick or deformed the client will look also is a difficult issue: Can the therapist bear it, and how should the therapist act?

Particular issues and concerns emerge for practitioners working with AIDS patients. Countertransference reactions can include unresolved attitudes and negative feelings about behaviors their clients may have engaged in such as their refusal to stop drug or alcohol use. Unresolved issues of racism, sexism, and homophobia frequently reemerge. Workers may be uncomfortable expressing these issues either with peers or in supervision. Other commonly identified issues with HIV clients are fears of contagion, fear of death, denial, overidentification, and anger. Because working with AIDS-affected adolescent clients requires so much support, clinicians should make use of support groups that optimally are available during regular work hours. These groups should be held routinely and should be designed to provide a safe place to explore and manage negative feelings, loss, and conflict. An important adjunct in managing countertransference feelings is participation in direct training to bind anxiety, reduce fear of contagion, and counter discrimination.

POLICY IMPLICATIONS AND RELATED ACTIONS

The immediate challenge for the clinician and educator working with AIDS-affected adolescents is to alter the view that AIDS is the disease of the "other." Research has shown that most U.S. residents, including teenagers, understand how HIV is transmitted and how they can avoid being infected. Therefore, confronting the belief that "it can't happen to me" should be an important focus of policy planning for public information and educational programs. Social workers, educators, and public health officials need to combine efforts to reach adolescents who are not getting the information and assistance they need to protect themselves from AIDS. Conveyance of information is complicated further by adolescent rebellion and distrust of adults as they move toward independence. Policymakers should strive to develop public information compaigns that include many youth-oriented materials. AIDS prevention education must become a standard part of contact with all adolescents. Mental health professionals play an integral role in the educational process; they may in fact be the first and primary source of AIDS prevention for adolescents.

Social workers and other members of the helping profession must become increasingly visible in educating policymakers. Policies should aim toward developing community-based, regional, and national prevention programs. Not all youth can be reached through the schools. Educational efforts should include street outreach; clinic-based education; counseling, testing, and referral programs; and programs that address the specific needs of runaway, incarcerated, migrant, homeless, and other youth in high-risk situations.

Community action is a very powerful weapon. The strongest educational and prevention efforts are those that involve all parts of the community: businesses, schools, civic and volunteer groups, religious organizations, and individuals. For example, the HIV Prevention Community Planning Initiative, a model developed by the CDC (1994) represents a step forward in the planning of culturally competent and scientifically sound HIV prevention services that specifically address unique community needs. Community planning is a process whereby the identification of high priority prevention needs is shared between the health department administering HIV-prevention funds and representatives of the community for whom the services are intended. In addition, the community planning process emphasizes the notion that the behavioral and social services must pay a critical role in the development, implementation, and evaluation of HIV prevention programs within a community. Many communities across the country have identified youth in high-risk situations as a group requiring intense prevention efforts. This kind of initiative strives to work in partnership with state and local health departments, national and regional organizations, and community-based organizations to address this need.

As the epidemic continues, repressive legislation and policies will continue to be introduced. Some of this legislation will be passed. Social workers and other members of the helping profession must become increasingly visible in educating policymakers, lobbying for appropriate policies, and pressing our professional associations to use their influence and resources to respond. The AIDS epidemic represents an opportunity for individuals, families, institutions, and systems to respond. Our responses must be coordinated and comprehensive; the resources and leadership potential of our social work institutions must be focused, committed, and consistently applied.

RECOMMENDED READINGS

Risky times: How to be AIDS-smart and stay healthy (1993) by Jeanne Blake. Risky Times Book Project, P.O. Box 15597, Kenmore Station, Boston, Massachusetts 02215.

Sex education in America: AIDS and adolescents (1993), by Media Works Inc. Media Works, Inc, P.O. Box 15597, Kenmore Station, Boston, Massachusetts 02215.

Programs that work (1994), by U.S. Centers for Disease Control and Prevention. Division of Adolescent and School Health. U.S. Centers for Disease Control and Prevention, 1600 Clifton Road, Mail Stop K-31, Atlanta, Georgia 30333. 404-488-5372.

REFERENCES

Cadwell, S., Burnham, R., and Forstein, M. (Eds.). (1994). *Therapists on the front line: Psychotherapy with gay men in the age of AIDS.* Washington, DC: American Psychiatric Press.

Centers for Disease Control (1985). Results of a Gallup poll on acquired immunity deficiency syndrome—New York City, United States. *MMWR 34:* 513-514.

Centers for Disease Control (June 1993). Surgeon General's Report to the American public on HIV infection and AIDS. Atlanta: Author.

Centers for Disease Control (December 1994). Adolescents and HIV/AIDS. Atlanta: Author.

Cole, A. B. (1992). Frame modifications with a dying client. *Smith College Studies in Social Work 63:* 313-324.

Macks, J. (1988). Women and AIDS: Countertransference issues. *Social Casework 69*(6): 346.

Montalvo, B., and Guiterrez, M. (1983) A perspective for the use of the cultural dimension in family therapy. In C. Falicov and J. C. Hansen (Eds.), *Family therapy collections: (6) Cultural perspectives in family therapy* (15-32): Rockville, MD: Aspen.

Pipher, M. (1994). *Reviving Ophelia: Saving the selves of adolescent girls.* New York: Ballantine Books.

Ryan, C. (1988). The social and clinical challenges of AIDS. *Smith College Studies in Social Work 59:* 3-20.

Media Works, Inc. *Sex education in America: AIDS and adolescents.* (1993). P.O. Box 15597, Kenmore Station, Boston, Massachusetts.

Simkins, L. and Eberhage, M. (1984). Attitudes towards AIDS, herpes, and toxic shock syndrome. *Psychological Reports 55:* 786-799.

Sunenblick, M. B. (1988). The AIDS epidemic: Sexual behaviors of adolescents. *Smith College Studies in Social Work 59:* 21-27.

Services to People with HIV in the Workplace

S. Michelle Martin

WHY DO THIS?
STATEMENT OF THE PROBLEM AND ISSUES

AIDS is the leading cause of death for Americans aged twenty-five to forty-four according to the Centers for Disease Control. More than half of America's workforce falls into that age category. Given these statistics, your workplace has probably already or will soon deal with AIDS/HIV.

Because the virus strikes people in all work settings, workplaces all across the country have been affected by HIV. As a result, employers have a great opportunity and responsibility to educate their workforce about HIV. Many companies have active HIV educational programs. Unfortunately, HIV education is not implemented at many work sites until an employee reveals that he or she is infected. Thorough and workplace-specific education is needed at that point.

Employees with HIV have some special needs at certain points of their disease progression. Employers have to be mindful of an HIV-positive employees' health and workload, as well as any adaptions the company will need to make for reasonable accommodation. Since 1990, the Americans with Disabilities Act, a federal law governing these types of adaptations has been in effect. Co-workers will be affected by both shifting work responsibilities and the emotional toll the disease may take on employees. Employers need to recognize the needs of both the infected individual and his or her co-workers, as well as management's needs.

IMPLEMENTING HIV EDUCATION IN THE WORKPLACE

A responsive HIV education plan includes several elements. First, the company must write a workplace policy on HIV. The policy will set standards for dealing with HIV across the company, provide support to employees who are infected with or affected by HIV, raise awareness and prevent infection among employees, help avoid a crisis when HIV becomes an issue in the company, and establish that the company will comply with legal responsibilities.

The policy can be quite extensive or a few simple paragraphs. The agency culture and management attitude will determine the length and extensiveness of the policy. Managers and supervisors should be involved in developing the policy. If this is not possible, they should be given the policy prior to other employees to become familiar with it so they may address employees' concerns.

When writing the policy, many issues need to be considered. The workplace policy should spell out how the company will treat and protect employees' confidentiality regarding HIV. As a social worker, you are keenly aware of the importance of confidentiality for clients. The same care and compassion should be extended to your workers with confidential issues. One way this point is illustrated is the manner in which health care claims are filed in your company. Many large employers have employees file claims with their human resource department. This means that any claims for reimbursement identify the presenting problem on the claim form or the medical bill. When these claims are turned in, the company personnel handling them will know the diagnosis of the employee. This situation might feel awkward and embarrassing for many employees, but it certainly affects employees living with HIV. The workplace policy should address this problem. A solution would be a recommendation to management to contract out the claims process to an external business.

The policy will also need to address the company's nondiscrimination policy related to HIV infection. Compliance with the Americans With Disabilities Act of 1990 should also be stated in the policy. The policy will need to address employee education and where to go for help within the company. As with many work assignments, if time and energy are invested initially, the implementation and effectiveness phases will be much smoother.

After your policy is written, it is important that it not be filed and forgotten. The policy should be posted in a common area so it becomes a part of everyday work life.

The next step to occur is the implementation of employee education. Decide what you need to communicate, how you intend to communicate it, and who will do the communication. The basic information to cover includes HIV transmission, HIV prevention, company policy on HIV, company benefits, and where to go for help, both within the company and externally. If the workforce has some occupational exposure to HIV, such as nurses, dental assistants, or emergency medical technicians, it is important to include information regarding universal precautions and the

Occupational Safety and Health Act of 1970 (OSHA). Clearly, these standards must be followed to avoid exposure. Managers and supervisors should be trained first as with the policy development. This will equip them to better answer questions and concerns that might arise. If you do not have an appropriate person within the company to provide education, your local chapter of the Red Cross or your area HIV/AIDS organization can usually fulfill this role.

Once the education component is initially completed, it should be offered again on a regular basis. Each new employee should get this information during their new employee orientation period. Hopefully, this will occur before the employee deals with HIV-related issues with clients or co-workers. Ongoing training for all employees should be implemented to reinforce the message of the HIV policy and the company's stance. Many employers schedule follow-up sessions every six months for all employees.

Each training session should include an opportunity for all employees to give feedback on the policy and training. This will give the employees a chance to discuss the usefulness to them of the training, and changes can be made based on this information. This will also give you information about the relevance of this for your employees. Some employees who have experienced HIV with family members, friends, or themselves might be upset with the subject matter. Keep this in mind and check in with your employees after the training session. Your role as a social worker can be very significant at this time. Employees needs might range from information and referral to simply listening to their story to help them access a mental health provider for ongoing help. All of these situations would call upon your expertise and knowledge as a social worker.

HOW TO HELP CO-WORKERS ADAPT TO HAVING A PERSON WITH HIV AT WORK

As with any life-threatening illness, HIV affects the infected person and those surrounding them. Since HIV tends to strike young adults, the impact on the work site is deeply felt. Co-workers will have different reactions and take various actions in dealing with an infected co-worker.

In the early years of the epidemic, fear of "catching" AIDS through casual contact was great. Although we now have much more information and know that you can not "catch" the virus in this way, some misinformed co-workers might react with fear of obtaining the virus from the infected co-worker. It is important to provide information to these co-workers and a safe place to talk about their fears. If this hysteria cannot be overcome, you might consider moving the employee to a different work placement where they will not have contact with a person known to be living with HIV. *Do not* relocate the employee with HIV unless they have requested a transfer. The person living with HIV should not be moved because this will reinforce the notion that he or she somehow might infect another or that he or she is the problem. If a co-worker has a problem, he or she is the one to be moved.

Since HIV assaults many people from typically disenfranchised communities, i.e., gay men, injection drug users, and sex workers, some employees might react judgmentally about other's lifestyles. These judgments can fuel circumstances that are already emotionally charged and sometimes result in blaming the person with HIV for his or her situation. Again, it is important to educate the co-worker. Many people believe that they do not know any gay men or injection drug users, but since there are often no outward signs of either, one would not know if the workforce did include gay men or drug users. Beliefs about sexual behaviors and lifestyles are often deeply held; such entrenched beliefs are difficult to challenge or change.

Because co-workers will see the progression of the disease on a daily basis, they may feel emotionally drained. The person with HIV will have good days and bad days due to the disease. Physical and possibly emotional changes will occur. Many people want to avoid these overt traits of terminal illness, but it is vital to the employees and the company that these issues are acknowledged. You might consider a retreat for the work group, a referral to an Employee Assistance Program (EAP), or utilization of company health benefits to obtain counseling or therapy.

Many work groups experience some of these nonsupportive reactions and emotions initially, but then the co-workers pull together to provide support and love during crucial times. Work groups can be of enormous assistance to people living with HIV and their loved ones. It will be up to you and your co-workers to strike the balance that is right for you. Whatever the outcome of the situation, growth and awareness will result.

Case Example

> Jess, a thirty-eight-year-old banker, became infected with HIV after receiving a blood transfusion in the early 1980s. He has tested positive for the virus after months of experiencing fatigue and weight loss. Jess continues to work, but approaches his supervisor about telling his entire department of his diagnosis. Rumors have already been circulating about his illness and sexual orientation. Some employees have declared that they will not work or share a bathroom with someone with AIDS. The bank hires an outside consultant to provide a workplace training and be present when Jess breaks the

news to his co-workers. The actual announcement of his illness and confirmation of some of the rumors is met with silence. A few co-workers privately offer their support; others now avoid him. However, the rumors and accusations stop. Jess is able to work a normal work week with periodic episodes of illness. Nine months after the initial announcement, he becomes too ill to continue to work. The employees of the bank organize to ask the bank management if they might share their sick leave with Jess. They also set up a rotating schedule of meal delivery and companionship for him. All these things help Jess die comfortably at home. Every year on the anniversary of his death, his co-workers take up a collection and make a contribution to the local AIDS service organization in his honor.

HOW TO PROVIDE REASONABLE ACCOMMODATIONS FOR PEOPLE WITH HIV IN THE WORKPLACE

Many businesses in America, large and small, for profit and not for profit, have productive employees who are vital to their companies, and these employees happen to be living with HIV. The fact that a person has HIV will not by itself affect the employee or the workplace. Supervisors will not have to make accommodations or adjustments simply because one employee has the virus. HIV will not usually affect work performance for employees. It is possible in some cases that the emotional toll of the disease might interfere with the employees' ability to do their work. Performance concerns should be addressed with any employee, regardless of HIV status, as soon as possible. However, at some point changes due to disease progression might affect work performance in various ways. In our case example, Jess was able to perform his job responsibilities but needed to shorten his work week by several hours. This change allowed him to pace himself and rest as he needed since fatigue was one of his major symptoms. Employers should check periodically with workers concerning how capable they feel about performing their work tasks. Supervisors should not assume that an employee cannot complete his or her job because of HIV. When considering talking to an employee living with HIV, remember to extend the same respect, dignity, and confidentiality afforded to any noninfected worker.

People living with HIV are protected from discrimination under the Americans with Disabilities Act (ADA). The ADA is a federal law that prohibits discrimination on the basis of disability in public accommodations, employment, public transportation, federal, state, and local government services, and telecommunications. Employees with fifteen or more employees are subject to ADA requirements. Employees with HIV must be given "reasonable accommodation" in the workplace. Reasonable accommodations are modifications or adjustments that allow a person with a disability to perform essential functions of their job. Essential functions of the job are defined as elements that are fundamental to successful completion of job tasks. An employer is not required to make adjustments that would result in significant expense or difficulty for the business. An example of reasonable accommodation would be allowing a person with HIV to have more frequent time off to attend medical appointments. Since the ADA is a recent law, many aspects and their interpretations are still unclear. Please consult your attorney or call the Equal Employment Opportunity office for further information.

Employees who are infected with HIV, in conjunction with their supervisor, may need to give some attention and thought to their job. Many factors will influence how this will occur and "what it will look like." The nature of the work, the previous relationship between the supervisor and employee, the extent of illness, and the desired workplace outcome will determine how this should be approached.

Work performance may change or suffer as the disease progresses. Work duties might need to be altered to accommodate these changes. For many people, work represents an important part of their identity. Some mangers might be uncomfortable as well and encourage the employee to resign or go on disability before it is appropriate. Retiring or obtaining disability might seem like the logical solution to many supervisors. However, this decision should be made by the employee when he or she is ready. Medical professionals can advise the person with HIV regarding work concerns and limitations and the affect of continued work on his or her health.

As discussed earlier, HIV disease is an emotional issue for family, friends, and co-workers. Obviously it is also emotionally charged for the person with HIV. Reactions of a person living with HIV will vary across the spectrum depending on disease progression and the outlook of the person living with HIV. A supervisor would be wise to deal with these issues as they arise. These emotions might be more evident when the employee is experiencing some crisis, such as initial diagnosis with HIV, significant drop in health status, or hospitalizations. The supervisor must bear these factors in mind.

Employee Assistance Programs

The utilization of employee assistance programs (EAP) related to HIV is often the easiest step an employer can take to ensure employees have the opportunity to address their mental health needs. An employee assistance program can help employees with a wide range of needs including HIV-related issues. To ensure that your employees get the best care possible, consider the following when choosing an EAP:

- Does the EAP have therapists who are trained and familiar with HIV, substance abuse, and gay community issues? Are the staff members trained in death and loss issues?
- Does the EAP have inservice trainings regarding these issues?
- Does the EAP maintain strict confidentiality regarding your employees sessions? Is this properly conveyed to the employee?
- Does the EAP make proper and appropriate referrals when sessions are finished?
- Can the EAP conduct both one-on-one and group sessions?

Since EAP programs generally provide a limited number of sessions that can be accessed and HIV is a long-term issue, the employees must have the opportunity to continue their mental health care. Employers should also examine the benefits of their group health insurance program. Many employees might need more than the limited number of sessions that an EAP provides. As someone living with HIV said to me one time, "This isn't a six-week thing. I need help for longer than that." Mental health benefits in a health insurance plan can make this possible. Furthermore, an employee might want to choose a provider. As a social worker, you are keenly aware of the importance of rapport. Someone dealing HIV must feel comfortable enough to explore and challenge themselves with a therapist.

In summary, the HIV epidemic is altering the psychological landscape of the U.S. workplace. There will be a day when all workplaces have encountered HIV/AIDS in some manner—whether the infected person is the spouse of an employee, a customer, or a valued employee. The practical tools given in this chapter will help prepare you for that time.

RESOURCES FOR ADDITIONAL INFORMATION

Business Responds to AIDS Managers Kit, National AIDS Clearinghouse, P.O. Box 6003, Rockville, Maryland 20849.

Equal Employment Opportunity Commission, Publications Helpline, 1-800-669-3362 (voice), 1-800-800-3302 (TDD).

Providing Services to Gay Men

Steven A. Cadwell

WHY DO THIS?
STATEMENT OF THE PROBLEM AND ISSUES

The general mental health, legal, medical, and financial issues described elsewhere in this book also affect gay men with HIV. However, gay men are uniquely affected by the epidemic because of its predominance within the gay community and because of the assault of homophobia that not only predated HIV but also has been exacerbated by HIV.

Since gay men continue to comprise the greatest number of people with HIV and since the epidemic has taken such a devastating toll on gay communities, most gay men in some way have been emotionally affected by the epidemic. Gay men can be emotionally affected in a range of ways: the trauma of actual infection, the anxiety concerning becoming infected, the demands of caregiving, and the grief over the loss of loved ones.

Beyond the sheer numbers affected, the epidemic has had particular meaning for gay men. Reacting to generations of oppression, the gay liberation movement of the 1970s aggressively asserted sexual expression of homoerotic love. The HIV epidemic has been like an unending scatter shot of terrorist bombs in the midst of the Gay Liberation Parade. Every gay man has to reckon with the emotional and personal meaning of this mix: making love can get confused with making sickness and death. Unless this concept is untangled, the mix can be devastating.

Because of the social stigma experienced by gay men due to the homophobia of the larger society, gay men with HIV often have unique challenges in getting legal, medical, and financial needs met. Homophobia can lead to isolation and self-destructive behavior, which makes HIV prevention in the gay community particularly challenging. For gay men with HIV, confidentiality in service delivery has been critically important for protection against multiple sources of discrimination that might result if information about HIV status *or* sexual orientation were revealed.

In certain urban areas, over the first decade of the epidemic, the gay and lesbian communities developed HIV service agencies to meet the particular needs of gay men. These agencies have evolved to meet the needs of all people affected by HIV and continue to offer vital services for gay men.

Although the gains made by these agencies have been substantial, gay men with HIV continue to need ongoing and broad-based social work advocacy.

An understanding of the way in which HIV has added trauma to an already oppressed group is necessary to prepare the social worker for effective interventions in policy and practice to meet the needs of gay men with HIV. This will include dealing with the social consequences of disenfranchisement, discrimination, and inequality, and the personal consequences of shame, isolation, and blame too often have been characteristic of the experience of gay men with HIV.

Indeed all gay clients have a vital need for social workers who are sensitive to their vulnerabilities to the assault of this epidemic.

EXAMPLES OF HOW THE ISSUE MAY PRESENT

HIV has affected the normative development of the gay client. HIV takes on particular meaning within the specific developmental stage of the client.

Studies have shown that gay men display the same range of mental health as the heterosexual population. Although no remarkable difference in distribution of mental health exists, one feature is very different. Critical in any gay man's development is reckoning with his sexual orientation—the process of "coming out." The stigma and shame of HIV may force the gay client to revisit the earlier critical developmental stage of coming out. Depending on where the client is in his own integration of his gay identity, having been diagnosed with HIV may either be a recapitulation of the old struggle or a fresh encounter with new experiences of stigma. He may have to deal with his own internalized homophobia concerning potentially being more publically perceived as gay, and he may have to deal with a second coming out—identifying as a person with HIV.

If he had hidden his homosexual identity in an isolating closet of shame, he may use the same isolating defense to deal with this other condition that society scorns. Often, moralistic feelings surface, which had earlier not been completely resolved. One gay client reacted to his HIV diagnosis by saying, "This is proof that I'm bad. The church and my family and society have been saying it all along. How can I see it any other way?"

Fear of AIDS forces a reworking of coming-out issues. Some men may go back in the closet, using the dissociative logic that if they disavow their gay identity, then they are not homosexual and not at risk for HIV. They may give up sex consciously, or become impotent, or entirely split off their sex life from their identity. They mix their homophobia with their AIDS phobia. Their shame of being homosexual and dread of getting HIV may isolate them again from either having sex or establishing relationships.

If we apply Erikson's "eight stages of man" as a model for understanding development, we can understand that the gay client who is negotiating the meaning of HIV in his life will be reworking dimensions of several earlier stages: trust versus mistrust, autonomy versus shame and doubt, industry versus inferiority, and identity versus role confusion. The renegotiation of these earlier issues is typical of any patient adapting to a chronic illness. A gay man's earlier developmental stages were already complicated by his sexual orientation. When he gets HIV, the renegotiation of earlier stages is also further complicated by these earlier phase-specific challenges. What was perhaps not fully resolved in the first round will be reexposed during this crisis.

A further complication is that many of these stage-specific conflicts are aroused simultaneously, creating a sense of chaos and disorganization. Normalizing the experience and focusing on each issue can help the client feel some sense of control and order and help him toward resolution. The type and degree of conflict of the client will be affected by his stage in the coming-out process, his developmental issues, his premorbid personality issues, and his stage of illness.

The gay client with HIV, who is generally in his twenties and thirties, is not only thrown backward to earlier issues but also catapulted forward into issues that are expectable in one's sixties and older. Some gay men may be panicked about finding an intimate relationship if they do not have one. Some may be reckoning with issues of generativity. Some men may be wrestling with the ultimate issue of life: ego integrity versus despair. Some may not have the ego capacity or the life experience to be dealing with these issues easily. Gradual loss in the normal course of life allows one to adjust to death. The unrelenting loss brought on by the epidemic assails multiple facets of a gay person's life. His own health, the health of his friends, and the cohesion of his community all may be collapsing simultaneously.

Addressing these dilemmas in therapy will be critical. Should the therapy focus on long-term characterological issues or focus on supportive work concerning accepting death and grief work? Should a man at age twenty-seven faced with an AIDS diagnosis pay off outstanding debts or go on a trip to Europe—perhaps his only chance to travel? Should a man at forty continue with his clinical practice of medicine or close shop and retire to his summer home? Should a thirty-two-year-old gay man who has always wanted a long-term relationship give up his aspiration for one upon learning that he has HIV? How does the gay man whose normal course of development has been radically affected by the news of AIDS diagnosis proceed with his life?

INTEGRATED ASSESSMENT MODEL

A multiaxial approach, which includes dynamics of intrapsychic and interpersonal, as well as person-in-culture issues, is especially useful to understanding gay men with HIV. Assessing medical, social, political, and psychological issues, we can better understand the meaning of the disease or the metaphor the illness represents. The gay client may experience HIV as a recapitulation of earlier conflict related to neglect, oppression, or abuse. Addressing the social stigma and internalized shame is critical. These issues may surface at any point in the course of a gay man's encounter with HIV:

> *In pre-antibody-testing counseling:* Mr. M., a thirty-five-year-old gay man who was abused in childhood and rejected at age fifteen by his fundamentalist family for being homosexual, anticipates that testing HIV positive would be further confirmation of his core "badness."

> *In post-HIV-positive testing:* Mr. C., a twenty-five-year-old gay man, confuses the tragedy of his infection with earlier abuse by his step-mother and alcoholic father.

> *In later stages of illness:* Mr. Z., a twenty-eight-year-old gay man, feels that his homosexuality caused him to get AIDS. His mother has never accepted his homosexuality. She also has been chronically depressed. He construes his diagnosis as contributing to more of his mother's depression. His guilt about his mother's depression inter-feres with resolving his grief over his real losses and his capacity to finish what business he can with his mother.

In any of these cases, individual treatment can be helpful. In addition, supportive group psychotherapy with peers can be valuable as the individual joins other members to learn new coping styles.

Other Sources of Support Should Also Be Assessed and Enlisted

Chosen family (lovers and friends who are chosen by the individual in adult life) and members of the family of origin are both potentially sup-portive, but in each case, specific issues should be explored. Ideally, the family can be a critical source of support. However, members of the family of origin may be struggling with their own homophobia or dynamic prob-lems that leave them ineffectual as an ally for the gay person with HIV. If they are willing, intervention can address some of the homophobia and shift the focus to real ways of assisting their gay family member. However, in some instances, the issues are too great to resolve and the autonomy of the gay man with HIV needs to be respected and his grief over the family's inability to be a resource addressed.

Although a potential source of support, the family may also be a hindrance. While always searching for resources and dealing with resistance to their use, the social worker must respect the autonomy and directive of the client. If the social worker does open the treatment relationship to include work with family members of the client, attention must be paid to preserving the primacy of the client-social worker relationship. Any change in the boundaries of the social worker's role must be negotiated for the relationship to retain its privileged, trusted status for the gay man with HIV.

FACTS THE SOCIAL WORKER
NEEDS TO KNOW BEFORE PROCEEDING

HIV arrived in gay life at the end of a decade of gay liberation and assertion, which ignited in 1969 when a group of gay men fought back against police harassment of a private gay bar, the Stonewall Inn, in New York City. In this period, one dimension of self-worth was expressed through liberated sexual behavior. With the onslaught of the HIV epidemic, homosexuality became linked with illness and death. In addition, the virus arrived during a time in which the larger culture was having a romance with medical care that seemed to promise extended mortality. Cancer and heart disease notwithstanding, belief in Western medicine's capacity to cure all ills was at a zenith. For most people, death was out of sight in their daily lives and thus out of mind. Death was taboo.

The majority "straight" culture met the news of AIDS as if it could dismiss the plight of the epidemic by labeling it a "gay plague" and thus dissociate from it. Unlike other lethal health problems such as heart disease or cancer, which also break the death taboo, the HIV epidemic has the added charge of breaking the sexual taboo as well. Accordingly, services with gay men must attend to all these levels of the epidemic: death phobia, sex phobia, and homophobia.

Gay men have been able to draw on their own growth and development as a community in discovering their capacity to care for one another. Gay men have been empowered as they have discovered other means to survive. The gay cities within the larger urban areas have proved their strength time and again, and rural gay networks have shown equal vitality. Service organizations have been developed to advocate for and support infected gay men. When the larger community failed, the gay community raised funds and developed services. Education and prevention were managed by the gay community itself as the larger public health system lagged behind.

Given the magnitude of the assault, it is not surprising that weaknesses are also evident in the gay community's response to the disease. The gay community has been further alienated and undercut by persistant lack of aggressive, assertive public support. National public health policy continues to vacillate and avoid a comprehensive approach to gay men's health needs.

On a personal level, the response to the assault can run the gamut. Within the context of stress overload and stigma, some maladaptive responses are understandable. Broadly, unsafe sexual behavior can be seen as a desperate or habitual and nonadaptive way of binding affect and self. However, this assessment of maladaption may be overly reductionistic. By definition, any repeated behavior that endangers health could be called compulsive. But now, no sex is totally risk-free. Consequently, if sex itself is a risky activity, then what degree of behavior change are we expecting from gay men to become safe? Abstinence? We must address the issue of the latent message we give when we talk about "safer sex." The challenge for gay men is to tolerate an intense level of uncertainty as they live with degrees of responsible risk that they consciously choose—alongside other risks such as driving a car or traveling by airplane. When we explore degrees of safer sex with this attitude we are joining them in their assessment of the quality of their life as reflected in their sex life.

Drug and alcohol abuse have already been shown to have higher incidence in the gay community. The disproportionate abuse may well be in response to the oppression and stigma in a homophobic society. Gay men in the midst of the HIV epidemic may again turn to these means of soothing pain.

Equipped with some of the general background of the gay experience, you now will need to know specifics about your gay client.

GUIDE TO ASSESSMENT OF GAY CLIENTS

Specific Background of a Gay Client

The following areas should be covered in a thorough intake evaluation of your gay client, including several issues specific to gay men and HIV.

- *Age*
- *Race/Ethnicity*
- *Religion*
- *Income Level*
  - Studies are now showing that differences in knowledge, attitudes, and behaviors often attributed to race or ethnicity are in fact related

to income and education. Significant differences are found between working-class and middle-class gay men in terms of attitudes about sexuality, community, and HIV disease. These differences are critical to developing appropriate HIV education interventions and developing effective HIV-related psychotherapy.

- *Risk Behaviors*
  - Sexual behaviors
  - IV drug behaviors
  - Alcohol and other drug abuse
- *Relationship Functioning*
  - Who else is in his life (friends, family, roommate, lover/partner)?
  - What does he call his primary relationship?
  - Who is his best friend?
  - What is his support network?
  - Whom can he rely on?
- *Point in Continuum of Coming Out*
  - Is the person out to himself, friends, family, or co-workers?
  - What is the gay man's support network?
- *Point of Impact of HIV*
  - Is the client HIV negative or positive, or is he debating being tested?
  - If he is HIV positive, where is he in the course of the disease?
  - In the client's words, what brings him to treatment?
  - What losses due to HIV has person suffered?
  - Are any friends and lovers ill?
  - Does he have friends and lovers who have died from AIDS?
- *How the Client Handles Crises (Particularly Illness)*
- *Preexistant Character Problems or Intrapsychic Conflict*
  - Has the client previously used mental health services?
- *Resource Referral*
  - Are services in place?
  - How much does he know about these?
  - Does he have a "plan to use them"?
  - Offer to help sort out his feelings about his options, which include individual therapy, group resource, therapy or support, couples therapy, family therapy, psychopharmacological intervention, and neuropsychological intervention.
- *Social Services Resources*
  - Disability
  - Welfare
  - Housing
  - Medical services

- *Medical Resources*
  - Are resources limited (especially in rural areas)?
  - Be creative, for example, by creating support groups over the telephone or a computer network.

KEY QUESTIONS TO ASK THE CLIENT

If you are doing case management for a gay client (1) ask his wishes about confidentiality regarding sexual orientation and (2) ask about his past experiences with homophobic services.

Sexual History

If offering mental health service, you should ask about a gay man's *sexual history*. A thorough sexual history includes the following general and HIV-specific topics: language, current sexual activity, current functioning, history of sexual experience, and history of coming out.

Language

The social worker should be able to speak about homosexual sexual practices directly and frankly. Capacity to be frank could save a client's life since the social worker has a critical opportunity to talk about safer sex with the client and may be able to explore the meaning of sex to help to ensure it is a functional and safe experience.

Always remember that clinicians' attitudes are important. A nonjudgmental stance is critical. Watch for indications of attitudes in body language, and adjust to the patient's vocabulary if needed.

The following are some tips about conducting this part of the interview:

- Progress from discussing general to specific information.
- Start by using professional terms. Be willing to adapt to the client's vocabulary.
- Acknowledge the patient's nonverbal communication; discuss the meaning of them.
- Invite the patient to comment on the process of taking the sexual history.

Current Sexual Activity

Cover material that will help make clear distinctions between gender orientation, erotic fantasies, sexual behavior, affectional behavior, and intimacy.

To begin, ask the following: "Tell me about your sexual experience?" (If client only gives homosexual or heterosexual experience, ask about the other. Estimates now indicate that 25 to 40 percent of the population are or have been bisexual.)

Regarding safer sex, ask the following, if he acknowledges sex with men: "Do you have anal sex?" "Do you receive the penis or insert yours?" "Have you let men come inside you?" "Do you know if anyone who you have ever had sex with has HIV?" "Do you know the HIV status of your present sexual partner?' "Do you have oral sex?" "Do you swallow cum?" "Do you swallow precum?" "Do you have anonymous sex?" "Are you currently sexually active?" "How often do you have intercourse?" "Do you have concerns about masturbation?" ("Do you have shame about it?" "Do you have the capacity to soothe yourself?") "Do you practice safer sex?" "What do you think is safer sex?" "How long have you been practicing safer sex?" "Have you concerns about earlier behavior that may have been risky?" "Have you ever had an STD?"

It is important to be specific, e.g., by asking when does client put on the condom and does he know how to use it, and what kind of condom does he use? Inquire if he uses latex condoms (not animal because lambskin condoms do not block HIV transmission). Also ask what kind of lubricant he uses (it should not be petroleum-based, e.g., vaseline, but rather water-soluble, which will not affect the latex.)

Studies show many people do not know how to use condom. Often they put on a condom too late—after some ejaculation has occurred—or do not leave room at end of condom for ejaculation and movement in intercourse. Ask if he unrolls the condom all the way to the bottom of the shaft of the penis when putting it on. Ask your client if he is careful not to tear the condom when opening the condom package. One study (Public Health Reports, 1990) showed 80 percent of 219 gay men studied were deficient in at least one of the four procedures just mentioned.

Ask about drug and alcohol use. Either can be a major disinhibiter and the cause of unsafe sex.

Additionally, you should ask if the client has concerns about sexual relationships outside of his primary one.

Current Functioning

Ask the client if he has any questions or concerns about his sexual functioning. Medication, illness, or emotional problems related to HIV may affect sexual functioning. Ask for a clarification of any mentioned problems, including duration, extent, ideas concerning the cause, and previous treatment. Ask if he has some question about sex he needs more information about. Has the client noticed any problems in his ability to have and enjoy sex? Does he have any concerns about his frequency of intercourse or lack of sexual desire? Determine if he has problems with relationships or with lack of orgasm. Does he have any concerns about sexual orientation?

History of Sexual Experience

History of sexual experience may need further detail depending on what has been initially identified. Areas to consider include experiences in childhood, adolescense, and adulthood.

Sexual experience in childhood. Attitudes about sex in the family, between parents, in one's religion, and in one's culture all affect our attitude toward sex.

Most children explore sexuality early on with peers. Ask your client what were his early sexual experiences and how did he learn about sex—from parents, school, or peers). Ask about your client's masturbation practices before he was able to reach orgasm at puberty.

Adolescence. Ask your client what puberty was like, as well as what his early experiences of wet dreams and masturbation were like? What were his early explorations with same-sex and opposite-sex partners? What was his first experience of intercourse with a partner? (Listen for rape or incest.)

Adulthood. Ask your client about his committed partnerships, extrarelational experience, changes in sexual functioning over time, and his sexual fantasies.

Sexual abuse and incest. Many people have been sexually abused or have questions about their early experience. Ask your client if he was ever abused. (This is *critical information* as studies are now connecting the repetition of unsafe sex as often being connected to a history of incest and sexual abuse. The gay man may be repeating early traumatic experience in his current unsafe sexual practices.)

History of Coming Out

Include a coming-out history. Be especially sensitive to whom he is out to and for how long. What was the coming-out experience like with his family and community? Determine how your client defines homosexuality. Just sex or is there a homoemotional element? Explore the meaning of HIV in his sex life. How has HIV affected his sexual expression? Is he more careful or less careful? Is he phobic? What has his experience been with gay bashing? What is his vulnerability to homophobia?

Symptoms. What are his coping strategies? Are they functional or dysfunctional? Is he isolated? Does he abuse drugs or alcohol? Is he sexually compulsive? Which of his needs are met through sex, intimacy, aggression, self-esteem, or control?

CULTURAL COMPETENCY CONSIDERATIONS

More about gay culture is included in the section discussing the general background of gay men.

Consider his community: is it urban or rural? Is he gay-identified or not? Are you familiar with gay terminology? If your client uses an expression you do not understand, ask! Become familiar with gay history, gay culture and current events, literature, music, film, businesses, and politics.

SUICIDALITY

Accessing and understanding suicidal ideation in gay men with HIV is critical. Gay men with HIV are at multiple risk. Because of oppression and stigmatization of homosexuals, gay men have often considered suicide as a way out of their oppression. The high rate of suicide among gay youth is severe testimony to this risk. Since suicide has been often considered as an option by gay men in crisis, the new crisis of HIV may precipate another bout of suicidality.

Different stages of the disease may present different triggers for suicidal feelings. Suicidal ideation as a response to recent diagnosis may be based on lack of information about the disease, limited emotional support, or a primitive way of coping with the news. In midstage, defenses may be down and thoughts of death may overwhelm the person. In the final stages of the illness, issues of pain, lost control, and dependency may trigger more thoughts of killing oneself. Over the course of illness different issues including discrimination, a personal history of losses due to homophobia, family rejection, legal problems, feelings of conflict over sexual identity, and lack of resources may all contribute to suicidal thoughts. Furthermore, personality factors and alcohol and drug abuse as disinhibiting factors may increase the risk. (See Jack Stein's Chapter on Clients who use Drugs.) Suicidal ideation may also be part of an acute grief reaction at the number of losses the person has had, unresolved bereavement due to unending losses, an inability to integrate the existential reality of mortality, or an identification with the social message that all people with HIV are unfit for life.

As ever in treatment, we must be vigilant about assessing the actual risk to the safety of the person. The expression of suicidality may be a metaphor of despair rather than an actual plan.

> Mr. A., a forty-year-old gay man with AIDS, having lost his career at its zenith as well as his health and his autonomy and also facing the loss of being able to see his ten-year-old son grow up, needed to express his despair—including frank talk about his suicidality. An AIDS activist, he struggled with the pull of the role of "the hero—the AIDS poster boy," and he railed against the difficulty of expressing his suicidality in circles where he felt it was not "politically correct."

As a powerful metaphor that deserves a safe place to be heard and understood, suicidal thoughts can be an expression of control and autonomy—a coping effort—rather than of anguish and depression. Social workers must therefore assess the risk of suicide and position themselves so that they can offer a safe place for clients to vent feelings and also step in more actively when they assess that a line has been crossed and the client is in danger of hurting himself. With the actively suicidal client, a firm contract needs to be made in which the safety of the client is paramount. If the client cannot assure his own safety within his alliance with the social worker, then steps need to be taken to ensure his safety through commitment to a psychiatric hospital. (The problem of distinguishing "self-deliverance" from suicide is discussed in the chapter "Ethical Issues in Clinical Practice" by Susan Patania.)

COUPLES

HIV has brought some gay couples together and has driven others apart. Couples may come into therapy seeking ways to continue their relationship. The therapist can help normalize the devastating challenges the couple may be facing in the epidemic.

HIV may affect a gay couple in a range of ways, including discovering their HIV status, negotiating their sexual needs, and dealing with the impact of the loss of their friends to AIDS. If a partner is sick with HIV, the couple's emotional and financial resources are bound to be strained. The intensity of their losses and their subsequent rage can be excruciating. Bearing witness to and often being the transference object of the couple's anger is a demanding function for the therapist. Most difficult can be the work of helping a couple facing dementia and severe physical disabilities.

(For more about working with couples and HIV, please see the chapter by Dennis Shelby in this book, as well as the film *Longtime Companion* and Tony Kushner's play, *Angels in America*.)

RACE

When Magic Johnson announced he was HIV positive, he got a supportive public response and further established that his superstar status cleared him of the racial barrier most African Americans struggle against. But he was extremely careful not to be identified as gay. Even so, the media and public reverberated with innuendo of his being a "faggot." Here is an example of the multiple oppression of gay men with HIV who are people of color. (See the powerful PBS documentary "Tongues Untied" by Marlon Riggs, an African-American gay man who died of AIDS.)

AIDS is increasing at a greater rate for blacks and Latinos than Caucasians. It is hard to determine the actual source of transmission because many black and Hispanic men would rather admit to abusing drugs than to having sex with men. The stigma, and thus the social consequence and internalized shame, can be even greater for black and Latino gay men with HIV. The level of denial can be greater; thus the pain can be more intense and the isolation more complete than among white men.

The possible isolation of a gay man of color with HIV thus becomes greater because he can be stigmatized on three counts: sexuality, disease, *and* race.

Among Latinos, the rate of infection is growing fastest, but their level of denial may be even greater than among black men. High-risk sex may be more prevalent but is often not identified with being gay. AIDS education thus hits an impenetrable wall of denial; their vulnerability may be denied because of their disavowal of high-risk behavior. The social worker needs respect the client's self-definition—whether "gay" or "bisexual."

Prevention and education efforts need to be better targeted—in the client's own language and in easily seen locations. Therapists, social workers, and counselors working with minorities should not collude with denial. The worker might want to help establish services within minoritiy communities. Additionally, the profession needs to recruit more minority workers.

BISEXUALS

Men who engage in sex with both men and women and are trying to hide their bisexuality are in a double jeopardy that can result in further isolation of their expression of homosexual interests. Rather than being direct about their sexuality, they may feel that they must be covert and seek sex in anonymous or paid sexual encounters, which are often higher risk for HIV exposure. In turn, they jeopardize the safety of their partners, both male and female.

The crisis of disclosure, the increased pressure on their sexual orientation issues, and their lack of a community of identity (neither straight nor gay) to buffer the stigma and confusion regarding HIV leave these clients isolated and very vulnerable to the impact of AIDS phobia and homophobia.

The social worker might want to form groups for bisexuals—or might want to read *The Bisexual Option* (Klein, 1993) to understand more about bisexuality.

Gay Youth

In a population already fraught with feelings of isolation and alienation, HIV is at once a paralyzingly frightening specter and an unreal issue that many youth, in a suspended state of belief in immortality, can hardly be expected to integrate. Gay youth struggle with deep feelings about their sexuality, including suicidal feelings. Very few socially sanctioned safe places exist in which a gay minor can explore his developing sense of self. If he is open about his orientation, he is apt to be alienated by his peers. To move into the older gay community would be premature. He needs time to try things out, just as his adolescent peers do. He also needs role models, which he rarely has. He is faced with a hard choice: either to be out and face the probable rejection of family and peers or lead a double life, which will cause disruption or delay in other developmental milestones.

Exacerbating his vulnerability further is the ambivalence our culture has toward teaching safer sex to any youth (let alone gay youth). Gay youth are more vulnerable to unsafe, impulsive, uninformed sexual expression. The San Francisco AIDS Foundation reports that as many as 40 percent of San Francisco's twenty- to twenty-five-year-old gay-identified men may now be infected with HIV. Some programs exist, such as the acclaimed seven-year-old "Project 10" program, a support group for lesbian and gay teenagers in one Los Angeles school district. Such programs, combined with a commitment to educate all teens about the full range of heterosexual and homosexual safer sex practices, could begin to address the needs of teenagers.

How can social workers help? Social workers in smaller urban, suburban, or rural areas should get information about programs that work in other cities. They should meet with youth leaders to develop programs.

Peer education groups are helpful. HIV speakers in high schools are helpful. Providing opportunities for teenagers to discuss worries about HIV exposure with other adolescents is a vital service that workers in a variety of settings can facilitate.

OUTREACH TO HIV-NEGATIVE GAY MEN: SURVIVORS

Largely overlooked because of the severity of the needs and demands of their infected peers, surviving gay men who are HIV negative comprise another vulnerable population in this epidemic. These men are in the midst of chronic trauma due to massive catastrophe and death. Their issues include shame at having "escaped" the disease and guilt about surviving. Phobic anxiety, hypochondria, and survivors' guilt are among the symptoms suffered by this group. Trying to make sense of the disturbing statistic that one-third of gay men in this country are now reported to be having unsafe sex, one observer, Dr. Walt Odets, has focused on the unconscious desire of this group not to survive "because of depression, loss, grief, guilt" (Odets, 1991, p. 45). Other contributing factors include "denial of fear about both safe and unsafe sex; plunging counterphobically into unsafe sex to master one's fear of it; poor self-esteem; and the experience of desirable intimacy in unsafe behaviors." Again, we must attend to the depression, anxiety, guilt, and isolation in the gay population.

For some gay men, gay life has merged with death. Some gay men's experience is that of soldiers in wartime or concentration camp survivors. Some of these men have lost their entire social network to AIDS. Their age and stage of development do not equip them to integrate this existential crisis. Dealing with their mourning is critical. The complication of emotional feelings concerning homosexuality and HIV can make the grieving process difficult. Differentiating between healthy and pathological grief is important. Because of the multiple losses a gay man may suffer, he may never completely finish grieving one loss when he suffers another loss. His grieving process may be disrupted while his actual grief is compounded. His problem of grief may be further complicated by the possibility that he may be facing his own HIV illness.

The worker can assess grief disturbance. Symptoms may include the following: demoralization, sleep disturbance, traumatic stress responses (such as panic attacks, nightmares, numbing, specific to fears about AIDS), increased use of sleeping pills, and preoccupation with one's own health.

Grief counseling may be critical. The tasks for the survivor are (1) to accept the reality of the loss, (2) to experience the pain of mourning, (3) to adjust to life without the deceased, and (4) to reinvest the energy devoted previously to the deceased in other relationship and endeavors. The gay man's grief needs to be acknowledged and normalized by the worker. Having a place to talk about the feelings is crucial. Individual therapy can be helpful in accomplishing these tasks. Also, peer support groups can be enormously effective, allowing expression of emotion, stages of grieving, and return to a more integrated life.

Differentiating as to how a client is coping with massive loss is critical. Two different phases of traumatic stress syndrome may be evident: (1) a numbed state of denial about the losses or (2) a state of repetitive and intrusive thoughts and feelings about loss. If the client is in a state of denial, he may need to be encouraged to experience his feelings as he tells the therapist about his traumatic losses. The therapist will need to actively pursue his denied affect, assuring the client that he is safe to express it. Often the client is rigidly fending off his tears out of fear that if he starts crying, he will never stop.

If a client is in a state of being overwhelmed by intrusive thoughts of loss, the therapist can offer a focused place for venting his affect. The structure of the therapeutic relationship can help contain the client's affect so that he does not feel it spilling over everywhere in his life. Gradually, the bereaved gay man may find that he can build new meaning in life through new investment in new projects and new relationships.

Rituals and remembrances may be important to develop. This whole subculture has needed a wailing wall. What the Vietnam War monument offered as expression of social grief over that war, the AIDS Quilt and Names Project has been for the gay community. Participation in this collective grieving is powerfully healing.

ACTION STEPS FOR SUCCESSFUL INTERVENTION

1. Assess the needs of the gay population in your practice area.
2. Investigate resources available. Make a resource list. Go to trainings or workshops provided by local gay health or AIDS organization.
3. Based on your interest and skill, offer yourself as a resource.
4. Get ongoing support! Get good supervision or join a support group for caregivers.

POTENTIAL BARRIERS TO SUCCESSFUL INTERVENTION

Within Yourself

What is your comfort level with gay clients? What is your countertransference? How do you deal with your own homophobia? It is best to refer to a gay-positive resource if you are not able to offer services without contaminating the work with your own homophobia.

If you are heterosexual, be sensitive to the gay client's experience of difference and discrimination.

If you are gay, watch out for confusion about your boundaries with your client. Are you too closely involved? Or alternatively, if your own personal life is saturated with HIV, are you positioning yourself too far away?

Supervision and support are critical to maintaining an effective empathic relationship.

Within Your Work Setting

HIV work with gay men is a highly charged area. Safe access for the gay client is vital. Try to alleviate shame and stigma induced by an insensitive institutional setting. How can people come to your service and not unnecessarilly lose confidentiality? This may be particularly difficult for rural gay men who may have more difficulty remaining anonymous if they pursue HIV services.

Make the environment gay friendly—*not* heterocentric. Have brochures that are gay-specific. In your waiting area, have periodicals such as *Out* magazine, *The Advocate*, and local urban gay/lesbian newspapers. And also include clinical literature relevant to gay practice in your bookshelf.

Within Your Client

Is the mode of therapy you offer reaching him? Although very useful to many clients, psychodynamic therapy identifies internal forces for troubling emotional states and may exclude the real external social forces that shape much of his experience. In addition to understanding the psychodynamic meaning of the client's experience, a cognitive-behavioral approach focusing on specific goals and objectives and teaching coping skills may be effective. Structured psychoeducational group work and use of humor may also help. Because the very act of coming to therapy may seem awkward and embarassing, the social worker must work at trying to normalize these reactions by predicting them and try to create a more active, welcoming relationship for these clients, serving as an advocate. If your client is of a minority ethnic background, determine if the therapy offered is sensitive to his needs?

If the client has characterological problems that preceded his HIV diagnosis, determine if you are a helpful resource. Watch for splitting between service providers. Offer as much containment as possible, and develop a good treatment team by communicating with other providers.

INFORMATION THE CLIENT SHOULD KNOW
BEFORE TAKING ACTION

One topic the client should have a thorough understanding of is confidentiality. The client should be alerted to the restrictions on confidentiality in the case of the therapist's duty to alert others if the client is a danger to himself or others.

The client should also determine his confidence in your level of commitment. Are you ready to see this work through, from office to bedside, health to sickness, living to dying? Will your agency or your private practice caseload allow for this continuity of care? Most important for gay men: Are you gay-sensitive?

POLICY IMPLICATIONS AND RELATED ACTIONS

While striving to meet the needs of our gay clients, social workers can continue historically proactive work dealing with homophobia—whether within the educational system, work settings, or in our clients. This is especially important for gay youth. We are often in vital positions in clinics and schools to reach youth who need to know that homosexuality is an orientation of which they need not be ashamed. Making the world safer for a gay man to come out and be out is a long-term goal for social work, especially in the arena of opposing oppression and upholding civil liberties. This means taking on the real pathology in our midst, homophobia, at all the levels in which it manifests.

On the policy level, our interventions can help expose stigmatizing policies and develop more protective policies for gay men with HIV. Conferences such as the Annual Social Work and AIDS Conference, the continued dedication to inclusion of gay issues on AIDS care agendas, the development of special resources such as the Living Well Program at the Fenway Community Center in Boston, and the commitment to political lobbying championed by NASW are examples of successful interventions.

RECOMMENDED READINGS

Therapists on the Front Line: Psychotherapy with Gay Men in the Age of AIDS, edited by Cadwell, Steven, Burnham, Robert, and Forstein, Marshall. American Psychiatric Press, 1994.

Carlton Cornett, *Reclaiming the Authentic Self: Dynamic Psychotherapy with Gay Men*, Northvale, NJ: Aronson Press, 1995.

Richard Isay, *Being Homosexual*, New York: Farrar, Straus, and Giroux, 1989.
Fritz Klein, *The Bisexual Option*, Binghamton, NY: The Harrington Park Press, 1993.

REFERENCE

Walt Odets, The Secret Epidemic. *Outlook*, Fall, 1991, pp. 45-49.

Providing Services
to HIV-Positive Women

Susan M. Gallego

WHY DO THIS?
STATEMENT OF THE PROBLEM AND ISSUES

The needs of women have always represented a unique challenge to the health care and service provision systems. Traditionally, these challenges have not been well met, and currently they are exacerbated by HIV. As a whole, women are at the bottom of the economic ladder. They endure more violence, are more vulnerable to crime, survive more rapes and incest experiences, have poorer health care, and die faster than men from most terminal diseases. It is also clear that women have different characteristics, problems, and service needs than men. This, along with the fact that HIV can present differently in women than men and that there has been limited research on HIV and women, makes it necessary to give special focus to HIV-positive women. Clearly, differences in hormones, genetics, sex roles, and socioeconomic conditions are all likely to influence exposure to the virus and the disease process itself.

Research indicates that the early symptoms of HIV in women are often gynecological in nature. As the disease progresses, symptoms are similar in both men and women. One U.S. study showed that women with HIV are three times more likely to develop cervical intraepithelial neoplasm, a precursor to cervical cancer. It was not until 1993 that the U.S. Centers for Disease Control (CDC) openly recognized the differences in HIV among men and women by changing their case definition of AIDS to reflect a female-specific disease manifestation, cervical carcinoma. Until then, women battling AIDS had been misdiagnosed or undiagnosed and, in many cases, had gone untreated.

Studies also tell us that infected women, as a whole, present much later in the disease process than do men. Some of this is due to the fact that many women have been misdiagnosed. We must also recognize that, for the most part, women in the AIDS epidemic have been described and considered mainly as vectors of transmission, infectors of unsuspecting men and innocent children. This early view of HIV-infected women prevented them from being viewed as individuals, themselves infected and "victims" of transmission. In addition, women have received some very strong societal messages, such as "good girls" don't get AIDS (nor do they even need to protect themselves from HIV), as opposed to the "bad girls" who do.

Exclusion from research and clinical drug trials has negatively impacted women's health and perhaps hastened progression of the disease for individual women. These studies often provide direct access to care, tests, and expensive treatments, which promote improved physical and emotional well-being. While this pattern is changing, it is important to note that in 1992, 1,151 women were involved in National Institute of Health (NIH)-sponsored HIV drug trials; at the same time, 13,628 men were involved in NIH drug trials.

Examining some statistics about women and HIV can help create a clearer picture for social workers. According to the Centers for Disease Control (CDC), since 1992, AIDS has been the fourth leading cause of death among women ages twenty-five to forty-four. From 1986 to 1990, the number of HIV-positive women in the United States grew by 600 percent, two and one-half times faster for women than for men. Forty-one percent of women with AIDS reported in 1994 acquired HIV through injection drug use and 38 percent through heterosexual contact with at-risk partners. Of the remaining 21 percent, 2 percent received contaminated blood or blood products and 19 percent had no specific exposure reported. In considering this last group, we must examine the impact of denial and fear on a woman's ability to see herself at risk for infection and her need to practice safer sex methods. Very few women think of themselves at risk for HIV due to their unfaithful partners, and even fewer heterosexual women consider the possibilities that their partners may be sexually active with other men.

Heterosexual contact is the most rapidly increasing transmission route among women. Women are at greater risk than men for acquiring HIV through heterosexual contact because virus transmission from men to women is more efficient than from women to men since women are the receptors of the man's semen. This is the "biology of the double standard." Another factor is that a greater proportion of men are infected, increasing the likelihood that women will have an infected sex partner.

If we examine these numbers further, we find that the incidence of AIDS for black and Hispanic U.S. women was approximately sixteen and seven times greater, respectively, than that for white U.S. women. Although black and Hispanic women make up 21 percent of all U.S. women, more than three-fourths (77 percent) of AIDS cases reported among women in 1994 occurred among blacks and Hispanics (CDC, "HIV/AIDS Prevention," February 13, 1995).

THE PSYCHOSOCIAL ASSESSMENT

Women with HIV face specific issues that can been determined through the assessment process. Included in this section are additional points to add to your current psychosocial assessment. Obviously, much of this assessment needs to take place over time and can only be completed after a clear and mutual level of trust and rapport has been established. Social workers need to reassess their clients on a regular basis. The constant physical, social, and emotional changes related to HIV necessitate an ongoing and thorough assessment and reassessment process.

Social workers must assess current and historic coping mechanisms and life circumstances. What were the challenges and how did they cope with problems before HIV? For example, is this a person who has had ongoing economic problems or is this person facing a new problem, perhaps resulting from having lost a job due to her HIV status. Understanding the present and past issues will help develop the most appropriate plans for interventions.

Drug and Alcohol Use

Include a drug use assessment as part of the overall psychosocial assessment. More effective risk-reduction and prevention counseling can be done once there is an understanding of substance use/abuse patterns. Education is clearly one role of a social worker. The fact that the social worker has a relationship with the client will aid in exploring some of the current risks and provide solid relevant information that may help reduce the risk of further infection or transmission. Social work ethics and training indicate the importance of assessing these issues in an open, nonjudgemental manner. A beginning point is simply to ask the client if she is currently using drugs or alcohol. Finding out if the client has a history of drug/alcohol use is also important. If the client is abusing drugs by injecting needles, one should determine if the client understands how to "clean her works" (disinfect her needles and equipment). If the client is abusing or misusing drugs (illegal or prescribed) and/or alcohol, these issues may also surface when you assess their present and past coping styles. Also, as we educate clients it is important to keep in mind that there is a great deal of controversy and unclear data on how drugs and alcohol affect the immune system and the progression of HIV disease. Advising clients that drug and alcohol use can impact the effectiveness of any medication they may use to treat their HIV-related conditions is useful, and certainly impacts their ability to make clear well-informed decisions. Research conducted through the National Institute on Alcohol Abuse (NIAA) clearly shows that risky behaviors, such as having unprotected sex, increase when people are under the influence of alcohol and drugs. The National Association of Social Workers' (NASW) HIV training curriculum for social workers contains information on drug use assessments, taking sexual histories, and risk-reduction counseling, which may prove to be a helpful resource.

Financial Resources

Women are less likely to have the energy to work outside the home and complete their daily household tasks or responsibilities once they begin to experience more symptoms related to HIV disease. HIV-positive women from lower socioeconomic levels often present with a lack of financial resources as their primary need. Examining their resources and their ability to access systems for applying for social security disability or short- and long-term employment disability is important. Keep in mind that the high costs related to HIV such as the costs of medicines, medical visits, and supplies, along with the loss of work time (unpaid sick leave, etc.) can quickly wipe out a person's savings account and resources. The majority of people with HIV struggle with the issues of diminishing financial resources.

Medical Resources

The many medical ups and downs of living with HIV necessitate a strong ongoing relationship with medical providers and the resources to obtain services. Encouraging and facilitating women's connection to ongoing healthcare is important. This will not only help in quality-of-life issues (such as early diagnosis and treatment of new opportunistic infections) and pain management, but it will also help establish the necessary documentation needed for medical disability applications (such as Social Security Income/Social Security Disability Income). Ideally, social workers can help women find physicians who are trained in and both comfortable with and experienced in gynecological conditions, internal medicine, and HIV/AIDS. Some women will want to examine nontraditional medicines, acupuncture, and the use of herbs with their physicians, so be prepared to help such women obtain information and form questions to ask the doctor. As the social worker begins to help with the resources for care, he or she should be aware that the need for the many (and expensive) medications may be met through a combination of state HIV medication assistance programs, Medicaid, and through compassionate use and indigent assistance programs administered directly through the pharmaceutical companies.

It is essential to have an ongoing dialogue with the client about what her understanding is of her current medical condition and symptoms. This will not only help assess how issues related to denial and lack of resources may be impacting her decisions, but also support her in seeking timely medical care. One example of this is a forty-seven-year-old woman we worked with who had been requesting extra sanitary napkins from our (AIDS services) food bank staff for over a month. The food bank assistant thought perhaps the woman needed some financial assistance to buy more so she referred her to a social worker. When the social worker spoke with the client, she found out that the woman was experiencing heavy ongoing bleeding and discharge, which the client believed had come about due to "the change." The social worker was able to bring in the nurse, and the three of them talked about menopause and HIV in women. During the discussion, the client also revealed that she had not discussed this with her doctor because she had not received her Medicaid card for the past two months (patients of this particular physician are told that they must present their Medicaid card in order to have an appointment). The social worker was then able to work on the Medicaid resource with the client and make a call to the physician's office and ask them to make an exception and see the client.

Legal

Some women are very fearful of disclosing their HIV status because they fear their children will be removed (by the child protective services in their state) or that they will be arrested because of how they became HIV infected (e.g., through sex work or illegal drug use). They may need legal advice about these matters. Recognize that exploring these issues may take time; thus, the social worker will need to pace the questions within the context of the relationship. Clearly the client must feel safe, understand the confidentiality issues, and have developed a sense of trust with the social worker. Within this context the social worker can ask if the client is currently involved in any legal proceedings or if she is on probation/parole? If she has children, she will need to examine plans for guardianship/custody. Has she made any plans for wills, durable medical powers of attorney, or directives to physicians?

Support System

Because of stigmas, such as the "good girl-bad girl" dicotomy that pervades perceptions about those with HIV, many women are afraid they will lose their support system once their HIV status is disclosed. They fear their partners will find someone else, leaving them for someone who is "healthy" and HIV negative. They are fearful that their parents will be afraid of getting infected, be angry about how they got infected, and then kick them out. They also fear that their grown children will be judgmental and ashamed and then turn their backs and not have any contact with them. It will be helpful to find out who knows that she is HIV positive and if there is anyone else in her support system who is also HIV positive. This is particularly important if the client has caregiving duties related to this person. It is not uncommon for HIV-positive women to be caring for their HIV-positive husbands and HIV-positive children. This caregiving role may prevent such women from following up on their own care and medical appointments.

Cultural considerations are important in this area. Is there an extended family, and can family members be counted on to help care for the individual when she becomes more ill? What resources within the community does she currently utilize or receive support from? An older Mexican-American woman needing a great deal of home care may not feel comfortable with either her husband or a home health aide from a local agency bathing her due to gender issues and values concerning respect. The social worker may need to work with the client to help her first voice her discomfort and then meet with the client's female relatives to assist with some of her more intimate care needs. This client may also be dealing with some guilt about her demising role as a caregiver due to her inability to cook, help raise grandchildren, and complete the tasks that a "good" woman does. She will need encouragement from the social worker to share some of these feelings and then to resolve the feelings.

Coping Skills: Present/Past

Knowing more about how the client deals and has dealt with challenges in her life will help the social worker anticipate and plan interventions more effectively. The client will utilize her specific coping style to handle her pain, anxiety, and depression as she deals with each new opportunistic infection or the latest test results that show a lowered CD-4 count. Determining how she spends her day may tell you that she is being isolative. Find out what she does when she feels sad or angry or what she did after she first found out she was HIV positive. This will give the social worker some clear information about her coping style. Thus, the social worker can begin to work with the client to build the support system, teach relaxation skills, and change old, less functional styles of coping and build upon the more functional ones.

Determining if there is a history of suicide, substance abuse, binges, etc., is also important. Keep in mind that the ups and downs of HIV increase the likelihood of relapse. One client we worked with binged on alcohol every time she was scheduled for an inpatient treatment or procedure. During her first visit with the social worker, she clearly advised her that she drank occasionally "to calm down." It then made sense when her anxiety and pattern of dealing with it brought her back to binge drinking prior to each planned hospital admission. Knowing this style of coping allowed us to anticipate the pattern, provide more support during the days prior to admission, and work on new more functional ways to lessen anxiety.

Another client who was very intelligent and had taught at a nearby university periodically became very hostile and demanding of staff time and agency resources. She demanded the latest medical journals, wanted copies of articles immediately, requested money to pay for long distance phone calls to researchers, and wanted immediate appointments with the nurse and wellness coordinator whenever she received "bad news" about her declining health. This was her way of coping with her fear and anxiety. Once we understood this pattern, we began working with her to anticipate the "good news" and "bad news" and helped her to express and deal with the feelings behind her anxiety. In many ways, being proactive and searching out information and research is a very positive coping mechanism; however, with this client it was creating more anxiety and isolation and less support.

View of Death/Dying

This can be impacted by your client's caregiver role. If she leaves behind children, a sick partner, an aging mother, etc., her sense of responsibility, fear of rejection, guilt, and denial may be increased. How does her religion or her sense of spirituality explain death? Death may clearly accentuate the grief issues, feelings related to "shattered dreams," and the multiple losses she is experiencing. You will find that some women will not want to discuss anything related to their death, which can be extremely challenging if guardianship decisions need to be made; other women, however, will be ready to videotape their good-byes to their young children. In all cases it is important to discuss what the client wants to do if/when she becomes bedridden or unable to think clearly and take care of herself. Does she want to go to a nursing home, to utilize a hospice program, or move to a relative's home? How she views death and dying will clearly affect this decision. One of my clients who was extremely fearful of being alone when she died opted to go to a hospice program in a small house staffed with twenty-four-hour care from very supportive and nurturing providers. The fact that I knew early on about her fear of dying alone helped me work with her to create an appropriate plan.

History of Family Violence/Rape/Assault/Sexual Abuse

These issues can clearly impact a woman's ability to receive medical care, practice safer sex, and ask for assistance. Some women have responded to childhood sexual abuse and violence by becoming involved in substance abuse, prostitution, and hypersexual activities. Once this woman begins experiencing the symptoms related to HIV, she may be less able to cope with her lack of sexual attractiveness and her inability to use her body as she once did. This can clearly create severe psychological problems and put the client into crisis.

The social worker must understand that continued violence and assault brings about shame, powerlessness, hopelessness, and self-destructive behaviors, and these coupled with dealing with HIV can be totally overwhelming. Research shows how violence and abuse affect self-esteem. Low self-esteem along with fear of violence and economic dependence may prevent a woman from insisting a man uses a condom or from leaving the house to go to a much-needed HIV-positive women's support group meeting. Assessing whether the diagnosis of HIV/AIDS will increase the likelihood of the client's exposure to abuse is also important.

We worked with a woman who had recently moved to our city to be with a man who was an assistant principal at a local school. They had met while he was on vacation and he had gotten to know her fourteen-year-old son. Her son was very intelligent, but according to her, he "needed a strong male role model." Both she and her partner were very worried about the type of boys her son was spending time with and their gang-related activities. She had told her partner "from the beginning" that she was HIV positive, and he "had no problems" with it. Upon moving here, she found that he restricted her activities: she had no car, no money, no job, and no medical care. She called our agency to inquire about our HIV wellness classes. When we tried to assist her with transportation through a volunteer, she indicated that her partner was "jealous" and such an arrangement would not work. We offered to have a social worker home visit, and her partner called us and told us he did not want any "AIDS people coming around." When she called us during the times he was not home, she told us that he became abusive and hit her when he got angry, but that he was "really good" to her son and that her son was doing much better here in his new school. She indicated that her partner refused to use condoms and did not want her to see any doctors unless she was "really ill." As we spoke with this client, we became aware of the fact that she had also been abused by her first husband. This pattern of abuse along with low self-esteem and a lack of economic independence affected her ability to seek and receive care and services. The social worker's first goals were not to work on safer sex issues or even to find a physician, but rather to work on obtaining support from other women (e.g., a women's support group phone line run by a center for battered women). The social worker also encouraged her to connect with her family, whom she described as very helpful, but she had moved away from them to live with her partner.

Mental Health Status

We must remember that women have a long history of misdiagnosed and undiagnosed psychiatric problems, which relates to discussions about the lack of research on women and the lack of women-centered providers. This pattern has been an issue in mental health concerns with HIV-positive women. Without question, receiving a positive test result or coping with the losses involving HIV can themselves bring about depression and a number of other psychological problems. The social worker must also be aware that the progression of HIV itself can impact a women's mental health. Therefore a mental health assessment must be done on an ongoing basis. Look for symptoms of dementia and depression, which may occur. Also, the side effects from some medications can cause some mental health problems. It is important to consult with the client's physician and, as appropriate, recommend a psychiatric evaluation. The client's mental health can be enhanced and supported by ongoing counseling.

SOCIAL WORK ACTIONS

1. *Become familiar with community resources for women and HIV/AIDS services.* Know what substance abuse treatment (inpatient/outpatient) is available for women. Sometimes, government-funded treatment programs make exceptions to long waiting lists for HIV-positive individuals so they enter these services more quickly. Team up and network with providers from AIDS service organizations, centers for battered women, and rape crisis centers; this will support both your work and the needs of your clients. This network may also help in following up with some of the policy suggestions listed later in the chapter.

2. *Anticipate multiple needs, which require a comprehensive mix of services and the provision of tangible services.* Prepare for exhausted women and families and look toward anticipating assistance in the home. The ups and downs of HIV/AIDS make planning very difficult,

but your assessment will make planning a bit more organized. Knowing the support system and the role of the woman (caregiver responsibilities) will help in making the appropriate referrals. This may mean that referrals for transportation and childcare will be at the top of the list. Delivering a bag of groceries is not only a tangible source of assistance for the family without food, but also helps in building trust and a sense of partnership.

3. *Be prepared to work with a wide range of emotions with your clients.* Many women will have a deep mistrust for the medical systems with which they are dealing, for reasons stated at the beginning of this chapter. This can cause resistance, noncompliance, and anger. In addition, many women are worried about their future and the family members they leave behind, and many are angry at those who might have infected them. Guilt, grief, fear, and exhaustion can envelop the lives of women living with HIV/AIDS. Social workers need to explore women's feelings of guilt and loss of control and then work to enhance support systems and access to care, which can minimize women's burden.

4. *Use an empowerment-based approach when dealing with women.* This perspective suggests that social problems stem not from individual deficits but rather from the failure of society to meet the needs of its members. Empowerment occurs on the individual, interpersonal, and institutional levels, where the person develops a sense of personal power, an ability to affect others, and an ability to work with others to change social institutions. Determine if your client will be best served by a female provider and whether she will benefit from a female role model. It may be very helpful to refer her to a HIV-positive women's support group or to a female therapist. As you work with her to create a partnership and a strong role as an advocate, problems can be partialized so that the social worker models one part (e.g., calling the social security disability examiner) and the client follows through with her part (e.g., getting the physician's report), all of which builds her sense of self-efficacy and control.

5. *Be open and prepared to discuss safer sex from a harm-reduction perspective.* This may mean you will need to access some support from providers who teach safer sex (e.g., HIV educators) or more information from your local AIDS service organization. Harm reduction is an ongoing type of intervention that recognizes the need to start where the client is and use appropriate interventions, which may help a woman reduce her risk of getting reinfected or of infecting a partner. This includes instruction for the woman who is an injection drug user (IDU) concerning using bleach to "clean her works" to using the female

condom or using Nonoxynol 9 with her diaphragm when having intercourse. It also means referrals to drug treatment, needle-exchange programs, if available, and instruction for her male partner on how to use a condom correctly.

6. *Be prepared to discuss pregnancy and family planning with respect and without judgment.* Statistics and information are constantly changing. The latest research from the 1993, National Institutes for Health (NIH) AZT clinical trial study (076) showed that only 8.3 percent of the women treated with AZT during pregnancy transmitted HIV to their infant. This is a reduction from the approximately 25 percent of HIV-positive women whose babies were HIV positive during the early years of the epidemic. Three-quarters (75 percent) of children born to HIV-positive mothers do not contract HIV before or during birth—even in the absence of AZT treatment. Current research indicates that pregnancy does not accelerate HIV, and at the present time, no one knows how to predict which mothers will transmit the virus to their babies. Much is still unknown and controversies abound, but social workers must understand and respect the importance of self-determination and the right that women have to make their own decisions. Ultimately, it is the woman's choice. Becoming pregnant, examining the options related to termination, deciding about medications, examining the woman's health and the baby's health, and addressing the long-term implications are all very complex issues. All of these issues must be examined with the client and within a biopsychosocial framework. Social workers must be aware that new research and information regarding HIV is constantly changing and that the "facts" we provide our clients with today may be different tomorrow.

POLICY IMPLICATIONS AND RELATED ACTIONS

A number of areas of advocacy for women with HIV can take the social work role beyond the individual level to the systems and policy levels, including the following:

1. Agencies serving women with HIV must incorporate and include women with HIV in all levels of programming, planning, education, and decision making, regardless of their sexual orientation, race, and education. This means being creative and flexible to find new ways to make this happen. Some programs provide taxi transportation so that women without transportation can more easily attend meetings; other programs have begun paying stipends to women who participate in programs.

2. Women with HIV need to be provided with education and training about their basic rights, including the right to have all medical procedures explained in a language they understand, the right to refuse treatment, and their rights under the Americans with Disabilities Act (ADA).
3. Childcare and transportation services need to be incorporated into all programs serving women so that they can take part in research, clinical trials, medical care, and social services, as well as participate on the planning and decision-making levels previously described.
4. "User-friendly/one-stop-shopping" type services need to be created. Women with HIV should be able to go to one place for their medical care and their child's medical care. The concepts of wellness can be incorporated in a way that supports women's health related to diabetes, cholesterol, family planning, breast cancer screens, *and* HIV. The colocating of services/agencies and a comprehensive holistic view of women's needs and issues will provide women more support and empowerment.

RESOURCES

1994 National HIV Frontline Forum Multimedia Self-Study Kit for Professionals Who Counsel People Living with HIV/AIDS. Video and discussion kit. NCM Publishers—Burroughs Wellcome Co. For free copies call 1-800-722-9292 ext. 54511, specify program BW-YO 5953.

1994 WomanSource HIV Multimedia Resource for HIV-Positive Women and Their Service Providers, Part I (Psychosocial Issues), II (Substance Abuse Issues), III (Focus on the Family). Videos and discussion kits. NCM Publishers, Inc.—Burroughs Wellcome Co. For free copies call 1-800-722- 9292, ext. 54511.

SEICUS (Sex Information and Education Council of the U.S.) Report, October/November 1993. At Issue with AIDS: About Women. Vol. 22, No. 2.

SEICUS Report, December 1990/January 1991. Women and HIV/AIDS. Vol. 22, No. 2.

Weiner, Lori S. (1991). Women and Human Immunodeficiency Virus: A Historical and Personal Psychosocial Perspective. *Social Work,* Vol. 36, No. 5, pp. 375-378.

REFERENCES

Centers for Disease Control (1995). Questions and answers. Draft guidelines for HIV counseling and voluntary testing for pregnant women, February, pp. 1-5.

Providing Services
to Elderly People with HIV

Gregory Anderson

WHY DO THIS?
STATEMENT OF THE PROBLEM AND ISSUES

Many of us in the fields of HIV/AIDS and aging had failed to notice that substantial numbers of older people were becoming infected and affected by HIV. While the prevention message was successfully reaching certain subpopulations and HIV infection rates were declining or stabilizing, the infection rate among adults over age fifty has continued to grow. While many still view AIDS as a younger person's problem, nearly 11 percent of all cases nationwide involve persons over the age of fifty, with 4 percent over the age of sixty (Centers for Disease Control, 1994). In addition, an increasing number of older persons are profoundly affected by HIV/AIDS as many of them are called upon to care for their ill and dying adult children and grandchildren.

The myth that older persons in our society become sexually inactive and therefore are not in need of HIV prevention and education has produced dreadful results. Likewise, the myth that older persons are not injection drug users has blinded us to the facts that a certain amount of drug use does continue in old age and that the cohort of older injection drug users is still very much at risk for HIV infection.

Recent research has shown that older persons have the same risk factors for HIV infection as do younger persons. To date, approximately two-thirds of all HIV/AIDS cases in the over-fifty population involve older gay and/or bisexual men. Increasingly, though, heterosexual transmission in the older population is seen as a growing problem. Research in the population has shown that older persons (between the ages of fifty and seventy-five) are one-sixth as likely to have used condoms during sex and one-fifth as likely to have been tested for HIV as have a comparison group in their twenties (Stall and Catania, 1994).

The problem of misdiagnosis continues to plague the older community. HIV/AIDS has been called the "great imitator" because many of the early symptoms of HIV infection mimic the aging process. Many physicians accustomed to working with younger gay men and drug users fail to diagnose HIV in their older patients. One sixty-three-year-old heterosexual woman who had received transfused blood during cancer surgery complained to her doctors for two years of chronic fatigue, weight loss, and increasing dementia. She was referred from one doctor to another, one of whom flatly refused to test her for HIV. Finally, her oncologist informed her that she had received tainted blood and tested her. By this time she had acute wasting syndrome, anemia, facial molluscum, and thrush. She, like so many older persons with HIV/AIDS who were diagnosed late in the disease process, was unable to benefit from early antiviral and prophylactic treatments. She lived for only two months following diagnosis. Researchers believe that the mortality and disease progression rate among older persons is higher than among younger persons.

The older person with HIV/AIDS is often isolated from the growing network of AIDS service providers because he or she feels "too old." Likewise, the tremendous resources of our aging network have not been utilized to provide age-appropriate HIV services to older persons. Older gay men and heterosexuals alike seem to suffer the stigma of HIV infection and are less likely to seek services other than primary care. The challenge to service providers is to develop competent services, outreach, and prevention and education strategies to serve the older community.

EXAMPLES OF HOW THE ISSUE MAY PRESENT

Professionals working with older adults in social service settings should always be on the lookout for changes in health status. The early physical symptoms of HIV infection, which are often easy to overlook in older adults, include the following:

- sudden weight loss or chronic fatigue unrelated to other organic problems or the aging process
- night sweats unrelated to other infections or immune suppression, such as in lymphoma
- chronic fungal infections unrelated to the side effects of prescribed medication
- shingles, which are common in older adults, may be HIV-related, not age-related
- dementia unrelated to Alzheimer's disease or other physical conditions such as stroke or arterial sclerosis

Accompanying signs of physical change can be signs of social withdrawal or changes in mental health status. The client who may or may not know he or she is HIV positive may be presenting with other problems common to older adults—housing, finances, health care, bereavement, retirement, or use of leisure time. In mainstream aging organizations, clients may be in need of benefits counseling, case management, or mental health services. In gay and lesbian social service agencies, older gay men and lesbians may present with the same age-related issues in addition to the problems of aging common to the gay and lesbian community—specific legal, medical, emotional, or institutional problems.

If you are going to successfully engage with an older client, you may need to demonstrate your willingness and ability to meet this client where he or she is at regarding his or her HIV status. Denial is a common defense mechanism for the newly diagnosed HIV-positive individual. As a social worker, you may need to recognize the force of denial in the older adult with HIV and be aware that those individuals may not be ready to disclose the true nature of their situation. A sixty-five-year-old client of mine asked that we refer at all times to his diagnosis as cancer rather than AIDS. The older client who is able to disclose to you may have very strong concerns about confidentiality and his or her need to manage the information.

FACTS THE SOCIAL WORKER
NEEDS TO KNOW BEFORE PROCEEDING

If it is your intention to organize services for elderly persons with HIV, it will be important to understand that you may be forced to contend with organizational resistance. The aging network is still in a great deal of denial regarding the extent of HIV in the elderly population. Aging service providers, fearful of alienating their non-HIV clients, may be unwilling to attempt to integrate HIV clients into the agency caseload. AIDS service providers, unused to working with older adults, may not see the need for age-specific services. Neither network may be ready to take on the task of providing service. Your attempt to organize for services is doomed to fail if you are without a sound educational strategy aimed at the hierarchy of your service organization. If you intend to create a new agency, you will need the cooperation of influential people in both the AIDS and the aging networks.

KEY QUESTIONS TO ASK THE CLIENT

When working with older adults, ascertaining their knowledge base about HIV/AIDS is very important. To assume that the older gay man is well informed because of his ties to the gay and lesbian community would be a mistake. It has been suggested that the more closeted a man is, the less likely he is to have internalized the changing sexual mores of the gay community. It would be equally unfair to assume that older heterosexuals know nothing about the epidemic. Many older adults, fearing for the safety and welfare of their children and grandchildren, have gleaned important information from the media. It will be important for the clinician to learn what the newly diagnosed client knows about treatment options, entitlements, and supportive services. Important questions to ask may include the following:

• What does the client's physician or geriatrician know about HIV disease?
• What does your client know about treatment options?
• What does your client know about mental health services, and if appropriate, would the client be amenable to a referral?
• What does your client know about entitlements available based on age and/or HIV status?
• What does your client know about long-term care options to meet his or her changing health status?
• What kinds of social supports are available to the client?
• What does your client know of supportive services available in the community, i.e., support groups for older persons with HIV?
• What does your client know about HIV risk-reduction practices to protect his or her sexual partners?
• Does the client have an alcohol or drug abuse problem that may impede self-care, and if so, would the client be amenable to an appropriate referral?

A successful gathering of information for comprehensive psychosocial assessment is essential for good treatment planning. It must be understood, though, that the older person with HIV may be quite reluctant at first to reveal important information. The clinician may need to be extremely patient in the information-gathering process to get an accurate picture of the client's specific problems and needs.

CULTURAL COMPETENCY CONSIDERATIONS

It is important to understand that older persons mirror the diversity in our society and that their responses to HIV will reflect that diversity. Many older gay men, for example, have a culture of their own that reflect a lifetime in the closet. They do not think, feel, and express themselves the way younger gay men do. In working with the elderly in cultural and ethnic communities, the social worker must understand the degree to which these elders have become assimilated by the dominant culture. Your agency may need to provide bilingual clinicians to provide competent service.

Because of the highly stigmatized nature of AIDS/HIV, it will be important to understand that different cultures have different values concerning the discussion of frank sexual matters, the use or nonuse of non-Western medical practices, and the role of religion and spirituality in times of crisis. Many elders in our society have profound distrust of mental health services. The Hispanic elderly, for example, are quite unused to going outside the family for help of any kind as they have a strong negative sanction against "airing one's dirty laundry in public." Creating an atmosphere that respects and values diversity in an agency setting is essential.

ACTION STEPS FOR SUCCESSFUL INTERVENTION

Whether you are attempting to provide HIV services for the elderly in an established AIDS program or in a service program for the elderly, or you are developing a new agency, certain action steps will be necessary to ensure that you will reach and serve the population. You may wish to follow the following outline:

1. *Do a community service assessment.* Examine your area aging agencies and area HIV/AIDS service programs to determine whether any programs are already serving the population.
2. *Develop an interagency council or task force to bring together professionals from the fields of AIDS and aging.* The outcome of this may be the identification of funding sources, political allies, and professionals willing and able to volunteer their services to augment your staff.
3. *Develop a realistic program of services to be offered.* If you are working within the context of an established agency, do not attempt a program that would put existing programs in jeopardy. If you are starting a new agency, be realistic as to how to best manage your financial and staff resources.
4. *Create a safe space where older adults with HIV/AIDS will feel comfortable and confident that their confidentiality will be maintained.* Intake and screening procedures may need to be altered to provide anonymity and confidentiality for the new client. The use of nonthreatening HIV/AIDS literature and posters in waiting areas along with postings of HIV confidentiality laws can demonstrate "safety" to the new client. Any program site for older adults or anyone who may be disabled by HIV/AIDS must be easily accessible.
5. *Develop an outreach strategy that reaches mobile and homebound seniors with HIV/AIDS.* The departments of social work at local health care facilities may be your primary referral sources until word of your

program reaches the community at large. Two model programs for seniors with HIV/AIDS, Elder/Family Services in Brooklyn and SAGE (Senior Action in a Gay Environment) in Manhattan, include information on their HIV/AIDS programs in all their published literature and receive many of their referrals from friends and relatives of persons with HIV/AIDS in the community. Caseworkers for agencies that provide meals for homebound seniors can be utilized to identify individuals in the community who may be dealing with HIV/AIDS but have been unwilling to reveal that information.

6. *Develop a program monitoring and evaluation plan to ensure quality control and to articulate a demonstrated need for potential funding sources.*

POTENTIAL BARRIERS TO SUCCESSFUL INTERVENTION

Older persons with HIV/AIDS often do not feel entitled to help. For example, older gay men may experience the sentiment that they have gotten "exactly what they deserve" and choose to isolate themselves. A sixty-seven-year-old gay man reported to his support group that a lifetime of "whoring" had gotten him infected and that he could not expect a lot of sympathy from his family and friends. Another gentleman in the group, age sixty-three, reported that he felt bad about using precious resources that should be going to younger people with HIV/AIDS. Older heterosexuals, so terrified of the stigma of HIV/AIDS, would rather not risk coming forward for assistance. It may be one of your responsibilities in working with this population to create an environment that will encourage older people to share in the work of surviving HIV/AIDS.

Older people often have a myriad of health problems associated with aging that may prevent them from fully participating in HIV/AIDS programs. An acknowledgment that this population may have special needs will help you adopt a flexible, accommodating program.

Your biggest barrier to success may be the unwillingness on the part of your colleagues and co-workers to overcome ageism and believe in your mission. Programs initiated with reluctance and reticence will send that negative message out to the community and reinforce stereotypes about older people and their lives.

INFORMATION THE CLIENT SHOULD KNOW
BEFORE TAKING ACTION

Older people with HIV/AIDS need to know that your agency will be a strong and clear voice of advocacy for their interests. They may need to be reminded that their need for confidentiality will be respected at all times. If they are unused to using professional supportive services, they may require special help understanding the dynamics of the client/worker relationship and the nature of collaborative work among professionals. Especially when there are adult children and grandchildren in the picture, the older client may need constant reassurance of your loyalty and of the presence of professional boundaries and agency ethics.

HIV Prevention and Older Adults

Until recently, the thrust of HIV prevention work has been aimed at younger persons. If we believe that HIV education is the first step toward HIV prevention, we must make state-of-the-art HIV/AIDS information available to all older adults. Again, Elder Family Services and SAGE have developed model programs to bring HIV education into the individual and family counseling sessions and to provide HIV/AIDS forums in senior centers. Comprehensive HIV education and prevention work require a long-term commitment on the part of individuals who work with older adults. In times of cutbacks and fiscal restraints, convincing program administrators of the necessity of this kind of work is very difficult. Just as we have learned with gay men who were heavily targeted in the 1980s, long-term risk reduction for older adults will not be a one-shot deal. Creating well-researched and well-funded educational models for older adults will be the next great challenge for the HIV/AIDS community.

POLICY IMPLICATIONS AND RELATED ACTIONS

Following the establishment of the Older Americans Act in the 1960s, a potent network of services for older adults in our society has been developed. Similarly, political action has led to the establishment of a social service network for people with HIV/AIDS. We will need to encourage these two vital networks to link their common interests and resources to work for older persons with HIV/AIDS. Rather than competing for resources, these two networks should acknowledge their common areas of interests, such as working for universal health care, and should be encouraged to work together. As the numbers of newly infected older persons grows and as the HIV/AIDS community ages in our society, an increasing need for good collaborative work between these networks will develop.

A further crisis is impending in the elderly community as the number of HIV/AIDS orphans continues to grow steadily in our society. In New York City alone, it is estimated that the number of HIV/AIDS orphans ages seventeen and under could reach 30,000 by the year 2000 (Levine, 1993). Many of these children are left in the care of surviving grandparents, who often are older women with limited financial resources and health problems of their own. A significant number of these children are HIV-infected themselves and will need excellent care if they are to survive childhood and their tumultuous adolescence with HIV/AIDS. We have yet to comprehend the enormous strain this additional burden could add to the lives of older caregivers and the social service networks that support them. I refer you to the chapter on elderly caregivers by Perkell in *HIV/AIDS in the Aging Population* (1996) for a more comprehensive look at this issue.

RECOMMENDED READINGS

Anderson, G. (1996). HIV/AIDS and the older gay man. In K.M. Nokes (ed.), *HIV/AIDS in the Aging Population.* Washington, DC: Taylor and Francis.

Perkell, J. (1996). The elderly caregiver. In K.M. Nokes (ed.), *HIV/AIDS in the Aging Population.* Washington, DC: Taylor and Francis.

Riley, M.W., Ory, M.G., and Zablotsky, D. (eds.). (1989). *AIDS in an Aging Society.* New York: Springer.

Stall, R., and Catania, J. (1994). AIDS risk behaviors among late middle-aged and elderly Americans. *Archives of Internal Medicine 154*: 57-63.

REFERENCES

Centers for Disease Control (October 1994). U.S. AIDS cases through September 1994. *HIV/AIDS Surveillance Report 6*(3).

Stall, R., and Catania, J. (1994). AIDS risk behaviors among late middle-aged and elderly Americans. *Archives of Internal Medicine 154:* 57-63.

Levine, C. (ed). (1993). *A death in the family: Orphans of the HIV epidemic.* New York: United Hospital Fund of New York.

Social Work Practice
with HIV-Positive People
in Rural Settings

Perry S. Sutherland
Jane K. O'Rourke

WHY DO THIS?
STATEMENT OF THE PROBLEM AND ISSUES

During the second decade of the epidemic, the second wave of acquired immunodeficiency syndrome (AIDS) has moved aggressively from urban to rural America. Resources readily available in urban settings either do not exist or are ill equipped to serve the growing need in rural areas.

People with human immunodeficiency virus (HIV) moving to rural settings may be returning home to families of origin or seeking respite in less stressful environments. For those coming home, the event is often mixed with feelings of shame, blame, and guilt. Their homecoming is particularly poignant once their health starts to be obviously compromised. Many families of origin learn of lifestyle choices and diagnosis simultaneously. The person with HIV is vulnerable emotionally and physically. For some, returning home is an admission of defeat, "the beginning of the end."

Others move to rural environments for other reasons, believing that services may be more available and easier to access than in the city and that life is simpler and can be lived at a slower pace. People who are HIV seropositive but not yet diagnosed with AIDS may be able to acquire services in rural areas that might not be available in urban epicenters (e.g., someone who is HIV seropositive may not be eligible for services at an urban AIDS service organization until they have been diagnosed with AIDS).

In addition, there are those whose exposure occurred in the rural environment and who feel at home in the rural community; thus, they do not perceive relocation as an option. The same risks outlined above may be magnified for these individuals who are likely to be known in the community. As a result, their ability to maintain privacy and control over their medical information is more challenging and more likely to be compro-

451

mised. For example, a client might decide to seek case management services in a different catchment area as a result of fearing disclosure.

Rural communities provide few support services, frequently rendering a feeling of isolation. Living with HIV is extremely stressful and provides a great many challenges; rural idiosyncrasies can exacerbate these challenges.

Stigma is an inherent factor in the HIV disease process, and it is experienced on many levels by those infected and affected throughout the course of the illness. Rural communities tend to be insulated from the hard realities of the epidemic and can be less than hospitable to people touched by this disease. A rural social worker can be the vital link in creating a supportive environment. As we integrate this work into our practice, we will serve as models to those around us, thus underscoring that this is everyone's work.

EXAMPLES OF HOW THE ISSUE MAY PRESENT

The social worker may receive referrals from a variety of sources, such as medical providers, AIDS case managers, priests, or ministers. The referral will likely be highly secretive and may be of an acute nature. There may be a dire sense of urgency as a great deal of difficulty may have transpired up to the point when the referral is received. An example might be a client who has moved from another community where he experienced job loss and abandonment from his social network as a result of the illness, fearing that the same might happen again.

People may also self-refer, and those who have moved from large urban epicenters may be familiar with social work and psychotherapeutic services but may be highly suspect of the quality or accessibility, given the rural setting. Family members may be the first to inquire about social work services, especially if they are acting as primary caretakers. They may be preparing for the return home of the loved one and need assistance in negotiating the maze of HIV services.

FACTS THE SOCIAL WORKER
NEEDS TO KNOW BEFORE PROCEEDING

Social work is ideally suited to this disease. However, social workers must be keenly aware of their own limits, personal fears about the illness, as well as their inherent biases, such as internalized homophobia. It is imperative that the social worker establish a level of comfort with people who are HIV seropositive, HIV disease, and the societal prejudices relating to both before proceeding. Due to the scarcity of resources, the social worker must provide case management as well as advocacy and family support services.

The social worker should identify the obvious referral sources first, such as AIDS service organizations, health care providers, spiritual leaders, teachers, and other social service agencies.

Learning medical information about opportunistic infections, such as pneumocystis carinii pneumonia, Kaposi's sarcoma, thrush, shingles, cytomegalovirus, as well as typical symptoms, including neuropathy, chronic fatigue, night sweats, and diarrhea is critical to the client-worker relationship. There is no typical course of HIV, but there are common signals to look for in understanding the disease progression of the client's illness.

Social workers need to have a working knowledge about the many medications that are specific to HIV disease, maintaining an awareness that the prescriptions will likely "out" the client to the local pharmacist. As these medications are usually very expensive, the social worker may need to assist the client in securing them directly from the pharmaceutical company through their "Compassionate Use" program, such as the Glaxo-Wellcome program for AZT.

You will need to assess the client's ability to access the office location given declining health. The client will not always be well enough to see you in your office, with likely alternatives being home or hospital visits. As a result, privacy and confidentiality may be challenged. Something as simple as a neighbor seeing the social worker in the driveway may lead to suspicion about the client's health status.

Some areas in which continuing education may be beneficial to the social worker include the following: epidemiology, disease specifics, financial and medical benefit programs, medications and access to them, safer sex protocols, death and dying, grief and loss, finding support for oneself, cultural issues, and dual diagnosis issues that may include chronic mental illness, substance abuse, or developmental delays.

Confidentiality will be of great concern—especially if it becomes widely known that you do AIDS work. Your reputation as an HIV service provider may lead to suspicion by others that all of your clients are dealing with HIV-related issues. Thought must go into the location of your office, as rural towns and cities are small and inopportunely intimate. Accessibility considerations should be made for those who are physically challenged.

KEY QUESTIONS TO ASK THE CLIENT

It will have taken the client a great deal of courage to seek out your services. They will fear risking disclosure for themselves, as well as their family. It will be important to ask the following on the phone:

- Is transportation an issue and will that determine the day and time of the sessions?
- Is mobility a problem and will they need help getting to the office?
- Are there any concerns about the location and people they may be afraid of running into?

In addition to a thorough psychosocial assessment, the following information is important:

- General health status, course of the disease, and primary medical providers
- CD-4 (T-cell) count, as well as viral load
- Previous hospitalizations for HIV-related illnesses
- HIV disease medications and side effects
- Participation in HIV drug protocols/research trials
- Premorbid experience with depression and suicidal ideation or attempts
- Release of information (medical providers and other support services)
- Impact of the disease on daily living
- Major supports
- Their "out" status with care/support providers
- Substance use patterns, both past and present
- Safety of living situation
- Mental status

CULTURAL COMPETENCY CONSIDERATIONS

Rural communities ascribe to being close-knit and friendly but often are experienced as closed and judgmental. The social worker must be vigilant about maintaining confidentiality to ensure the safety of the client. Many rural communities are less than enthusiastic about diversity and frequently can be homophobic, including members of the helping professions (doctors, dentists, nursing staff, counselors, etc).

Substance use and abuse is frequently a common and often accepted coping mechanism in many parts of rural America. There are three predominant areas of concern: (1) the reality of intravenous drug use in rural communities, (2) unsafe sexual practices resulting, in part, from substance use, and (3) the client struggling with HIV and using substances to escape the pain and reality of the disease. It is extremely important that the social worker have a working knowledge of substance abuse and its interplay in the epidemic of HIV.

Sources of education and information about the epidemic are quite limited. The media and community centers such as schools and churches can filter information in a skewed and intolerant fashion. There is limited availability of current information for the general public to increase their awareness or knowledge base.

Public transportation is most often fragmented at best and unavailable at worst. Most rural communities do not have a well-developed public transportation system. Consequently, clients may need to rely on family, friends, or neighbors. This may present another concern if the client does not want anyone to know he or she is receiving social work services. Depending on others contrasts with the often stoic, self-sufficient ideals of rural America.

It is often very difficult to ask for assistance, and this may prevent the client from seeking help or accessing the benefits and/or entitlements s/he may be eligible for.

ACTION STEPS FOR SUCCESSFUL INTERVENTION

Providing necessary social work and therapeutic services in rural areas brings forth the ultimate challenge of a social worker's skills. Establishing the clear demarcations of confidentiality is paramount in the provision of rural clinical services. Completion of a comprehensive biopsychosocial assessment of the client and the client's family system is imperative; a fine example of such an assessment is provided by Compton and Galaway (1979). Included in this process is, as previously mentioned, an identification of available community resources. A social worker must be willing to actively advocate for the provision of services for their clients with HIV in light of fear, resistance, and active discrimination.

The social worker should also determine the availability of specialized services in accessible urban areas. Such services may include clinical trials of medication as yet unavailable by prescription, clinics that may specialize in the treatment of certain HIV-related illnesses, more comprehensive medical consultations, etc. These resources may be most readily accessed through AIDS service organizations in urban centers.

POTENTIAL BARRIERS TO SUCCESSFUL INTERVENTION

Many barriers exist to adequate provision of services for persons with HIV in rural areas. With few exceptions, underlying or overt discrimination and homophobia may create an extraordinarily hostile environment for both the client and the social worker. Denial and fear of the presence of drug use in the community may also create difficult obstacles within the existing network of services. Though prejudice reduction and homophobia training may not be acceptable avenues of direct response to oppressive attitudes, the inclusion of the impact of homophobia on service provision is paramount to a successful training on HIV disease. Experts who can comfortably and safely move trainees and service providers through the complicated web of substance use, abuse, and dependence should also be engaged in the training process.

Fear of contagion and ignorance of HIV and its process may well be the foundation for limited access to services. With the perception that the cost of treatment and support services is significantly expensive, there may be worries that a rural service network might not be able to afford to respond. In many cases, jobs in rural areas do not provide health insurance benefits, either because they are part-time or the businesses are small and family-owned. In an effort to combat these fears and misperceptions, the social worker may want to engage the support of a physician or medical facility that may take a leadership role in providing accurate education to the community and its service providers about HIV disease. Again, the social worker's coalition-building skills may prove invaluable in moving the community attitudes and beliefs from oppressive to proactive and compassionate.

Lack of confidentiality in small communities and within social service networks may become a major barrier, potentially preventing the client in need from engaging the system in the first place. Fear of retaliation or discrimination by neighbors, merchants, churches, medical providers, etc., is real—though there have certainly been many exceptions. Gossip and small talk in both rural and urban settings are at times difficult to manage, and nearly impossible to control. All trainings should continuously highlight the importance of confidentiality, reminding providers that professional codes of ethics dictate the maintenance of an individual's confidentiality. Many states also have civil laws that limit the exchange of HIV-related information while at the same time allowing for the "protection" of the public through existing public health laws. Social workers should also be aware of and inform their clients about the difference between anonymous and confidential HIV antibody testing, as well as the accessibility to both.

Physical isolation from adequate medical care and supportive groups may lead to difficulty in making an adequate treatment plan operational. Emotional isolation and lack of a supportive, empathic network of family and friends may sabotage the best of clinical efforts. Again, this is a difficult barrier to overcome within the rural environment. Assisting the client in accessing more comprehensive services in urban and suburban areas will likely be a part of the service plan. Assistance with transportation may be necessary. The social worker should contact the AIDS service organization in the urban center to ascertain existing options, i.e., support group members already commuting for services may be willing to have others carpool with them. Within the rural setting, use of innovative technologies may prove helpful, such as utilizing conference calls as a support group.

The social worker may also experience a similar lack of community support for his or her efforts, often feeling isolated and overwhelmed. It is imperative that rural workers establish networks of support for themselves, even if such networks are created via telephone or computer. A connection with the nearest AIDS service organization may prove to be an emotional lifesaver for the isolated rural social worker. Attending the National Social Work and AIDS Conference may also provide a forum for support and increase knowledge.

INFORMATION THE CLIENT SHOULD KNOW BEFORE TAKING ACTION

Clients need to be aware of the risks of loss of anonymity and confidentiality if and when acquiring services in rural areas. Clients should also be aware of the scarcity of reliable resources and the potential for discrimination. The social worker should teach clients how to carefully and assertively advocate for themselves and then encourage them to do so. Historically, persons with HIV have been the ones to "teach" the social and medical services systems about the disease, how the systems should act, and how people with HIV should be respected and treated. Clients who choose not to act in this capacity should be assisted with other alternatives, such as having a family member, their partner, or the social worker advocate on their behalf. Though it certainly may not be the best or most acceptable of solutions, many people with HIV continue to relocate to more urban or suburban areas as rural communities continue to struggle to establish the necessary services.

POLICY IMPLICATIONS AND RELATED ACTIONS

First, social workers should provide themselves with the opportunity to learn about HIV and AIDS. Such learning can be accomplished by several avenues, including reading, attending conferences or training, or visiting an AIDS service organization and learning of their services, protocols, and available resources.

Second, social workers need to advocate for and create HIV/AIDS training opportunities in rural communities. Through collaboration with agencies representing the HIV continuum of care, training or conferences may be made available on a communitywide basis. Another effective method is to offer and/or arrange inservice trainings for community agency staff and providers. This option is often preferred because costs are contained and trainings can simply become a part of the staff development process. Preexisting resources and agencies in more urban areas are often very willing and able to assist in the provision of needed trainings and consultations. Also, some states have formed statewide alliances in an effort to ensure availability of direct services and community education.

From a clinical perspective, it is imperative to utilize a social casework model of service provision, including in the assessment process the client, the client's family and friends, and available and needed community resources.

Engaging the client's support network must, of course, occur only with the client's permission. The client's partner/spouse and friends are typically the people most easily engaged as needed. Many relatives, however, may be resistant to engaging in any way with the client, for the myriad of reasons noted earlier in this chapter. However, with finesse and compassion, the social worker may be very successful in positively engaging members of the client's family into the network of support. A willingness to reach out to family members is imperative, even if they are actively hostile toward the disease process or newly discovered information about the client, such as his or her sexual orientation, drug use, etc. It is also likely that a community "needs assessment" should be completed, utilizing one of the many assessment frameworks that have already been completed in some rural and many urban areas by organizations such as local divisions of the United Ways or by AIDS service organizations which have developed planning capacities.

RECOMMENDED READINGS

AIDS Resource Pathfinder
http://www.nnlm.nlm.nih.gov/pnr/etc/aidspath.html
    Provides online links to National Institute of Allergy and Infectious Diseases (NIAID) Gopher, WHO Programme on AIDS, CDC National AIDS Clearinghouse, Detroit Community AIDS Library (DCAL) Homepage, HIVNET/GENA (Global Electronic Network for AIDS), AIDS Patents Project, CHAT: Conversational Hypertext Access Technology—The AIDS Information System.

Compton, Beulah Roberts, and Burt Galaway. (1979). *Social work process.* Homewood, IL: The Dorsey Press.

HIV Database, Los Alamos National Laboratory
http://hiv-web.lanl.gov
New sequences presented in GenBank format, alignments of all HIV-1, HIV-2 and SIV genes, analyses of genetic sequences, including phylogenetic trees, related cellular protein sequences, and diskettes in GB or EMBL format.

Maine AIDS Plan
Maine AIDS Alliance
39 Green Street
Augusta, ME 04330
207-621-2924

National Social Work AIDS Network
c/o Harlem United: Community AIDS Center
207 West 133rd Street
New York, NY 10030

National Network of Libraries of Medicine
http://text.nlm.nih.gov/cps/www/cpstoc.html
Infectious Diseases: 24. Screening for Infection with Human Immunodeficiency Virus

NLM Agency for Health Policy and Research Guidelines
http://text.nlm.nih.gov/ahcpr/ahcpr.html
Clinical Practice Guidelines: 7. Evaluation and Management of Early HIV Infection Consumer Guides: 7a. Understanding HIV: Consumer Guide, 7b. HIV and Your Child: Consumer Guide.

Shernoff, Michael (March 1996). Returning with AIDS: Supporting Rural Emigrants. *Focus, 11*(4): 1-4.

Tartaglia, Alexander (March 1996). AIDS and the rural church. *Focus, 11*(4): 5-6.

Providing Services to People with Preexisting Mental Illness

Emily Leavitt
Patricia Sullivan

WHY DO THIS?
STATEMENT OF THE PROBLEM AND ISSUES

Preexisting mental illness may refer to those individuals with histories of psychotic illnesses—for example, schizophrenia, schizoaffective disorder, and bipolar affective disorder with psychotic features—as well as those with preexisting conditions that are exacerbated by HIV/AIDS, such as severe depression.

These clients can present complicated challenges to social workers and other providers. The common treatment concern is that the mental health condition significantly impairs the client's overall functioning.

EXAMPLES OF HOW THE ISSUE MAY PRESENT

Social workers in all settings may encounter HIV-infected clients with preexisting mental illness. For example, a case manager at a housing program notices a resident who generally isolates himself from others and mumbles to himself. A medical social worker observes extreme mood changes in one AIDS patient from visit to visit. A family reunification worker finds that a previously high-functioning young mother who is HIV positive is forgetting to feed her children. In all of these cases, staff might quickly assume that the observed behaviors stem from HIV, overlooking the possibility of preexisting mental illness. It is often the social worker with a biopsychosocial framework who realizes that psychiatric and/or substance abuse issues need to be assessed and treated along with the HIV.

FACTS THE SOCIAL WORKER
NEEDS TO KNOW BEFORE PROCEEDING

In working with clients who are "dually diagnosed" (i.e., HIV and mental illness), social workers need a basic understanding of medical and psychiatric disease processes, including the following:

- There is a high prevalence of mental illness, often undiagnosed and untreated, in our society.
- Substance abuse frequently coexists with mental illness.
- Mentally ill individuals are at high risk for contracting HIV due to unsafe sexual behavior, substance abuse, impaired judgment, and poor access to education and prevention services.
- Social workers need a basic understanding of the routes of HIV transmission and the course of the disease.
- Social workers need a sound understanding of how to assess and diagnose major mental illness, and of the impact of HIV on psychiatric conditions.
- Social workers need to have familiarity with symptoms of CNS (central nervous system)-related conditions, such as HIV-associated dementia complex or toxoplasmosis, and they need to know when and how to advocate for further medical workups.
- Social workers need to know mental health and substance abuse treatment options for HIV-infected clients.
- Social workers need to know how to utilize local crisis services and state laws regarding involuntary hospitalization.

KEY QUESTIONS TO ASK THE CLIENT

A crucial aspect of providing services to clients with preexisting psychiatric conditions is gauging their psychological and social functioning. Clients with preexisting conditions often have previous evaluations and reports that are available to the social worker. Though this information is helpful, it is often useful for you to complete your own assessment, especially when the evaluations are dated or there is a discrepancy between the evaluation and the current clinical presentation.

In performing a clinical assessment, key questions such as those utilized in diagnostic psychiatric interviewing are important. Prior to beginning the interview, you should note whether the client has self-referred or has been referred by another agency or provider. A typical assessment would include the following:

1. *Identifying information.* Name, age, gender, etc.
2. *Chief complaint or presenting problem.* What does the client state is wrong?
3. *History of presenting illness (HPI).* This section describes the frequency, duration, and severity of the presenting symptoms.
4. *Family/social history.* This section describes family of origin information (including any family history of psychiatric or substance abuse issues), significant relational history, school history and level of education, former or current occupations, and current means of financial support.
5. *Medical history.* This section includes the client's understanding of his or her disease, the current diagnosis (e.g., AIDS, symptomatic HIV), history of disease, the CD-4 count, current providers, medications and treatment, and any other medical conditions.
6. *Psychiatric history.* This section includes any previous treatment or history of psychiatric conditions. Reference should be made to any past or current suicidal ideation, history of violence, paranoid ideation, and visual or auditory hallucinations.
7. *Substance use history.* This section includes the frequency, amount, and type of any past or current drug or alcohol use and/or abuse (including prescription medications); how long has the client used; if there is any previous history of treatment; if the client is undergoing any current treatment; and how long has the client been clean and sober if in recovery.
8. *Mental status exam.* This section should comment on appearance, behavior, speech, mood, affect, thought, cognition, judgment, and insight.

From these interview questions, you can form your *diagnostic impression.* In addition to the DSM-IV diagnosis, this may include a brief summary of general impressions and a prognosis. Based on the diagnosis, *treatment recommendations* and interventions are developed.

It is often helpful to the client to end the interview by asking the client if he or she has any questions. Clients are often curious or anxious about the process and what "is wrong with them." Discussing your impressions and possible treatment recommendations can be reassuring to the client.

In working with clients with HIV, it is not uncommon for clinicians to become focused solely on the client "post HIV." Recording a full psychiatric history can help remind the clinician that all clients have a history, including previous ways of coping with, responding to, and conducting one's life.

CULTURAL COMPETENCY CONSIDERATIONS

Culture encompasses many aspects of an individual, including ethnicity, gender, class, educational experience, sexual orientation, religion, regional upbringing, level of acculturation, and life experiences in North American culture. There may also be a "culture" of being HIV positive or of being mentally ill.

When working with individuals with mental illness and HIV disease, you must recognize the client's cultural fabric as well as possible expectations of your role. It is helpful to ask yourself the following questions:

- How is mental illness viewed within the culture?
- How is seeking help (outside the family) viewed?
- How are issues of sexuality and substance abuse able to be addressed?
- What are the dormant strengths of the culture that can be of help to the client?

The importance of cultural competency and sensitivity in HIV social work has been increasingly recognized over past years, and we must maintain a constant awareness. However, in crisis situations, we are bound by our ethical and legal responsibilities, regardless of a client's particular background. For example, if a client consistently talks about guns, bullets, and silencers, this must be evaluated in terms of danger to self or others, regardless of the role guns may have played in his upbringing/culture. Also, in the "culture" of AIDS service providers, we expect and encourage discussions about suicide; however, we must still respond within our legal and ethical boundaries as mental health practitioners.

ACTION STEPS FOR SUCCESSFUL INTERVENTION

It is true that these clients can be difficult to work with and to treat. They may have serious problems complying both with medication regimens and appointment schedules. In addition, they may exhibit substance-abusing and drug-using behavior; have difficulty localizing and describing symptoms; and engage in obtrusive, inappropriate, and disinhibited behaviors.

In treating clients with preexisting conditions, the following guidelines are helpful:

1. Resolve any immediate crises, such as suicidality or grave disability.
2. Depending on your clinical assessment, identify key areas to be addressed. (For example, if a client is often noncompliant with medications, consider a linkage to a mental health case management program.)
3. Work with the client to establish these treatment goals (both short-term and long-term).
4. Establish any necessary contracts to reach these goals.

5. Refer to other providers for any special services (e.g., substance abuse services) and work to agree upon a common treatment plan for the client.
6. Assess client on an ongoing basis to determine whether other psychosocial concerns need to be addressed and to monitor the client's progress in achieving goals.
7. Renegotiate goals and the treatment plan as necessary.
8. Obtain all necessary releases of information.
9. Document all services provided and sessions conducted.

POTENTIAL BARRIERS TO SUCCESSFUL INTERVENTION

The primary barrier to successful treatment for this population is lack of adequate treatment for mental illness, substance abuse, and other medical problems in our communities; however, even when resources do exist, coordinating care can be very difficult.

Traditionally, mental health and medical programs have not worked closely together; even within a single hospital, relationships between the departments of psychiatry and medicine can be distant. In such settings, the care of patients who require both medical and psychiatric expertise may be compromised.

Mental health clinics, day treatment programs, and psychiatric residential facilities frequently lack knowledge, awareness, and perhaps willingness to work with patients who have HIV. These programs are not designed to deal with patients with declining health or chronic medical problems such as fevers, diarrhea, acute pain, or wasting syndrome. Inpatient nursing staff may be unfamiliar with infusion or other HIV-related medical procedures. Psychiatrists may lack knowledge regarding HIV-related medications—especially when used in conjunction with psychotropic medications.

HIV risk assessment is critical in psychiatric settings. Mental health providers may be hesitant to discuss risk factors for a variety of reasons, including the fear that the topic may distress patients or increase suicide risk (contrary to evidence), the reluctance to deal with the ethical and legal implications of patients practicing unsafe sex, and staff discomfort in taking sexual histories and discussing sexual practice.

Medical settings are usually not well equipped to work with patients with serious mental illness. These patients often lack primary or preventative medical care and may be initiated into the health care system as a result of their HIV. Medical providers, often reflecting the general indifference of society toward chronic mental illness, may lack awareness and sensitivity, for example, by believing that all psychotic patients are dangerous and should be institutionalized. Medical providers frequently fail to investigate and treat complaints of depression or anxiety, believing that "of course he's depressed—he has AIDS."

Another potential barrier is our own discomfort with our clients' terminal status. Facing and discussing death and dying is one of the most challenging tasks for health care professionals and terminally ill patients. The stress and anxiety for both can be magnified when patients are mentally ill, and in response, providers may overlook spiritual and counseling needs. But, a psychiatric diagnosis in no way negates a patient's very real fears of decline and death. One actively psychotic patient stated shortly before he died, "It's not that I want to go on living. It's just that I'm afraid to die." Even the most disturbed patient—unable to articulate her feelings—can be acutely aware of losses, bodily changes, and pain, and will need to share fears and concerns.

INFORMATION THE CLIENT SHOULD KNOW
BEFORE TAKING ACTION

The client needs to know who you are, what your agency is, and what you do. Dually diagnosed individuals probably have a variety of ideas about why they are seeing "the social worker," and these ideas may not relate at all to your job description. Therefore, it is your job to clearly and concretely explain your purpose and what you can and cannot do. Because of the nature of mental illness, it may be necessary to repeat this explanation over time. Obviously, unless a legal hold is involved, clients can refuse your assistance, no matter how much you think he might benefit from it.

Many clients with mental illness have a minimal or incorrect understanding of their psychiatric and medical diagnoses and the role of medication. Psychoeducation becomes an important role of the social worker, as we often find ourselves teaching our clients about their treatment as well as "how to use the system."

POLICY IMPLICATIONS AND RELATED ACTIONS

Just as social workers should play a key role in assessment and treatment of clients with preexisting mental illness and HIV, we must also become involved in policy, program development, and education in this area.

Social workers continue to advocate for increased funding for mental health and health care for all, and this is particularly critical with Federal

CARE funding (The Ryan White Act). Social workers can advise or act as policymakers in developing a nationwide health care system that addresses all aspects of patient care, including psychiatric and substance abuse treatment.

HIV-infected patients with preexisting mental illness benefit from programs that can address both their psychiatric and medical needs, and there are successful residential programs in various communities that provide medical, mental health, and substance abuse services. Ideally, new adult day health programs—traditionally developed to respond to the needs of the elderly—will now address the complicated physical and psychological needs of HIV-infected patients.

On-site mental health services can have a tremendous impact on HIV-related outpatient and inpatient medical care, both through direct patient contact and through consultation and training for staff. Specialized inpatient psychiatric units can provide treatment and discharge planning for the patients with concurrent HIV disease and mental illness, and all psychiatric facilities should be encouraged to incorporate HIV-related risk assessment into their intake procedures.

Social workers have always provided informal consultation to other staff regarding the psychosocial aspects of HIV disease. Social workers have the expertise, particularly in psychosocial and systems theory, to also provide formalized training to physicians and nurses in medical and psychiatric settings.

RECOMMENDED READINGS

Dilley, J., Pies, C., and Helquist, M. (Eds.). *Face to face: A guide to AIDS counseling.* Berkeley: Ten Speed Press, 1989.

Odets, W., and Shernoff, M. (Eds.). *The second decade of AIDS: A mental health practice handbook.* New York: Hatherleigh Press, 1995.

Winiarski, M. *AIDS-related psychotherapy.* New York: Pergamon Press, 1991.

HIV Services in Correctional Facilities: Negotiating a Complex Environment

Robert J. Battjes

Peter J. Delany

WHY DO THIS?
STATEMENT OF THE PROBLEM AND ISSUES

The AIDS epidemic has emerged as a major public health problem within correctional facilities, currently constituting the leading cause of death among men and women in custody of the correctional system. Given high rates of injection drug use among correctional populations, HIV infection and AIDS within correctional facilities are found largely among injection drug users (IDUs); however, HIV disease among men who have sex with men (MSM) and among noninjecting heterosexual partners of IDUs are also of concern. Though some HIV transmission occurs within prison, most individuals are infected prior to incarceration. Unlike in the general population, women in correctional facilities tend to have higher rates of HIV infection than men based on higher rates of IDU among female offenders.

Due to the increasing number of inmates admitted to correctional facilities who are infected with HIV, corrections and public health officials are concerned that prisons and jails are becoming reservoirs that may amplify HIV infection as inmates are released back to the community. Thus, HIV services provided in correctional facilities will have a major impact not only on the well-being of inmates themselves, but also on the future course of the epidemic in the larger society.

Given that correctional facilities will continue to house significant numbers of HIV-infected people, or who are at high risk for infection, corrections-based interventions represent a significant opportunity to engage infected persons and those at risk in interventions that may limit opportunities for exposure. Interventions within correctional facilities also offer important opportunities for protecting the sexual and injecting partners and future children of infected male and female inmates after they are released back into the community.

Within correctional facilities, a range of medical and psychosocial interventions must be considered, including the following: HIV prevention, drug abuse treatment, medical care for HIV-related diseases, counseling/grief resolution for terminally ill persons and their significant others, prerelease planning and postrelease follow-up, HIV education for correctional and medical personnel and inmates, and systemic/organizational interventions. The remainder of this chapter will provide the social worker with a basic understanding of the context in which practice takes place as well as an overview of possible intervention strategies that may be effective with this population.

THE PRACTICE CONTEXT

In the past fifteen years there has been a tremendous increase in the number of individuals remanded to the custody of prisons and jails, and much of this increase is due to individuals incarcerated for drug-related offenses. A major factor has been tougher policies, including policies stemming from the "war on drugs," which have led to mandatory sentences and the restriction of cases that could be diverted to alternative punishments. Many of those incarcerated for drug-related offenses will cycle through the system again and again.

The impact of overcrowding and the increased percentage of individuals within the system who are HIV-infected create real safety and health problems for corrections officials charged with the care of these people. Though tremendous strides have been made in improving conditions within our prisons, it is not difficult to imagine the difficulty for correctional health care workers to adequately detect and treat HIV infection, sexually transmitted diseases (STDs), and tuberculosis in a timely manner. Additionally, corrections officials and health care workers, just as their colleagues in the community, face a great deal of ignorance about HIV— how it is transmitted and how to reduce risks.

The types and mix of HIV/AIDS services appropriate for correctional facilities will vary depending on a number of factors, including type of facility, institutional population, and geographic location. Regarding geographic location, rates of HIV infection and AIDS among IDUs are substantially higher on the East Coast and in Puerto Rico than elsewhere in the United States. Thus, programmatic elements that focus on currently infected and ill persons will be much more central to program efforts in these areas; elsewhere program efforts will be focused more largely on prevention efforts.

Social workers can contribute much to services for people at risk or who are infected with HIV in prisons and jails. The unique nature of the correctional environment requires a systems approach that takes into account both the individual's need for concrete services and needs of the institution in terms of safety and security. In addition to considering the needs of the correctional facility, the social worker also needs to consider influences from other settings, including the family, social networks, and the surrounding community.

EXAMPLES OF HOW THE ISSUE MAY PRESENT

Most social workers are more comfortable with the notion of beginning where the client is and moving externally if clients cannot negotiate the system on their own. However, the nature of HIV and AIDS among offender populations requires the social worker to rethink the question of "Who is the client?" In this case, the client includes not only the individual inmate, but also the correctional setting, the family/social network, and the community that will be serving the individual upon release. Thus, social workers may find themselves confronted with a number of multiple and sometimes conflicting tasks related to the demands of each setting. For example, corrections officials, charged with the responsibility of maintaining offenders in a safe and secure setting, may view HIV prevention programs as secondary to their primary mission. Family networks may not be ready or willing to handle a diagnosis of HIV infection. Social networks may actually be antagonistic toward an individual's changing behaviors, especially where a drug-using lifestyle is central to the relationship. The community may be reluctant to accept the responsibility of a high-risk individual, both in terms of financial and political resources. The benefit of intervening proactively in each of these settings is that it increases the linkage of services and resources that can support real behavioral changes.

Some Key Areas to Consider in Developing Action Steps in Multiple Settings

As with any intervention, it is important that to understand the nature of the problem and the resources available to intervene within each setting. The social worker will need answers to many of the following questions before proceeding.

1. What is the nature of the problem?
   - What is the prevalence of HIV infection in the institution and in the surrounding community?

- What is the type and magnitude of the drug problem, particularly the IDU problem, among both the inmate population and the surrounding community?
- How do the issues of family, friends, gender, race, and cultural issues—including sexual orientation—impact this problem in the correctional setting, the family/social setting, and the community setting?
2. What is the knowledge level about HIV/AIDS in each setting?
   - What is the understanding of HIV/AIDS, including how it is transmitted and how to reduce risks?
3. Who are the key players within each setting—correctional, family and social network, and community?
   - How do those involved think it should be handled?
   - What background, experiences, and resources can be brought to bear on this problem within each setting?
4. What key issues must be addressed for persons at risk?
   For persons at risk, social workers need to assess the types of risk (drug use, unsafe sexual practices) and behavioral changes that need to be made to reduce or eliminate exposure, including HIV counseling and testing, drug treatment, and counseling about relationships and behaviors that put one at risk.
5. What key issues must be addressed for persons infected with HIV or who have AIDS?
   When a person is infected with HIV or has AIDS, social workers must still assess risks and the behavioral changes necessary so as to limit reexposure and exposure of others. As important, they must assess the health and social needs of clients in order to help them manage their illness and address life and systems issues related to a terminal illness. Some of the key issues to be addressed are discussed using the following case summary.

ADDRESSING KEY ISSUES

Case Study

William S. is a thirty-two-year-old married male who was referred to the social work department by the prison health clinic after testing positive for HIV. Mr. S. has been incarcerated for the past six months following a conviction on charges of possession of narcotics and solicitation. He acknowledges an addiction to cocaine, describing a pattern of injecting cocaine and smoking crack that had increased markedly during the year prior to his arrest. Mr. S. states that he prefers to inject cocaine and that he was shooting up daily with "friends" before his arrest, oftentimes sharing equipment without cleaning it. He also smoked crack several times a week. He supported his habit mostly through selling drugs, committing petty crimes, and occasionally, prostituting himself. Although Mr. S. reports that he always used condoms with men he did not know, he never used condoms with his wife or any other woman that he slept with "because you can't catch AIDS from a woman." He has two children, a four-year-old who lives with his maternal grandparents and a one-year-old who, he believes, is in foster care. His wife, Mrs. S., is currently in treatment for her own cocaine addiction. He has not seen either his wife or children in over a year and has no knowledge of their HIV status.

Partner Notification

Encouraging infected persons to notify sexual partners as well as helping to reach out to their drug-using network is important in terms of prevention and treatment. Knowledge of Mr. S.'s HIV status may convince his wife and injecting partners to be tested and to monitor their medical situation. Mr. S. may also want to notify the grandparents and foster care so that his children can be tested.

As indicated in this case study, effective partner notification requires sharing accurate information about HIV transmission risk, helping clients recognize their responsibility for others who may be infected, and helping them contact individuals whose whereabouts are unknown. Local public health officials can assist in partner notification efforts where a contact's whereabouts are unknown or when a client prefers not to directly interact with a contact. Local public health officials can also make available counseling and testing, treatment, and other social services.

Medical Care

Medical intervention is critical to maintaining clients' current well-being and extending life expectancy. The role of the social worker is to facilitate the identification, planning, and targeting of individual medical services with prison medical staff and Mr. S. Where resources are insufficient to meet the needs of Mr. S., the social worker may act as an advocate with medical and administrative staff to obtain these services—in house when possible, but certainly from the community if necessary.

In a larger sense, the role of the social worker is to work at the system level to ensure that medical providers, administrative staff, court referral personnel, and local public health providers are providing adequate procedures for identifying and targeting individuals in need of medical intervention, both during and following incarceration.

Grief Work

For newly diagnosed persons and for persons who have been living with HIV and AIDS for some time, the social worker can play an important role in dealing with grief resolution for individuals and their significant others. In addition to providing for material services such as medical care and living conditions, the social worker may find it useful to provide some support for Mr. S. to examine just what his diagnosis means in his life. Encouraging Mr. S. to work through the grieving process that is normal with a diagnosis of HIV seropositivity may help him to take a proactive approach in the management of his care when he is symptom-free as well as help to reduce risks for reinfection. Optimally, this process will also be preventive in nature by helping Mr. S. take steps to plan for managing the physical, emotional, and social fallout that occurs when he does become symptomatic.

A parallel issue relates to how to best address the issues of grief and the feelings and emotions associated with finding out that a family member or friend has been diagnosied as HIV positive. If Mr. S. agrees to notify his wife and those taking care of his children of his medical status, referrals for support services may be given at the time of referral for testing. However, if "compassionate release" policies do exist, or if Mr. S. is released to another facility for treatment, further consultation and referrals will most likely be needed to aid family and friends in coping with what may be a long-term illness. Initially, this may focus on the provision of material resources such as financial aid, but helping Mr. S. and his family and friends with the transition from one environment to another may also require referrals for support groups and counseling.

Finally, ongoing care of the staff is critical if the quality of care is to be maintained. As Mr. S. and his family and friends need to work through the grief and stress, so do the staff members who interact with these individuals. This includes the medical, correctional, administrative, and social work staff. Taking care of staff members includes providing regular training in HIV- and AIDS-related issues and regular opportunities to unwind and discuss feelings without fear of reprisal. It may be helpful to provide the services of a trained critical-incident debriefer from a local community, especially if a patient dies of AIDS or an AIDS-related illness while in custody. Ongoing superivision for all personnel is crucial for staff members charged with the care of HIV-positive individuals.

Discharge Planning

For persons with HIV facing discharge, prerelease planning and post-release follow-up are essential. The primary role of the social worker will be to assist Mr. S. in making contact with key treatment and social service agencies in the community before his release. Being an ex-offender, a drug addict, and HIV positive creates a number of barriers that require a very proactive, even aggressive approach in order to ensure some level of service continuity as Mr. S. transitions from the prison setting to the community.

One approach that has had some success is the Assertive Community Treatment (ACT) model developed by Dr. James Inciardi at the University of Delaware and modeled on the Assertive Case Management method, which was developed for work with the chronically mentally ill. In this model, the social worker focuses on reconnecting Mr. S. to his community through the provision of material, interpersonal, and moral support in such areas of housing, education, use of leisure time, and self-care in dealing with daily living and medical needs.

In the ACT model, Mr. S has access to the social worker twenty-four-hours-a-day. Further, the social worker would actively track Mr. S., going to him rather than waiting for problems to arise. Instrumental support such as rent and food money, transportation, and access to medical and drug treatment and support services are available to Mr. S. through the social worker. Above all, this approach stresses the continuity of care for Mr. S. in moving from the institution to the community and while in the community.

Education

Education for Mr. S. and other clients with or at risk for becoming HIV seropositive is critical. This education must include not only information about the disease itself, and its transmission, but also training in how to change behavior to reduce risks. Though there is some controversy about teaching such behaviors as "safer sex," the policy deserves some discussion if we are to have any significant impact on the transmission among this population (see the section on policy implications and related actions as well as references by S. Coyle (1993) and F. Rhodes (1993)).

Additionally, it can be very helpful for professional staff to receive cross-training in critical areas such as corrections and drug treatment. An important role for the social worker can be to create opportunities for cross-training to encourage sensitivity to the missions and demands of each profession. This type of experience may also be helpful for community contacts to help understand the constraints within which people in each setting operate.

ACTION STEPS FOR SUCCESSFUL INTERVENTION

Effective interventions that involve multiple systems within multiple settings require patience and a long-term outlook. Understanding critical settings and how they interact allows the social worker to plan and coordinate strategies aimed at changing targeted behaviors at the individual, institutional, and community level. Further, it helps to identify and integrate new norms that reinforce the development of healthy behaviors.

1. *Create a planning group utilizing key actors.*
2. *Using the key issue questions, assess the needs of the client systems in each setting.* What types of services are needed for which people in each setting? Where will the planning group get information to create accurate assessments? Can these needs be categorized into immediate, short-term, and long-term needs?
3. *Develop an initial strategy for intervening within each setting.* What types of interventions will be used—reducing risks and/or enhancing protective factors (HIV testing and counseling, education, medical care, individual case management, coordination of services between settings, support for family members, etc.)? Who will be responsible for each intervention? What is the payoff for participation; that is, what will each player/organization gain from the intervention?
4. *Incorporate process and outcome evaluation into the activity plan from the beginning.* Has the intervention been implemented as planned? If not, why not? What is the definition(s) of success for each intervention—abstinence from drug use, increased access to services within and across settings, reduction in risky behaviors? How will these be measured? How will the feedback be used to improve the intervention? How will information about the program be disseminated?

POTENTIAL BARRIERS TO SUCCESSFUL INTERVENTION

Historically, a lack of coordination has existed both within and across settings that serve people infected with HIV and those at risk for becoming infected. Several barriers to implementing interventions aimed at improving coordination of services at crucial linkage points can be identified. These include such concerns as losing control of resources and personnel, inadequate funding for service expansion or coordination, regulations that limit opportunities to work across settings, and inadequate training for corrections and service personnel. Although these are complex issues, working within a planning group framework is a useful strategy to identify where conflicts exist; thus, problem solving can be employed to create new opportunities for interaction.

POLICY IMPLICATIONS AND RELATED ACTIONS

In the past, primarily three policy options have been pursued in relation to HIV and AIDS in correctional setting, namely control strategies, prevention strategies, and drug abuse treatment strategies. These policy options and some of their implications are discussed below.

Control Strategies

Approaches to control HIV-infected inmates have generally included mandatory testing and/or segregation. Some institutions may institute mandatory testing for all admissions while others mandate testing only when histories indicate drug use, homosexual contact, or sexual contact with IDUs. Although these approaches may identify many infected individuals at the time of admission, HIV antibody tests may not reflect infection for up to six months. Thus, there is a danger that mandatory testing may create a false sense of safety and decrease risk-reduction behaviors within the institution. Mandatory testing programs also assume that confidentiality of results can be maintained and that individuals will act responsibly once a diagnosis is known. With either mandatory or voluntary HIV screening, careful consideration must be given to issues of confidentiality and safety within the institution, adequacy of counseling that accompanies testing, and the provision of HIV-related medical care and drug abuse treatment where indicated.

A second policy option that some prisons and jails have implemented is to segregate seropositive inmates and/or persons with AIDS. Some prisons have dormitories set aside for seropositive inmates, including hospital facilities to treat inmates with AIDS and AIDS-related conditions. Several court decisions have upheld segregation when it is voluntary and if additional services have been provided to meet the needs of those who are segregated. An important question that needs to be addressed is not how many can be identified and segregated, but how many will not be identified who are at risk and need to be convinced to change behaviors to protect themselves and others.

Prevention Strategies

Preventive interventions are essential to reducing HIV transmission within institutions, and protecting inmates and/or others following release. Interventions need to target persons infected with HIV, persons at risk, and their significant others. Brief interventions are effective in assisting many MSMs and IDUs reduce their high-risk behaviors while more intensive and repeated interventions are needed for some high-risk individuals who are resistant to change or relapse (Coyle, 1993; Rhodes, 1993). Preventive interventions must include not only information concerning how HIV infection is transmitted, but also how it is not transmitted (e.g., casual contact) and how to reduce risks to prevent exposure, reexposure, and transmission to others.

Providing information focused on key concepts of risk is not enough. Many individuals who meet the criteria for high risk (IDUs, MSMs, having multiple sex partners, or having a sex partner who is an IDU) clearly understand the basic concepts related to HIV. Prevention must also include information and interventions that focus on techniques for changing risky behaviors and protecting oneself. Since frank discussions about risk reduction can be controversial, social workers in correctional settings must discuss the importance of prevention with medical and management officials and obtain their support for these interventions. Medical and social history taking, which gathers specific information on lifestyle (IDU, sexual contacts, condom use), provide opportunities for brief preventive interventions or referral to more intensive interventions. Among IDUs, many have attempted to reduce their risk for HIV infection by cleaning their syringes with bleach. Yet, the bleaching practices actually implemented are often inadequate to kill HIV, and other paraphernalia that may also transmit HIV, such as cookers, cottons, and rinse water, are often ignored. Thus, information provided as part of prevention efforts must be thorough.

Research has shown that interventions need to be sensitive to gender and race. For example, many women will use condoms with their irregular sexual partners, but not necessarily regular sexual partners who may be IDUs. Additionally, many high-risk women are financially or emotionally dependent, which inhibits implementation of safer sexual practices. In conducting preventive interventions in correctional facilities, social workers must remember that men who engage in sex with other men within institutional settings often do not self-identify as homosexual; therefore, they may consider interventions that target gay men as irrelevant to themselves.

For lockups and booking facilities, where time and staffing generally do not permit individualized interventions, a videotaped intervention is available (see National Institute on Drug Abuse, 1995, in the resources). Development of community referral sources for these facilities is another potential approach.

Drug Abuse Treatment Strategies

Though preventive interventions focused on risk behaviors have proven effective with many IDUs, many others continue to engage in high-risk behaviors in spite of involvement in prevention programming. These people are also often the least likely to enter treatment. Prison-based drug abuse treatment provides an important opportunity to initiate the recovery process, and prison-based treatment models exist that have proven effectiveness, especially when combined with postincarceration continuing care. Although the number of correctional facilities that have drug treatment programs is growing, a substantial number of institutions are without treatment programs, and social workers should consider systemic initiatives to encourage development of programs where none exist.

Harm-Reduction Policies

The previous policies are aimed either at managing the infected person or eliminating the behaviors that place a person at risk for infection. What has received less attention in the practice and research literature are policies focusing on harm reduction. These include the distribution of condoms and clean needles/syringes to inmates who continue to use substances while in prison. Condom distribution has played a major role in HIV prevention strategies since early in the epidemic, and in recent years an increasing number of communities are implementing legally sanctioned needle-exchange programs to make sterile syringes available to IDUs. Certainly, these are options that engender strong reactions, especially as both sex between men and drug use in a correctional setting are illegal. However, as these options become increasingly accepted outside of correctional settings, it seems advisable to discuss how such policies may impact within these settings.

CONCLUSION

This section has presented a systems approach to working with HIV and AIDS in correctional settings emphasizing three primary settings: the correctional setting, the family/social setting, and the community setting. This approach addresses the critical need for developing coordinated services that move between settings and rely heavily on social workers' skills for organizing and coordinating often disparate actors. Resulting from its perspective and training, the social work profession is in a unique position to identify areas of overlap and fragmentation in services for people with HIV and AIDS.

RESOURCES

Health Resources and Services Administration (1995). *Progress and challenges in linking incarcerated individuals with HIV/AIDS to community services.* Rockville, MD: Author.

Rivers, J.E. (1993). Substance abuse and HIV among criminal justice populations: Overview from a program evaluation perspective. In J.A. Inciardi (ed.), *Drug Treatment and Criminal Justice.* Newbury Park, CA: Sage Publications, Inc.

The following may be obtained by contacting the National Clearinghouse for Alcohol and Drug Abuse Information at 1-800-729-6686.

Coyle, S. (1993). *The NIDA HIV counseling and education intervention model: Intervention manual,* NIH Publication No. 93-3580: Rockville, MD: NI4.

National Institute on Drug Abuse (1995). *Drug abuse treatment in prison: A new way out,* NCADI VHS74 ($8.50 recovery fee for shipping and handling of videotapes).

Rhodes, F. (1993). *The behavioral counseling model for injection drug users,* NIH Publication No. 93-3579: Rockville, MD: NI4.

SECTION IV:
ECONOMIC SUPPORTS
AND HOUSING

Economic Supports and Advocacy

Jay Laudato

As we all do, people living with AIDS and HIV (PWA/HIVs) have health, emotional, and concrete needs. In assisting PWA/HIVs, regardless of the focus of the intervention, social workers should be familiar with the available economic supports and programs that provide access to health care and concrete services for their clients. Awareness of benefit programs can enhance social workers' ability to provide psychotherapeutic services and assist in creating stability in their clients' lives. Through entitlement assessment, referral, and advocacy, social workers can have a profound impact in the improving the quality of lives of people living with HIV/AIDS and their families.

This chapter is intended to provide social workers with a basic understanding of how to conduct an assessment of financial needs, available public and private entitlements for PWA/HIVs, and advocacy strategies. This chapter is not exhaustive on the kinds of entitlements or benefits available to PWA/HIVs (particularly local programs) or the specific eligibility criteria established for those benefit programs. *Accordingly, social workers using this text should consider this chapter as a starting point for gathering locally specific entitlement information to assist clients in securing resources to meet financial and material needs.*

HOW TO CONDUCT AN ECONOMIC ASSESSMENT

Conducting an assessment is the starting point and basis for all future activities and interactions with your client. The following discusses the areas for which information is needed to assist a client in making a referral to the appropriate entitlement programs. Much of the following information is adapted from a system established by the financial advocacy unit at the Gay Men's Health Crisis in New York City, where I was the coordinator for several years.

Introduction to the Assessment

In order to assist your client in accessing entitlement programs, you will require detailed information about their income, assets, and expenses.

Clients may be uncomfortable about sharing explicit information about their financial affairs. You should explain that you are requesting only necessary information to assist them in accessing financial assistance and that the information will be kept confidential.

Confidentiality is not only a hallmark of a professional in human services, but in the case of HIV, is strictly legislated. Each state has different HIV-related confidentiality laws. Social workers should familiarize themselves with these laws and the applicable policies of the organization in which they work. If you are assisting a client in applying for benefits or advocating on their behalf, you may need to obtain a separate consent form before contacting another agency and disclosing a client's HIV status.

Before gathering financial information, you should spend some time determining the current emotional status of the client. Very often, assessments are conducted with clients at the time of a crisis, such as the first hospitalization for HIV-related causes or a client's decision that he or she is too sick to continue to work. Clients are particularly vulnerable at these times, and requesting necessary information about, for example, the cash-in value of their life insurance policy can precipitate an emotional crisis. Social workers working with any client, but particularly PWA/HIVs and benefits/entitlements, should keep two things in mind: (1) timing is everything, and (2) everything is a process.

Timing Is Everything

While a client may be at a very vulnerable point because of his or her emotional status, you may be encountering the client on the last day to stop his or her health insurance from being canceled or to stop an eviction from his or her apartment. Therefore, you must obtain from the client enough information—even during an emotionally vulnerable episode—to ensure that his or her living situation, health coverage, and income are secure.

Everything Is a Process

Conducting a full assessment of resources and entitlement needs at a time when the client is confronting a life-threatening diagnosis or some other personal loss is grossly insensitive. It should also be understood that the assessment process is also an educational process for clients and that you will be providing them with information on which they will be required to take action. Providing clients with current and accurate information about eligibility and the application process for available entitlements will begin to empower them to take control over their financial circumstances and living situation. Therefore, a social worker should make a determination if the assessment should be postponed and emotional issues addressed first in order for the client to be able to receive and act on the entitlement information.

Conducting the Assessment

The following are key areas in which to gather information and their implication with regard to private and public benefit programs.

Basic Demographic Information

Get the client's or family's basic demographic information. If the client gives you permission to act on his or her behalf with an entitlement agency, that agency is very likely to ask you for the client's date of birth, social security number, address, and telephone number—every time you contact them. It is worthwhile to have in the client's file, his or her health insurance policy number, utility account numbers, and the basic demographic information of all *collateral* or *dependent* family members. In general, public entitlement programs include the income and assets of collaterals (legally married spouses) and dependents (children under the age of eighteen years for whom the client is the legal guardian) in determining the eligibility for entitlement programs. The income and assets of the parents and siblings of adult clients are usually not considered in determining the client's eligibility even though he or she may be living in their household.

Determining if your client is a citizen or has some other resident standing in the United States is also important. Immigrants to the United States are generally ineligible for any type of public assistance entitlement. PWA/HIVs who must apply for benefits to secure needed health and financial assistance jeopardize their residency within the United States. No person with HIV infection is currently accepted for permanent residency within the United States without a special waiver, which can be very difficult to obtain and should not be attempted without the assistance of an attorney who specializes in this field. The Immigration and Naturalization Services is identified when any immigrant applies for a public benefit, unless they have become a naturalized citizen. Immigrants who must apply for public entitlements are generally required to leave the country once their health is stabilized if their residency is undocumented or their visa expires. For people who are seriously ill, including PWAs, there are waivers to remain in the country to receive medical care. Such a waiver is called a *voluntary stay of departure*. Applying for this type of waiver should only be done with the assistance of an immigration attorney with experience in this process.

Health Status

Knowing the client's specific diagnosis is important because most entitlement programs have eligibility criteria based on an HIV-related diagnosis. For example, the Social Security Administration finds persons with AIDS automatically eligible for benefits with the exception of those with nondisseminated Kaposi's sarcoma (KS). Some non-HIV-specific social service agencies, such as Cancer Care in New York City, provide assistance to clients with certain diagnoses.

Living Status and Household Members

This area includes both the information regarding the client's physical living situation (i.e., house or apartment) and the people with whom the client lives and their legal relationship to the PWA/HIV (e.g., spouse, dependent minor). Both have a major impact on the entitlements for which a client may be eligible.

Understanding the client's living arrangement includes knowing if the client rents or owns his or her apartment or home and if he or she is required to pay for utilities, heat, and water. In most states, owning the home you live in is considered an *exempt resource*, which means that while the property is an asset, it does not count against a client's eligibility for entitlements. However, in most states people who own their own residence and receive *asset-tested benefits* (benefits available only to people with income and assets below prescribed limits, such as public assistance or Medicaid) likely to have a lien put against their property by the state. The state will seek to recoup the entire amount of any entitlement provided to the client if the client seeks to sell the residence or when he or she passes away. Additionally, if the client owns any other property including a vacation home or a share in a family home in which he or she is not a full-time resident, these assets will make him or her ineligible for asset-tested benefits.

In addition to gathering information about a client's living status, you should find out who is living with the client and their legal relationship to the client. As stated in the basic demographic section, almost all means- and asset-tested benefit programs will request to know who is living with the client to determine if these persons can assist in supporting the client.

In general, adults are responsible for themselves. An adult client with AIDS can live in his or her parent's home without having his or her eligibility for entitlements effected as long as the client is responsible for paying for part of the rent and other basic expenses of the household. Children who are younger than eighteen are generally considered dependent on a related adult, whether that is a parent, grandparent, aunt, or uncle. Clients who are legally married are considered to be responsible for the financial support of the other spouse. Therefore, in a case in which one spouse is a PWA/HIV and is married to another person who is working, the income of the working spouse is *deemed* available to the PWA/HIV, which generally makes that person ineligible for means- and asset-tested entitlements. It should be noted that many states have special provisions in which the working spouse can keep all his or her income and need not contribute to support of the ill spouse if that person must be institutionalized in a long-term care or nursing facility. Any clients in that situation should be referred to an attorney specializing in these matters. Social workers can contact the local bar association or legal aid society for referrals to free or low-cost legal services to secure this exemption.

This is the one area in which gay and lesbian spouses find the law working to their advantage. Gay and lesbian unions are not currently recognized by law in any state and therefore, the income of a gay or lesbian spouse is not deemed available for the support of a PWA/HIV. This includes those states and localities with *domestic partnership* ordinances, which enable gays and lesbians to be eligible for their spouse's health insurance benefits or rights to an apartment or home after the death of their spouse.

Assessing the entitlement eligibility of families can be extremely complex even for eligibility specialists within entitlement agencies. In general, entitlements (as will be described more fully) have been developed so that eligibility for one entitlement provides access to another. For example, if a client is eligible for public assistance, he or she is usually eligible for food stamp benefits and is not required to fill out a separate application for this benefit. The converse is also true—if you lose eligibility for public assistance, you also lose your eligibility for food stamps. For families with multiple members, some eligible for certain HIV-specific benefit programs and others not, assessing and maintaining eligibility can be a full-time job.

Disability benefits and benefit programs available to PWA/HIVs oftentimes are considerably higher than the comparable benefit for nondisabled individuals. Accordingly, when assisting families to secure benefits and live within a budget, the social worker should be aware that when the client with AIDS passes away, the entire family may become ineligible for some benefits and may lose housing subsidies or medical coverage. Preparing families for this eventuality requires sophistication with both entitlements and also the psychosocial issues related to life-threatening diseases. A social worker is an appropriate professional to assist clients and families dealing with AIDS to address issues of death and dying and preparation for the future living circumstances of all family members. However, estate planning is a legal matter, and it requires an attorney to establish a living will/medical directive, to establish guardianship for a dependent minor, and to develop a legally binding will. Social workers involved with clients with HIV/AIDS should develop a referral relationship to a legal services entity to assist clients in securing these services (see the section on estate planning).

Income and Other Assets Information

It is important to gather information about your client's sources of income and other assets before assessing his or her eligibility for any entitlement program. In the next section, a general overview will be provided of the various private and public entitlements available to PWA/ HIVs. Very few public entitlement programs are not means- or asset-tested. Therefore, it is important to know if clients have sources of income such as work or union pensions; taxable assets such as stocks, bonds, interest-bearing saving accounts or property; or a financial interest in a business. In general, personal property such as jewelry, antiques or art work does not count toward entitlement eligibility. However, the value of an automobile does count as an asset for entitlement eligibility.

During the application process, entitlement agencies generally have to accept your word on reported income and accompanying documentation (bank records). However, these agencies have very sophisticated means of accessing information about clients' personal finances, including computer matches with IRS information and access to bank reporting to the federal government on interest income from different assets. Entitlement agencies will, in general, penalize applicants for any transfer of assets within a specific time period prior (a look-back period) to date of application for a benefit by withholding the benefit for a certain period. In New York State, a transfer of assets not disclosed during the application process will make a client ineligible for twenty-four months from the date of the application. It cannot be stressed enough that efforts at concealing or dispersing income and assets will almost invariably be uncovered and will be disastrous for the PWA/ HIV and professionally damaging for the social worker.

Clients who have assets and must spend-down those assets because they have no source of income or means of accessing health care other than public entitlements should be counseled to spend these funds in a "responsible" fashion. Public entitlement agencies will find spending of assets on gifts or luxury items as opposed to bills and living expenses to be "irresponsible" and done simply to qualify for entitlements, and as with a transfer of assets, will withhold benefits for a prescribed period.

Health Insurance Information

It is vitally important to gather specific information about the client's health insurance benefits. Unlike public entitlements, health insurance for most persons comes from employment and is subject to different regulations than public entitlements are. PWA/HIVs who have left their employment have a very short time after their last day of employment in which to apply to retain their health insurance. As will be described, PWA/HIVs (in most states) can apply to extend their group coverage for eighteen months after their last month of employment and in some cases during an additional eleven months, thus totalling up to twenty-nine months. However, neither the insurance company nor the employer is required to provide an application to the client nor request payment for monthly premiums. Social workers working with clients who have left their employment should advise clients to immediately contact their employer or health insurance company about extending their coverage. All correspondence with health insurance companies, including all monthly premium payments, should be sent by certified return-receipt-requested mail. Some health insurance companies are very reputable and seek to assist their plan members, but others consider only the extensive financial liability presented by PWA/HIVs and will look for any opportunity to rescind their coverage.

Documentation

All entitlement agencies will request certain documents to verify the client's identity, citizenship, income, assets, and household composition. It is worthwhile for social workers (particularly case managers who have an ongoing relationship with the client) to compile a file of client's documents. All clients should keep their own original documents and be encouraged to maintain their own document file. The following is a list of documents that clients should gather to facilitate the application process and social workers should consider in maintaining a document file: birth certificates, original social security cards, tax returns including W-2/W-4 forms (from at least the past two years), bank savings and checking statements (approximately last six months), mortgage documents, apartment lease, deeds to real property, savings bonds, stock/bond certificates, health insurance policy and premium bills, utility bills, and documentation of HIV-related diagnosis from a physician. For families, the clients should gather the same documents from their legally married spouses and dependent children. In addition, for dependent children, documentation of school attendance is almost always required by entitlement agencies.

ADVOCATING FOR BENEFITS AND ENTITLEMENTS THAT ARE AVAILABLE TO PWA/HIVS

After you have gathered information about the client's health status, living status, household income, assets, and health insurance information, you will have sufficient information to provide a client with a referral or to assist him or her in applying for the appropriate entitlements. This section is intended to provide a brief explanation of (1) the major public entitlements and broadly available private benefit programs, (2) general eligibility criteria, (3) the application process, and (4) advocacy strategies.

To provide detailed information about all these entitlements by individual state and locality in this chapter would be impossible. To obtain specific information about these entitlement programs, social workers should contact local AIDS service organizations, which generally have detailed information about all of these programs. Please remember that this chapter is intended to give social workers basic information about these programs, which should be a starting point for gathering specific and current information about these programs in your area.

Social Security Disability

What Is Social Security Disability?

Social Security Disability (SSD) is actually considered to be an insurance program by the federal government. SSD payments are based on your entire earnings history. If the award is below a certain level established by each state and the client does not have other assets or income, the client may also be eligible for Supplemental Security Income (see the following section). All clients who can no longer work should be encouraged to apply for SSD. The Social Security Administration (SSA) will determine if the client has enough paid quarters of coverage, through Federal Insurance Contributions Act (FICA) taxes, to be eligible for the program and meet the health-related requirements for disability. Many other public and private entitlement programs will request to know if the client has applied for SSD/SSI before processing their applications, including public assistance, short-term disability, and extension of COBRA private health insurance benefits.

SSD benefits are not paid until the sixth month of disability. Therefore, the client may be eligible for short-term disability (discussed later in this chapter) from the state or SSI during the interim period. PWA/HIVs who receive SSD automatically receive Medicare on their twenty-fourth benefit month or the twenty-ninth month of disability.

What Are the General Eligibility Requirements for SSD?

In order to qualify for SSD, the client must have paid FICA or social security taxes for at least twenty of the preceding forty fiscal quarters (if the client is thirty years old or older) and be considered disabled under the regulations established by the Social Security Administration. SSD is not a means-tested or asset-tested entitlement. If the client meets the eligibility requirements for SSD, he or she can receive this benefit regardless of the other benefits or income he or she may be receiving.

Applying for SSD

Most states allow for PWAs to apply for SSD through a Teleclaim number. A Social Security representative will complete the application over the telephone with the client and mail the completed form. The client must sign the form and return it with original documents (such as a birth certificate, social security card, latest W-2 or income tax return, etc.) to SSA for processing. All original documents are returned to the client. The Teleclaim system is generally very efficient and reliable.

Advocating for Clients with SSD

In general, the only time a client will need advocacy assistance with SSA will be during the application process or a continuing disability review. There are only two eligibility criteria for SSD: an earnings history documenting paid FICA taxes and a permanent disability.

In general, if a client is found ineligible due to insufficient earnings history, little can be done—unless the client can prove undocumented FICA tax payments. FICA tax records are obtained by the SSA directly from the IRS. SSA will share these records with the client if a dispute concerning previous earnings or tax payments arises. If the records are incomplete, the client may have W-2s or W-4s documenting previous tax payments or may be able to obtain these from past employers. Without this type of documentation, it will be very difficult to change SSA's determination.

Disagreement with a finding of disability is a much more likely occurrence. Most clients with an AIDS diagnosis will not have a problem in being found disabled for SSD. Clients with HIV-related illness, however, must prove that their condition is disabling. SSA considers disability to be the inability to perform full-time work rather than solely a measure of the severity of the illness. In general, clients must have their treating physician document that their condition prohibits them from engaging in full-time work. SSA bases all disability findings on their Disability Report form. Social workers should convey to the client's physician that, despite clients' fluctuations in physical functioning, the functional assessment areas of the report should be completed given their lowest or worst level of functioning not their best.

Advocating with SSD

Any time SSA sends correspondence to a recipient regarding their payments or disability finding, they inform the client of his or her rights if he or she disagrees with SSA's finding on the matter and the time period for appealing the decision. Clients may request an *informal conference*, a *reconsideration*, or a *fair hearing*. An informal conference is an appointment with a SSA representative in which the representative explains to the client the determination of SSA. No SSA decision can be changed at an informal conference, and in general these appointments are not useful, since an SSA representative can explain a determination over the phone.

A *reconsideration* is a formal request to SSA to review its decision. Clients can submit documentation in support of their position to be reviewed during the reconsideration. A reconsideration must be requested before a fair hearing can be requested. In general, reconsiderations are not done in person. Clients should request a reconsideration of any decision that they believe to be incorrect. A reconsideration can take about two months.

If after a reconsideration is conducted and SSA still gives an unfavorable determination, the client may request a fair hearing. At this point, the client should be referred to a legal or other specially trained advocate in this area. Fair hearings are conducted by an administrative law judge and are as much concerned with the legal process of the determination as with the specific circumstances surrounding the decision. Most legal service organizations have specially trained lawyers and paralegals who work on disability issues. Fair hearings take about two to three months to schedule and an additional three months to receive a decision.

Again, it is important to remember that timing is everything. If the client receives an unfavorable determination, the client may request *aid to continue* (if he or she is already receiving benefits) pending the reconsideration or fair hearing decision, as long as it is requested prior to the date of the planned action. "Aid to continue" means that the client continues to receive his or her benefits during the time of the appeal process. If the deadline for appealing a decision is missed, the client can always request a reconsideration, in general, but he or she cannot request aid to continue. Given that the reconsideration and fair hearing process can take up to nine months to resolve, failing to secure aid to continue can be a great hardship. Sometimes SSA will reinstate benefits pending a hearing if the situation is a compelling one. However, an effort such as this should be done with the assistance of a legal or other specially trained advocate.

Supplemental Security Income

What Is Supplemental Security Income?

Supplemental Security Income (SSI) is a program designed to provide disability and retirement benefits to persons who did not have a long enough earnings record to be eligible for SSD or social security retirement benefits. Unlike SSD, SSI is a means- and asset-tested benefit program that pays a flat amount to all recipients. SSI payments are based on a federal standard and are supplemented by each state.

There is no initial five-month waiting period for SSI benefits as there is for SSD. Therefore, if the client has applied for SSD and is without income or assets, he or she should apply for SSI benefits to bridge this waiting period. SSI recipients are usually automatically eligible for Medicaid benefits; therefore, they do not have to apply separately for this benefit. SSI beneficiaries are not eligible for Medicare benefits until age sixty-five.

What Are the General Eligibility Requirements for SSI?

In order to be eligible for SSI due to HIV status, a client must be disabled and meet the income and asset criteria of the state in which he or she resides. Different states have different income criteria and asset criteria for their SSI programs. However, all states consider the following areas for income:

- earnings from any employment
- money that is received as a gift
- money from interest-bearing bank accounts or investments
- any type of pension and any other government or private benefit

SSI can be added to other benefits. For example, a client may receive a minimal SSD award and still be eligible for the difference between his or her award and the state's SSI payment level. Assets that can effect eligibility for SSI include the following: checking/savings or any other bank account, automobiles worth more than a certain value, any life or disability insurance policy with a cash-in value, and burial funds worth more than a certain value.

Applying for SSI

Clients can apply for SSI in the same manner as they apply for SSD—through the Teleclaim system, as previously described.

Advocating with SSI

In general, SSI can refuse or reduce payments to recipients because they are ineligible for benefits due to disability status or because of an overpayment due to excess resources or income. The process for advocating with SSI is the same as one previously described for SSD. In general, it is easier to get "aid to continue" with SSI recipients than with SSD because the Social Security Administration recognizes that SSI is a program designed for persons with limited income or assets whereas SSD is not.

What Is Short-Term Disability?

Many states have mandated that employers provide short-term disability (STD). STD is a program designed to assist persons who have left work due to a disabling condition and cannot work temporarily or are pending SSD benefits. In general, STD is administered by individual state's Department of Labor-Worker Compensation Boards. Like unemployment insurance benefits, STD usually provides six months of benefits at 50 percent of the gross pay of the applicant up to a certain capped amount.

What Are the General Eligibility Criteria for STD?

In general, STD is available to full-time employees who are not part of a union or who do not work in governmental agencies. Employees in those types of jobs are usually eligible for some other type of income assistance, such as an extended sick leave or employee benefit program similar to STD. In order to qualify for STD, employees must apply within a certain time limit.

Applying for STD

In most states, employers are required to provide STD coverage to full-time employees; thus, clients seeking this benefit should apply directly to the personnel department of their employer. Again, most PWA/HIVs who are part of a union are not eligible for STD, but they are usually covered under some other benefit program. A physician's statement attesting to a disabling condition is required. Applicants do not have to have a permanent disability to receive STD. STD is a program offered in many states but should not be confused with SSI and SSD, which are federally mandated programs available through the U.S.

Advocating with STD

Persons applying for STD usually do not encounter difficulties in receiving this benefit if they are covered by their employer. STD is not worker's compensation, in which an applicant is seeking to show that they were hurt or disabled because of their job. STD as a program is administered in a manner similar to unemployment insurance benefits. If a claim is rejected, applicants can have a hearing before an administrative law judge. Hearings can be requested by calling a state's Worker's Compensation Board. Legal advice or representation is a good idea.

Public Assistance

What Is Public Assistance?

As most people know, public assistance is a program designed to provide cash assistance to people who are not disabled but cannot find employment. Public assistance eligibility usually provides recipients with automatic eligibility for Medicaid and food stamps. Public assistance is only likely to be an option for a PWA/HIV if the client does not meet the disability criteria for SSI/SSD or has no other means of support while pending these or other disability benefits. However in some states and cities, PWA/HIVs can receive both public assistance and disability benefits (SSI/SSD) as a subsidy in meeting rental and nutritional expenses.

Public assistance is also available in most states as an emergency assistance benefit. Clients who are facing eviction or utility shutoff can apply for public assistance to meet these onetime expenses.

What Are the General Eligibility Requirements for Public Assistance?

Public assistance programs have stringent eligibility requirements with regard to both income and assets. Most states require that applicants for public assistance enter either a work training program or work placement program unless they are single adults caring for young children. PWA/HIVs are likely to exempted from this requirement, but they will be required to apply for SSI or SSD.

Applying for Public Assistance

Clients who need to apply for public assistance must generally do so in person at the local Department of Social Services office. (Although, this may vary from state to state.) Clients are screened for eligibility on their first appointment and are usually given a second appointment within one week of the initial appointment to bring in documents verifying identity, income, and expenses. The process can be expedited if the client brings to the initial appointment the following documents:

- a birth certificate
- social security card
- a lease or mortgage statement
- all utility bills
- copies of all recent bank account statements

If more than one person lives in the household and that person is legally responsible for the care of the PWA/HIV or is legally dependent on the PWA/HIV, proof of that person's identity, income, and assets is also required. For legally dependent minors, proof of school enrollment and evidence of support or lack of child support from an absent parent is required. Generally, public assistance will make a determination within thirty days from the date of the application and benefits will begin shortly thereafter. Some states have provisions for immediate or expedited benefits. Usually these programs provide a very small cash grant and food stamps to clients pending benefits who have no other means of support.

Advocating with Public Assistance

Public assistance programs are regulated by individual state's social service laws. In some states, clients who dispute a planned action of the Department of Social Services are eligible for "aid to continue" pending a fair hearing. Having a legal or other specially trained advocate in this area is a good idea. However, unlike SSI or SSD, fair hearings on public assistance benefit issues often result in the problem being remanded (sent back) to the local center for reevaluation. That is not to say that a fair hearing should not be pursued if a client has a problem with his or her benefits. Rather, public assistance (and food stamps) offices in general have a greater latitude to rework and resolve issues at the center level than SSI/SSD offices do. Case workers or their supervisors are more able to reopen closed cases and issue backpayments to recipients than other public benefit programs. Therefore, it is suggested that social workers attempt to work with the public assistance caseworker to resolve problems. Also, social workers should not be timid about asking to speak to supervisors who generally have a more in-depth understanding of public assistance regulations and have a greater ability to expedite benefits than line staff.

What Is Medicaid?

Medicaid is a health coverage program for individuals and families who either receive an income- or asset-tested public entitlement such as public assistance or SSI or who have income equal to or below these benefit programs and have a medical need. In general, Medicaid programs pay for inpatient care, doctor's visits, and prescription medications. Please note that Medicaid programs vary widely from state to state both in terms of the medical benefits offered and the eligibility for the program. Social workers may be familiar with the basic Medicaid program within their state, but may not be aware of enhanced benefits or operational procedures for PWA/HIVs. For example, several states have applied to the federal government to expand the benefits offered under their Medicaid program to meet the needs of PWA/HIVs. These states are New Jersey, New Mexico, Ohio, Hawaii, South Carolina, Pennsylvania, and Washington. In addition, North Carolina and Illinois include PWA/HIVs under a broader category for expanded benefits for disabled people. Other states have expanded their Medicaid program to include the payment of private health insurance premiums to assist otherwise eligible Medicaid recipients retain access to their private health care providers. Social workers should contact the Medicaid program in their state for the specifics of these programs.

What Are the General Eligibility Requirements for Medicaid?

In general, Medicaid is available to persons who receive one of the two federally qualifying public benefits—Aid to Families with Dependent Children (AFDC) or SSI. Some states have expanded eligibility of the program to persons receiving public assistance programs other than AFDC and disabled individuals. Some states have expanded eligibility to include PWAs who meet certain financial criteria. Other states permit persons who have large ongoing medical expenses into the Medicaid program under what is usually called a "medical spend-down program."

Applying for Medicaid

Medicaid is most easily accessed by receiving a federal public assistance program—AFDC or SSI—which include Medicaid coverage automatically. If the state in which the client resides permits persons not receiving these benefits to qualify for Medicaid, an application must generally be completed with an eligibility specialist in a local Medicaid office. Often if the client is an inpatient or requires home care services, hospital or home agencies can complete an application for the client so that he or she does not have to travel to the local Medicaid office. All applicants (excluding those on AFDC and SSI) will need to supply documents verifying identity, income, assets, and health status, as described earlier in this chapter.

Advocating with Medicaid

As with most other government benefit programs, if the client disputes a decision made by the Medicaid program in relation to his or her eligibility for the benefit, he or she can apply for a fair hearing with "aid to continue." As with other fair hearings, representation by a legal or other specially trained advocate is a good idea. Most often, problems with Medicaid will center on eligibility for the program and not on what services are covered.

However, PWA/HIVs may encounter problems when the Medicaid program will not pay for a therapy or service because of its experimental nature or because the product is being used in a manner for which it is not approved. For example, many PWA/HIVs utilize nutritional supplements, vitamins, or alternative therapies such herbs. If these services are denied, a Medicaid recipient should first have his or her doctor contact the prior approval office at the local Medicaid center. Usually the prior approval office is staffed by a physician or other clinically trained staff person with whom the client's doctor can speak to explain the benefit of the prescribed therapy. If the prior approval office refuses to allow payment for the therapy, a fair hearing may be requested. It should be noted that clients often prevail at fair hearings in securing services (such as increased home care hours) or traditional therapies (such as nutritional supplements). However, securing payment for alternative therapies is less likely.

What Is Medicare and Who Is Eligible?

Medicare is a benefit that is provided to persons who have been receiving SSD benefits for twenty-four months or have reached age sixty-five.

Medicare has two components—Part A and Part B. Part A covers inpatient hospital stays and limited home care services and is provided without cost to all SSD or Social Security Retirement recipients. Part B covers doctor's office visits, most injectable drugs, and durable medical equipment such as canes and wheelchairs. Medicare does not cover prescription drugs. Medicare recipients are generally required to meet a yearly deductible and copay for outpatient services.

Applying for Medicare

No application is needed for Medicare. The Social Security Administration generally sends a letter to an SSD recipient about three months prior to their twenty-fourth benefit check and informs them that they are eligible for Medicare. The client is requested to select if they want only Part A or both Part A and B. All recipients must accept Part A, even if they have private health insurance that covers hospitalization and home care. In general, private health insurance companies require that new Medicare recipients drop their hospitalization coverage. The insurer generally offers the client a "Medi-gap" or "Medi-sup" policy that will cover expenses not covered by Medicare. Clients may retain their major medical or outpatient coverage through the private insurer, but Part B—if they choose to obtain it—is considered the primary insurance by most insurance plans. Part B has a monthly premium that is deducted directly from the recipient's SSD check. Medicare recipients can also receive Medicaid benefits, if eligible. If the client receives both Medicaid and Medicare, the Medicaid program will pay for the monthly Part B insurance premium and no deduction will be made from the client's SSD benefit check.

Advocating with Medicare

Disputes with the Medicare program are usually resolved by making phone calls to the program or through written letters. The Medicare program generally provides a telephone line for recipients to contact if they have questions or problems concerning their Medicare benefits. In general, recipients who cannot resolve issues with agency staff on this help line can request a fair hearing. Obtaining legal advice or a specially trained advocate is strongly suggested.

COBRA

What Is COBRA?

COBRA is a federal law which mandates that people who are covered by group health insurance through their employer may retain their health insurance for the same total cost and at the same coverage for eighteen months after they leave their job. (The term COBRA actually is an acronym referring to a number of laws put forth by Congress as part of the federal budget process.) In some states, COBRA coverage is extended an additional eleven months for persons who leave their job because of disability in order to provide them coverage until their Medicare benefits begin.

What Are the General Eligibility Requirements of COBRA?

In general, COBRA is available to all persons who are working in a job that is covered by group health insurance. However, exceptions do exist, including most people working in unions, governmental agencies, and agencies owned or operated by religious organizations.

Applying for COBRA

Clients should optimally complete the application for COBRA benefits before their last day of employment. In most cases, the client can complete the application for COBRA benefits within the thirty days after he or she leaves the job. Please be aware that, in general, neither the employer nor the insurance carrier need inform the client that he or she is eligible for COBRA. Accordingly, do not wait for an application from the employer or insurance company. In addition, the health insurer is allowed to drop the client from COBRA coverage if any of the monthly payments are late.

To apply for the extended COBRA coverage for disabled persons, the client must only apply for SSD benefits within the first eighteen months of coverage, and the onset date of disability must be on or before the client's last day of work.

All correspondence with the insurance company or the employer, particularly the initial application and all payments, should be sent by certified, return-receipt-requested mail. When completing the return receipt, write on the card the purpose of the correspondence, e.g., monthly premium payment. Copies of all correspondence, bills and canceled checks for payments or premiums, and copayments should kept in a file by the client. The client's written correspondence and canceled checks are the only acceptable proof of complying with the terms of the client's COBRA agreement.

Advocating with COBRA

Advocating with COBRA on eligibility for benefits usually always requires an attorney or specially trained advocate's assistance. Advocacy is usually done with a private insurance company that is regulated by federal and state law as well as the terms of the group policy contract held by the company with the insurer.

Advocating for payment of a covered medical expense can be initiated by the client or the social worker and can be conducted directly with a claims representative of the insurance company. For disputed claims regarding the necessity of the treatment, it is suggested that the client's treating physician contact the insurance company and speak to a clinically trained staff person or case manager to explain the necessity of the treatment in question. If the claim still cannot be resolved, the social worker should make a referral to an attorney or specially trained advocate in this field.

Managed Care

What Is Managed Care?

Most people think of managed care as insurance plans that require little or no payment (copayments) for medical services. Managed care organizations market themselves by advertising their generous provisions for preventive care services, such as physical checkups. Some even cover the costs of physical fitness programs, stress management, and smoking cessation programs. All these efforts are geared to maintaining the health of the plan's enrollees, hence the term health maintenance organizations (HMOs). Also, in general, HMO monthly premium costs to employees are very low. As such, these plans are often attractive choices to people when selecting a plan through their employer.

While the emphasis on primary and preventive care does keep people healthier and does keep costs down, HMOs principally make their greatest profits by "locking in" enrollees in fixed networks of doctors and hospitals. These physicians and hospitals have, in general, accepted discounted payments based on the volume of visits and admissions to be generated by this locked-in population.

In addition, HMOs have strict guidelines for approving the use of specialty and inpatient care services. The use of these expensive services are controlled by primary care physician gatekeeping and utilization review and management staff. Primary care physician gatekeeping means that the doctor the client selects when joining the HMO must approve all the specialty, diagnostic, and inpatient services. This means that clients enrolled in the plan cannot simply make appointment with specialists but must go through their primary care physician if they want the plan to pay for those services. As an incentive, primary care physicians in HMOs are generally rewarded with bonuses if they keep the use of these expensive services low.

Utilization review and management at the HMO staff follow all doctors' patterns of making referrals for expensive services and if one doctor appears to be making a greater number of these referrals than other doctors in the plan, the staff investigates these referrals and works to bring the physician in line with the practices of other plan physicians. Utilization management staff members also work with hospitals to expedite the discharge of patients, thus saving costs.

While utilization review and management has a focus on cost-containment, it can also be seen as a good thing. Nobody wants to undergo diagnostic tests or stay in the hospital if it is not necessary. It should also be noted that if a patient is found to have a serious condition, HMOs usually have utilization review personnel who are specially trained in that health area and can provide an important resource to the primary care physician in accessing appropriate care, including greater access to specialty care.

Therefore, while some HMOs have a bad reputation for denying care services to people with serious health conditions, others do an excellent job of maintaining the health of well persons and delivering appropriate health services to people with serious health problems.

Advocating with Managed Care Companies

As stated, managed care plans, due to their low premiums, are attractive choices to employees when selecting a health plan. In addition, many states are now requiring Medicaid and urging Medicare recipients to join managed care insurance plans. Accordingly, many PWA/HIVs may be solicited by these insurers. Before joining a plan (or if the client is already in an HMO), he or she should find out the following information:

- What services are covered in the plan, and are there limits to these services? (Limits on services are most often applied to mental health, substance abuse treatment services, and home care services.)
- How many board-certified infectious disease- or HIV-experienced providers are part of the network? Can these doctors be selected as the primary care provider?
- What is the plan's policy on specialty referrals, and can standing referrals be made by the primary care provider? A standing referral means that if, for example, a patient has been diagnosed with cancer, a standing referral is made so that the patient can see an oncologist (a speciality provider) as often as needed without getting a referral from the primary care provider.
- Is the patient's hospital or are hospitals known for HIV-related care services part of the network?

- Are out-of-network services covered and at what percentage? (Out-of-network means that patients can choose to be treated by a physician or at a hospital that is not part of the HMO's network because of the experience that provider may have in treating a specific condition. Plans that allow out-of-network services are usually called point-of-service plans).
- What is the plan's policy and does it pay for investigational treatments, other clinical research options, or alternative therapies? (In general, most insurance companies do not pay for these services, but some are starting to pay for some alternative therapies such as acupuncture. More important, does the plan pay for medical care that may result from the use of an experimental treatment. For example, if a client is enrolled in a drug trial that causes him or her to require hospitalization due to an adverse side effect, will the plan cover that hospitalization?)
- What is the grievance process if the client has been denied a service, and how long does the process take?
- If available, request to know if other PWA/HIVs are part of the plan and how do they rate their satisfaction with the plan's services? (Some states require that insurance companies monitor patient satisfaction and some plans evaluate subpopulations of patients. This information should be available from the plan.)

If the client is part of an HMO, he or she should work closely with his or her primary care physician as much as possible to obtain approval for all needed services. Gatekeeping of services is a central responsibility of physicians in managed care organizations, and the provider should be able to facilitate access to treatments by demonstrating their medical necessity. This is particularly true of alternative therapies.

If the client encounters an issue with approval for a service, the first step is to contact the services office of the plan. Member services will take the client's compliant or grievance and render a decision on the issue. When contacting member services, the social worker should obtain the name of the plan representative working on the issue and the expected date for a decision on the grievance. As previously stated, if the issue concerns the medical necessity of service, the primary care physician should be requested to speak to the prior approval/utilization review office or provider relations.

Advocacy efforts with managed care plans will most likely be required to secure payment for services provided outside of the network of providers. These out-of-network services are generally consultative examinations by specialists or sophisticated diagnostic examinations and treatments. Again, the physician/gatekeeper should assist in demonstrating the medical necessity of this service and the inability of the network to meet the patient's need. In many urban areas of the country, HIV-related treatment advocates are available to assist PWA/HIVs and their physicians and social workers in documenting the effectiveness of specific treatments to substantiate their case for payment. These groups are a valuable resource, and social workers should become familiar with the group in their area.

Both managed care and indemnity insurances generally have proscribed caps on both mental health and substance abuse treatment benefits. In general, once the annual cap on these services is met, clients must pay for these services or seek out the care from public facilities. Advocacy is most likely to be required to secure payments for mental health providers that are not part of the panel of providers but have a particular expertise which may facilitate the client's treatment. This may be a demonstrated experience in mental health issues related to HIV/AIDS, lesbians and gays, or persons with addiction histories. The social worker will need to demonstrate the need for the specific service and the absence of providers in the network who could deliver that specialized service. Social workers should consult the insurance board in their state regarding legislation related to regulation of insurance companies or assistance in advocating with these companies. Again, seeking specialized legal counsel in these matters is advised.

Food Assistance Programs

What Are Food Stamps?

Food stamps are coupons that can be used to purchase food at grocery stores. The program is intended to help individuals and families on limited budgets purchase food for a nutritious diet. Food stamps are provided through a federal program and are available throughout the country. However, the amount of food stamps for which a client is eligible will vary from state to state. In some states, enhanced food stamp benefits are available to homeless persons and persons with ongoing unreimbursed medical expenses.

What Are the General Eligibility Requirements for Food Stamps?

Food stamps are available to all persons who meet income and asset criteria, which are generally equivalent to the limits set for public assistance programs. All persons receiving public assistance and SSI are usually automatically eligible for food stamp benefits. While automatically eligible for food stamp benefits, SSI recipients may be required to complete an application for this benefit, unlike for Medicaid.

Applying for Food Stamps

In most states, persons receiving public assistance should not need to fill out a separate application for food stamp benefits. If your client is receiving a public assistance benefit and is not receiving food stamps, you should contact his or her caseworker at the public assistance office. SSI recipients are also automatically eligible for food stamp benefits and should receive a letter after they have been accepted into the program that informs them where to apply for this benefit. There is generally a separate section in local social services office that processes food stamp applications for SSI recipients. SSD recipients are not automatically eligible for food stamps and should be directed to apply for them at a local Social Services office.

Advocating with Food Stamps

Clients often believe that their food stamp award is incorrect because other persons with the same source of income are receiving more or less benefits than they are. This occurs because food stamps are the only public benefit that considers actual monthly living expenses in the calculation of the benefit amount. In general, other public benefits such as SSI and public assistance do not consider actual living expenses (rent, utilities, etc.) in determining benefit amount.

If you believe that the food stamp benefit is incorrect or the benefit has ceased for any reason, you can contact the local social services office and speak with a food stamp representative, but generally a worker will not be assigned to a case. However, if the client receives public assistance, you should contact his or her public assistance caseworker to resolve any issues with this benefit. If the client's living situation has changed in any manner such as a rent increase or higher utility costs or unreimbursed medical expenses are incurred, the client may file a new food stamp application at any time and have his or her benefit reassessed. Should the issue be unresolvable with the worker, a fair hearing can be requested. Again, obtaining legal assistance or the assistance of a specially trained advocate is strongly advised.

Additional Supports and Issues

Private Disability Insurance

Some clients may have private disability insurance that they received through their past employment or had privately retained. In general, these programs are regulated by the individual state's insurance board. Advocacy efforts on these matter are usually best handled by an attorney or other specialized advocate.

ADAP

ADAP is the acronym for the AIDS Drug Assistance Program. ADAP is available in all states and is funded in part by the Ryan White Care Act. The scope of the benefits under the ADAP vary greatly from state to state. At a minimum, the ADAP program provides free HIV-related medication to persons who have limited means or insufficient insurance coverage. Some states have funded their ADAP program to cover a wide range of medications as well as home care, mental health treatment, and primary medical care. Medicaid recipients are generally not eligible for ADAP programs. Medicare recipients, however, are generally eligible. Referrals to ADAP programs can be obtained from local AIDS service organizations or your state's department of health.

Utility Subsidies

Many states and cities offer utility and telephone subsidies, which are credited directly to the account of PWA/HIVs who must pay for their own utilities. These program are not AIDS-specific but are usually intended for the elderly and disabled. Social workers should contact the local utility company's community relations office for more information.

Food Programs

Most communities provide food programs in which persons with limited incomes can either receive groceries, ready-made meals, or free meals in a community setting. These programs can be a great assistance to clients with HIV/AIDS who are living on a fixed budget.

Recreational Programs

These community programs can provide PWA/HIVs with free movie passes, theater tickets, or tickets for other social events. All of these things can help PWA/HIVs extend their monthly budget and develop a support network of other people living with HIV/AIDS.

Life Insurance Benefits

A variety of for-profit companies, called viatical settlement companies, will purchase the life insurance of PWA/HIVs or other terminally ill people. These companies generally offer the client a percentage of the total value of their life insurance based on a physician-assigned prognosis. The amount of the settlement increases as the prognosis decreases. Social workers need to be mindful that if a client receives these funds, the funds must be used in meeting their normal living expenses if the client will need income- and asset-tested entitlements. If the settlement is spent on gifts and vacations, public benefit agencies may determine that the client spent-down his or her resources in an irresponsible manner and may withhold benefits for a protracted period of time. Social workers counseling clients on this situation should review the section on income and assets earlier in this chapter.

Estate Planning

Estate planning is a matter that should be handled by an attorney or legal advocate. Social workers can assist clients with AIDS in addressing their diagnosis and mortality in a sensitive and supportive fashion. Estate planning is an important matter that should include guardianship of dependent children, living will/medical directive, and bequests of possessions and resources. In general, if a legally binding will has not been drawn up, authority for deciding the estate usually reverts to the closest biological relative, which may not be the wish of the client. Also many PWA/HIVs develop neurological problems in the late stages of the disease, and then can no longer be found competent to complete estate-planning activities. Social workers can assist clients in a sensitive manner to address these issues, and reinforce for the client the sense of control and continuity with cared for persons in their life that this action provides.

Housing for People with HIV

Jeffrey S. Austin
Margaret Smith

WHY DO THIS?
STATEMENT OF THE PROBLEM AND ISSUES

By the early 1980s, it had become clear to the pioneers of AIDS-related services within the initial centers of the nascent epidemic—New York, San Francisco, and Los Angeles—that housing would become a critical need for people struggling with this frightening, new, and not-well-understood disease. Thus the Shanti program in California, New York City's Bailey House, and several other important early housing efforts were created. Fifteen years later, there are now more than 200 AIDS-specific housing programs in the United States.

Other than perhaps the tuberculosis sanitariums of another era, what real precedent is there for disease-specific housing? The development of the AIDS housing field has been, in essence, a triumph of improvisation, borrowing variously from existing models of inpatient hospice facilities, residential drug treatment programs, therapeutic communities, and geriatric residential care facilities. Program structures can range from relatively loose (our experience) to extremely rigid.

In this chapter, we are going to draw from our experiences as founding executive and clinical directors, respectively, of Sunrise Community Housing in Providence, Rhode Island. Incorporated in 1989, this program has evolved from an inner-city rooming house with minimal program structure, to a multilevel housing agency, providing a continuum that ranges from housing referral and assistance, a twenty-one unit scattered-site program, a home-based personal attendant care program, and a congregate residential care facility, serving between seventy and one hundred persons each year.

Our intent is for the information, experiences, and opinions shared herein to be useful for social workers making referrals or working directly with residents of such programs. We have chosen to use extensive case examples in this chapter for several reasons. We believe these examples will provide the social worker with insight into the complex, multilayered,

509

and complicated issues that arise both for those who are residents of the housing models we describe and for staff working within this complicated subfield of social work practice. We have come to realize that the experiences we had as we developed this program have been our best teachers. Our professional training had prepared us for *some* of what ensued, but we were unprepared for the intensity, depth, and breadth of the issues we encountered.

Fundamentally, all housing program models must address a host of complex clinical issues and decisions. The presenting issues of persons with *long-term housing instability or homelessness* may include the following:

- lack of income
- chemical addiction
- psychiatric personality disorders
- history of criminal activity and incarceration
- domestic violence

Concomitantly, an AIDS housing provider may, under the same roof, be trying to provide a suitable and pleasant living environment for clients who have maintained stable housing throughout their adult lives, but now present with needs for specialized housing due to sharply reduced income, illness-related disabilities, or overburdened family care systems. It can be a very difficult balancing act in terms of operating policies and consistent treatment of the client population as a whole.

At best, HIV housing programs can dramatically improve the duration and quality of life of residents. Our experience is that by providing a stable housing setting, clients are far better able to regularly access and adhere to medical treatment, as well as maintain productive patterns of rest and nutrition. Congregate settings offer the added advantage of social interaction and peer support for persons in advanced stages of illness.

COMMON TYPES OF AIDS-HOUSING PROGRAMS

At the most basic level, many organizations, either AIDS-specific or not, offer housing financial assistance, either on an emergency or ongoing basis, and housing advocacy/referral. Our concern in this chapter, however, is those programs that operate and manage housing units. These programs fall under two general categories: scattered-site apartments and community/congregate residences.

Scattered-Site Apartments

Scattered-site apartment programs for individuals and families with HIV are operated in many locations throughout the United States. Program designs vary. *Tenant-based* subsidies can take the form of vouchers, or contractual agreements that are allotted to the client rather than tied to a specific apartment unit; conversely, with *project-based* rental subsidies, an agency identifies and leases dwelling units, which are then, in effect, sublet to the client. Some agencies will place two or three unrelated persons together in a single unit; however, our experience suggests that such an approach would create a fertile ground for interpersonal and territorial conflict, perhaps causing more problems than it would solve.

Supportive service components may range from minimal (agency monitors timely rent payments and basic cleanliness) to intensive (agency provides on-site supervision). The norm falls somewhere in the middle. Perhaps the greatest advantages to this type of housing derive from (1) allowing persons with HIV to reside within a normalized community environment, thus avoiding any sense of "ghettoization," and (2) services may be delivered on an individualized, as-needed basis.

An important determination prior to referring a client into such programs is an assessment of the client's capacity for independent living, in terms of medical stability and basic living skills. Particularly with clients with histories of chronic homelessness, the social worker should ascertain if the client knows how to budget money, shop for and prepare meals, and maintain basic activities of daily living.

Supported apartments best suit those clients still able to maintain a high level of independent functioning, and they may be the only workable option for those who lack either the social skills or the desire to live compatibly with others in a congregate setting.

Depending upon individual circumstances, it can be possible to maintain clients in supported apartments throughout the duration of their illness and death. The key factors in such instances are the presence of a "primary caregiver" and strong family or social networks of care and support. With those in place, hospice and home care services may be brought into the apartment, allowing the client to remain in his or her own home throughout the course of illness and death.

Additionally, programs that accept the principles of harm reduction, have found it possible to safely house some clients still actively involved with drugs and alcohol. It must still be noted that in unsupervised apartment programs, behavioral, emotional, and physical problems can emerge and flourish without the social worker's timely awareness.

The real difficulty in providing and coordinating services for clients in supported apartment programs is that HIV/AIDS is rarely the primary problem in their lives. A distinct and constant challenge to the social worker is focusing on achievable goals and recognizing that successful outcomes must be judged from the perspective of the client.

The following are two very different case examples that illustrate the value of housing placement in scattered-site settings.

Case Study: Arthur

Arthur is a forty-year-old gay man. Despite a very low CD-4 count, he remains highly active. Arthur is charming and gregarious. Prior to his illness, he lived in many different cities, supporting himself through working in restaurants and selling antiques. At the time he was referred for independent housing, however, circumstances had forced him to move in with the family of his older brother. Lacking a car, he was essentially trapped in a small suburban house. While this situation provided a roof and bed, it offered Arthur a poor quality of life, punctuated with friction and conflict within the family. Arthur became severely depressed, hopeless, and lethargic.

Provided with a centrally located one-bedroom apartment, Arthur's life has changed dramatically. Using castoffs and salvage, his apartment is decorated with tremendous flair. He has cultivated friends from the neighborhood, and he has occasionally been able to work "under the table" at a local restaurant. Most important, his sense of independence and quality of life has, we believe, allowed Arthur to bounce back from several harrowing bouts of illness and surgery.

Case Study: Gloria

Gloria, a thirty-nine-year-old African-American woman was homeless and five months pregnant at the time of her referral to Sunrise's apartment program. She had another child, nine-months-old, in foster placement. Apart from prenatal care offered through a community health center, Gloria was receiving no medical attention for her HIV, and she was linked with no other HIV social service organizations.

Gloria had extensive history of both alcohol and injectable drug addiction. Prior to entering the Sunrise program, she had completed a short-term treatment program and was remaining clean. The stress of homelessness, however, and the company of other persons actively using placed her at high risk for relapse.

Upon admission, Gloria was referred to several local agencies for additional services. She was initially placed in a one-bedroom apartment, prior to the impending birth of her baby, with the plan of moving into a larger unit, so that she could petition for the return custody of her other child.

Within a week after the giving birth, staff members began noting behavioral changes. She became isolated, secretive, and (a telling symptom of problems within any housing program) late with her rent.

Gloria resisted all attempts at intervention by Sunrise staff members. It was reported from the community that she was again using drugs and supporting that through prostitution. The state's child welfare agency quickly stepped in and assumed custody of Gloria's baby.

Not surprisingly, Gloria became submerged in despair. Over a period of weeks, however, she began to gather her internal and external resources, voluntarily joining a women's day-treatment program. After one week, it was clear to Gloria that she needed not just to use the support of that program but also to physically distance herself from the drug-using associates who had come back into her life.

At this writing, Gloria remains in a residential treatment program. Her apartment is being held for her, and she maintains contact with Sunrise staff members several times a week. If she is able to demonstrate a prolonged period of recovery and stability, Gloria may be able to successfully petition to regain custody of her children.

Thus far, we consider this a success story. Concrete housing proved to be Gloria's point of entry into "the system," and Gloria, for all her difficulties, has maintained connections to the support networks that offer the best hope of reconstructing her life.

Community/Congregate Residences

This category of housing represents the greatest challenge, but occupies a critical niche in the spectrum of need. For many persons in late-stage illness, supervised community residences may be the only option for appropriate housing and services.

On a national basis, such programs offer many differences in terms of scale, program structure, and level of care. Additionally, state regulations for licensure differ widely. Overall, a well-conceived and operated community residence is able to offer patients highly individualized care throughout the full course of illness. Most facilities allow residents to die at home. Depending upon the model, medical management may be handled through internal staff or outside providers—or some combination of the two. In general, such facilities almost invariably offer more individualized care, a more homelike atmosphere, and a higher level of autonomy and personal identity for the client/resident than traditional skilled nursing facilities or other institutional settings.

Our experience is that congregate/community residences offer two particular challenges for both provider and resident: (1) managing the dynamics of "family" (biological family, extended/affilial family, and the family-like role often assumed by the provider), and (2) issues of death, dying, and recurrent loss.

The Family Issue

It is clear, and probably desirable, that at Sunrise House, both staff and residents have a sense of belonging to a "pseudo-family" system. In our setting, the executive and clinical directors (by virtue of gender and role) tend, for better or for worse, to be perceived as parental figures. With direct care staff acting as benevolent aunts and uncles, the residents inevitably assume roles of children and siblings. This may allow residents to regress then, through membership in the nonthreatening "pseudo family" system, consolidate psychological gains and come to terms with their own problematic roles in their families of origin.

The overwhelming, ever-shifting tension in most congregate housing programs is recognizing and balancing between:

- the resident's need, desire, and *right* to function and be treated as an adult; and
- the same resident's need to periodically regress, to be taken care of, and to adhere to the structure of group living.

At Sunrise House, it is our desire and stated mission to provide our residents with maximum personal dignity, autonomy, and identity. Many residents, particularly those who have struggled with addiction, do not consistently display adult behavior in response to adversity, interpersonal conflict, or internal distress.

Ultimately, we are not a family. The last thing we wish to do would be to replicate what many of our clients have experienced as family. We are, however, a "pseudofamily," selectively providing love, tenderness, respect, discipline, and separation as appropriately as we can.

Death and Loss

The fundamental, inescapable issue of providing congregate housing to persons with AIDS is death and dying. It reverberates in distinctly different ways for staff members and for residents as groups—and obviously on an individual basis.

Interestingly, few congregate AIDS housing programs consider themselves to be "hospices," yet virtually all such programs embrace at least some philosophies of hospice care, and many work cooperatively with and access services from outside home-based hospice providers. Potential distinctions might include the factors such as age, an association of hospice with providing strictly palliative or "comfort" measures only, and a tendency for inpatient hospice operations to be conducted and formulated according to medical/nursing traditions rather than social work practices.

This discussion of hospice/not hospice illuminates a common challenge: the client's ability and/or willingness to accept living in an AIDS residence as "the final stop." Social workers seeking an appropriate and necessary housing placement for people with AIDS will commonly encounter client resistance such as, "But that's a place where people go to die," or "I just don't think I'm ready for that yet"—even when the client is clearly in end-stage disease. Pragmatically, at Sunrise House, we have often agreed to accept a resident on a "temporary" basis while recognizing that the duration of stay will be permanent.

Case Study: Penelope

Penelope (nicknamed "PP"), a thirty-year-old African-American woman, was first referred to Sunrise in the summer of 1991, at which time she had been hospitalized with high fevers immediately after her release from the Rhode Island Adult Correctional Institution. At that time, Sunrise House had no appropriate room for Penelope, and she felt ambivalent about living at Sunrise; thus she was discharged to the shelter system.

As has been the case with many clients, Penelope had been rejected by her family and was on the streets by the time she was adolescent. In another respect, her history was unusual in that for the previous decade, she had averaged ten arrests per year, in effect, using the state prison as a shelter. Remarkably, she claimed to have never been on general public assistance, having opted instead to be caught at shoplifting or "loitering for indecent purposes" when she was in need of food or a place to stay.

In the fall of 1991, Penelope again underwent an extended hospitalization, this time with a cytomegalovirus, an AIDS-related infection which would require that she receive daily infusion therapy. While Sunrise at that point had a room for her and would be an appropriate place for the management of her at-home infusion therapy, Penelope, when referred, became tearful and angry, charging that Sunrise was "only out to take money from sick people," and that "my family loves me, and they'll take care of me!"

Refusing Sunrise, it appeared that Penelope would have to be transferred to a state-run medical institution. At the eleventh hour, however, a cousin willing to take PP into her home in Providence was located. Penelope was then admitted to a home-based hospice program, allowing her a period of stability and level of family support that been denied her for most of her life.

In the fall of 1992, Penelope was again hospitalized and referred to Sunrise. Her family caretaker, now pregnant, had become exhausted from the demands of caring for a needy and periodically difficult individual. Feeling burned out, as well as alarmed by PP's occasional periods of mental confusion and disorientation, the family member refused to bring her back home from the hospital.

This time, Penelope was willing to entertain the notion of living at Sunrise House. Through the cooperation of the hospice organization, Sunrise staff, and PP's primary physician at a local hospital, a transfer was arranged.

Sunrise staff experienced some trepidation that PP, because of her moodiness and occasional hostility, might have a difficult time adjusting to Sunrise's congregate living environment. Experience proved the contrary.

With only a single instance of interpersonal conflict, related to some bad prison history with another resident (which was soon resolved), PP seemed to be at home and at peace from the moment she came in the door in the middle of October. The ragged-haired, wild-eyed person first encountered in 1991 had assembled a stylish wardrobe and an array of cosmetics and hair-care products.

Extremely frail, but defiantly independent PP was capable of rallying her energy for shopping trips and changes of hair-color and style. Her infusions (twelve hours overnight and two in the morning, five times each week) tended to keep her tethered to her bedroom; nevertheless, she still found ample time to smoke and "hang" with the ongoing Sunrise kitchen table coffee klatch. She was tremendously buoyed that her cousin's unborn child (determined as female by ultrasound) was to be named Penelope.

In the second week of December, Penelope began to exhibit mental status changes. She would be confused with regard to time and date, and sometimes slept with one arm raised in the air. Her deterioration was noted with anxiety by the resident population, all of whom had grown fond of her.

Thursday evening the tenth, PP became increasingly agitated. She was at one point discovered half-fallen from her bed in the course of trying frantically to locate her shoes and some hair attachments that she had purchased recently but misplaced. Asked why, she announced to a staff person that "Jack said I'm getting out of here soon." When asked who Jack was, she shrugged and replied "Some guy."

Friday morning the eleventh, PP was unresponsive, with racing pulse and labored breathing. She died at 9 a.m.

Case Study: Robbie

Robbie was a thirty-nine-year-old Caucasian male. While much of his early life history is unclear, Robbie spent much of his childhood in an orphanage and foster placements in the South. One foster home in particular had subjected him to extreme physical abuse. He alluded to having a sister, but neither knew her address nor wished to locate her.

Robbie, of predominantly homosexual orientation, had various brushes with crime, alcohol, and drugs in his adolescence. Probably falsifying his age somewhat, Robbie enlisted in the Army and was sent to Vietnam. While there, Robbie's drug use extended to the extremely potent marijuana of Southeast Asia and soon thereafter to heroin. His addiction recognized by his superior officers, Robbie was jailed, given treatment, and discharged from the service.

The next decade of his life remains cloudy—although it can be gathered that Robbie drifted around the country, sometimes being known under different names. He described periods of time in New Orleans and the Midwest, and seems to have been an exceptionally heavy drinker and cocaine user.

In 1987, Robbie surfaced in Rhode Island. Hospitalized after being found unresponsive on the State House steps, Robbie was diagnosed with HIV and syphilitic encephalitis. Robbie became a client of a local multiservice AIDS organization and developed a complex, often difficult and intense relationship with the staff of that agency.

The agency was experimenting with providing housing. Robbie had formed a love relationship with another client, Freddie. They began living together in a subsidized apartment. One year before his death, Freddie "took to his bed," with Robbie caring for Freddie through the end of his life in that apartment. Robbie was also doing some drug-dealing from the apartment at that point, to help make ends meet.

Freddie was a passive and dependent person, yet he possessed a certain magnetism that drew a wide range of people to him. Robbie, on the other hand, was rough, brusque, and crude. After Freddie's death, the support system that had developed for Freddie found Robbie impossible to tolerate, and it soon evaporated. Since neither he nor Freddie had paid their rent for ten or eleven months, the agency that provided the apartment evicted

Robbie and he was referred to Sunrise House. He moved in in December 1991.

Robbie's early days at Sunrise did not go well. Along with his own unpleasant demeanor, the dynamic and composition of the house at that particular time (in terms of both residents and staff) were far from ideal. When internecine conflict of various types would erupt, Robbie tended to be either the focus, instigator, or cheerleader.

Gradually, however, the situation changed, and it changed to a stunning degree. As other residents with whom Robbie had difficulties either died or moved on, a new group came in with whom he was able to make a fresh start. Relaxing in his environment, his defensiveness and combativeness waned. A Robbie of an entirely different character began to emerge.

Over time, Robbie began to assert himself as a figure of authority among the resident population. As he made himself better-known and understood, certain personal attributes not previously displayed, such as kindness, charm, and intelligence, began to evidence themselves.

Robbie's physical condition, however, steadily deteriorated. Kaposi's Sarcoma (KS) lesions on his face, torso, penis, and legs had progressed to the point of exceptional disfigurement. As his lymphatic system ceased to function properly, his legs became grossly swollen, draining constantly onto the floor. Fungus and dead skin tissue created a foul smell, which was only somewhat alleviated by frequent dressing changes.

Both emotionally and physically, Robbie had his good days and bad, receiving massive doses of intravenous morphine through a portable pump. He did not leave the house for the last year of his life, but busied himself with naps, cigarettes, and kitchen table gossip—and his Nintendo Gameboy. A talented cook, he would stump around the kitchen, preparing elaborate meals for other residents. Unless propped up in the recliner in his bedroom, Robbie spent all of his time, day and night, at the kitchen table, smoking and drinking coffee. He feared that if he used his hospital bed, he would die.

He developed his own coterie of friends and visitors, including several priests who visited regularly. Most significantly, Robbie formed an intense bond with another resident, Liza. Liza, a twenty-plus-year heroin and cocaine addict, was well known and liked in the IV drug community. Robbie and Liza became the "Ma and Pa Kettle" of Sunrise. They bickered like an old married couple. Liza cut his hair and changed his leg dressings. They became utterly devoted to one another.

Robbie began to fail rapidly. Staff and residents were in the process of emotionally coping with his impending loss. He had by now begun to sleep in his bed, from whence he played out fully the role of a dying elder statesman. He preplanned his funeral and burial arrangements—something unusual for our population—and seemed in peaceful control.

Then, suddenly and unexpectedly, Liza died. As experienced as staff and residents were with death, the loss of Liza without warning stunned and devastated the entire house. Robbie rallied. In the face of his own loss, it was he who truly consoled everyone. Not surprisingly, his "rally" was not of long duration. Weeks later, he began again to lose ground medically. Robbie had made a choice early on to seek no treatment whatever for his KS beyond palliative care and pain management. At the very end of his life, it was not possible to adequately control his pain. He was "maxed out" on morphine, having developed a tolerance for truly staggering doses.

After several punishing days of witnessing Robbie, clearly in agony, chain-smoking as though each cigarette was binding him to life, he finally gave up.

Robbie's funeral remains legend. He died maintaining significant body mass. His weighty casket was carried by struggling staff into the church. . . and became wedged in the entrance door. After a service built around country singer Conway Twitty's recording of "The Rose," staff and residents followed him to the cemetery, tossing packages of cigarettes into his gravesite as they themselves shoveled in the earth.

* * *

A common question is, How do you *do* it? It has been our experience that few pursuits within the helping professions offer as much opportunity for truly effecting positive change in a client's existence than providing AIDS housing—we get to "make a difference" in distinct and often dramatic ways, by providing comfort, kindness, and stable, dependable client-provider relationships that are mutually fulfilling. Certainly, this depth of relationship and human interaction *can* take place in other care environments; most AIDS residences, however, are programmatically designed so that it *will*. There is triple benefit to this process: (1) the client can experience authentic, consistent emotional support from the provider while maintaining as much autonomy as possible at a time when autonomy is severely threatened; (2) the provider receives professional and human satisfaction; and (3) for other residents, the dying process is observed and demystified, with an assuring implication that their own death will be experienced in an atmosphere of caring and dignity.

For both providers and residents, the process of dying and death is usually longitudinal in nature. Recognizing the inevitable, we are often able to take part in an "anticipatory grief" process.

Our experience has been that the difficult deaths to assimilate—for both residents and providers—are those that happen suddenly and unexpectedly. On occasion, we have also experienced the deaths of residents who were not particularly, or even remotely, likable, which elicited a peculiar guilt based on lack of sorrow or even relief. Perhaps the worst experiences with death have occurred in the rare instances in which the most advanced and aggressive pain management therapies have proved inadequate, and "the good death" became a prolonged ordeal.

Overall, having experienced scores of deaths at Sunrise House, we have noted that this environment has helped all parties concerned grasp and calmly accept the idea of death as an experience that awaits us all.

CULTURAL COMPETENCY CONSIDERATIONS

To a much greater degree than in apartment programs, congregate living providers must grasp and accommodate a startling range of cultural competency issues. There is ample room for conflict, misunderstanding, and judgmentalism between residents, between residents and staff, as well as between residents, staff, and outside persons, i.e., volunteers. Our experience, however, has been that problems with diversity are rarely overt and explosive, but are instead subtle, and subversive to the self-esteem and comfort of whomever is being targeted. It should also be noted that in group living, someone always has to be a scapegoat, a role most easily assumed by anyone "different."

Sexuality and Its Cultural Expression

It is worth noting that we have been aware of very little overt sexual activity on the part of our residents, probably due to incapacity and shifting priorities in the face of illness, and some lack of propinquity.

We have occasionally witnessed the tragedy of gay men and lesbians whose families have been unable to make reconciliation concerning issues of sexuality. More commonly, when sexuality has been a problem in this and similar programs, the root of conflict has been religion-based.

Staff members with fundamentalist religious backgrounds have had to either adjust their beliefs regarding sexual morality—or surrender them at the door. More troubling has been the internalized judgment of dying gay men concerned about their prospects of heaven or hell. In this instance, the intervention of supportive and experienced clergy is absolutely imperative.

Rarely have we encountered homophobic attitudes and behaviors on a resident-to-resident basis. Upon admission, when a presumably heterosexual male is questioned about his attitude toward gay men, the predictable reply has been, "so long as they don't come after me." It must also be considered that many clients, through their experience of street life and prison, have seen it all, twice. On the infrequent occasions when we have had lesbian clients, we have noted and had to address some discomfort and judgmentalism on the part of female staff.

Issues Concerning Race/Ethnicity/Social Status

One must marvel at the manner in which HIV/AIDS housing serves as a medium for bringing together, in shared living quarters, a staggeringly diverse range of populations. Our experience has been that tension and conflict rarely erupt in direct confrontation or aggression. Rather, we have observed, endured, and occasionally been drawn into complicated dramas played out sub rosa. Here, however, is a troubling case history that was anything but under the surface.

Case Study: Frank

Frank was a forty-four-year-old African American. A native of New York City, Frank had been referred through the local Veterans Administration medical facility. In late-stage illness and in need of regular transfusions, Frank would typically make the four-hour drive from his apartment in Queens to Rhode Island for medical treatment.

Frank had been, by his own description, a "sleep-in-the-subway junkie." Successfully rehabilitated by an intensive residential program in New York, Frank was transformed. He became a successful optician and long-distance runner. This was an intense, intelligent, and extremely rigid individual, who was unswerving in his belief that if he could turn his life around, so could and should everyone else. His judgment of any individual who did not meet his standards of behavior and propriety was swift and unyielding. (Frank, clearly, serves well as a example of errant admission-planning for a congregate housing program.)

Frank could tolerate no structure other than that which was self-imposed. His narrow and judgmental view of existence created conflict at every step. He was particularly suspicious of any person not of color. In Frank's eyes, any action or situation that did not meet with his approval was a pointed and deliberate expression of racism. He ably pitted staff against each other according to skin color.

Frank's residence in the program was an ongoing nightmare. He was on the verge of being removed from the house until his health crashed, and he was diagnosed with aggressive toxoplasmosis, resulting in significant cognitive deterioration. Another infection landed him in an intensive care unit. This intensely dignified individual was in an open unit, his tall frame inadequately covered by a hospital gown. Asked by his social worker whether he wished to remain in the hospital or return to Sunrise to die, he said that he wanted to go "home to Sunrise," which he did.

What conclusions can we draw from this case? In Frank's charges of racism, was there some underlying thread of truth? Was there a way that the objectionable behaviors of his fellow residents, most of whom were still rooted in the mores of the street and drug life, might have been made less personally threatening to him? We do not know.

Alternatively, we have experienced occasional challenges in serving Latino persons. Language barriers sometimes intervene, if not with the resident, then with family. We have had non-Latino residents who would persist in calling a Latino "Jose" or "the Spanish guy."

Fundamental differences from person to person regarding ideas about volume levels in music and conversation, cleanliness, and cooking habits are a constant theme in any group living environment. These small conflicts can, however, be subtly cast within a racial/ethnic context that is difficult to address in any concrete fashion.

Issues of diversity (and potential for problems) also abound in staff members. Presently, Sunrise House has on staff a spirited blend of individuals. We have gay, lesbian, and straight people. We have Christian fundamentalists, Muslims, agnostics, and Irish Catholics.

To our relief, however, any obstacles presented by this diversity have been short-lived. To the extent that it is communicated and continually reinforced that prejudicial and discriminatory attitudes about race, ethnicity, and religious affiliation are not tolerated, conflict has generally been kept to a minimum.

KEEPING YOUR SANITY WHILE THOSE AROUND YOU ARE LOSING THEIRS

Residential services for people with AIDS can be like a minefield. One social worker characterized the work as dealing with "the fire and the flood at the same time." As with all intense clinical work, supervision provides essential support and perspective into the many difficult issues presented in these settings. Particularly in the congregate living setting, it is difficult for the staff (from the executive director on down) to balance the relationships between themselves and residents. On one level, weekly supervision may be needed between line staff and the clinical director. On another level, senior staff should obtain support and supervision outside the setting. Administrative and clinical staff of scattered-site programs need similar support.

POLICY IMPLICATIONS AND RELATED ACTIONS

1. *Do your homework.* Be well informed of the admission criteria and policies of the housing provider. Know your client, and be aware of any history that may influence housing placement. Get a release to disclose information. We need to rely on your impressions and experience, and we value our relationships with referral sources who understand our criteria.

   The admission criteria for Sunrise, as an example, is fairly simple, but has considerations that are both objective and subjective. Objectively, one must be HIV positive and have a low income. Some gray area exists concerning drug and alcohol use. Clearly, if a client is using heavily and constantly, living in this kind of housing is not going to work. There can, however, be extenuating circumstances, and we are happy to have people linked with methadone treatment, if necessary.

   Most subjectively, we need to assess whether or not a client is going to be willing or capable of living cooperatively with others. We need to know how the client handles conflict, anger, frustration, and grief.

2. *Do more homework.* Visit the program facilities so that you may give your client an informed sense of "what it's like."

3. *Know how financial and logistical issues work regarding housing.* Social workers may be involved in housing as planners, administrators, or direct service workers.

4. *Determine what the client wants.*

CONCLUSION

In this chapter we have presented two housing models for people with HIV/AIDS: a congregate living facility and scattered-site apartments. We have described and discussed many of the issues that may arise for residents and staff in these programs and what facets on which the social work practitioner may wish to focus in training and practicum experience. Although it is difficult and sometimes emotionally draining work, it is some of the most concretely and spiritually rewarding social work to be found within the HIV/AIDS epidemic.

SECTION V:
CARING FOR THE PROFESSIONAL CAREGIVER

Caring for Ourselves: Understanding and Minimizing the Stresses of HIV Caregiving

Kitsy Schoen

WHY DO THIS?
STATEMENT OF THE PROBLEM AND ISSUES

All human service and health care providers face the challenge of coping with stress and burnout. Now, when we must work with increasingly complex client needs in an era of diminishing resources, the challenge is greater than ever. This creates the classic conditions for stress—when the demands exceed an individual's ability to respond.

As a group, professional caregivers are often vulnerable to, as one HIV provider described it, "heart fatigue." We may be better at addressing clients' needs than our own. The lesson many of us have to learn is that preserving our own well-being is essential to effective caregiving. With so much focus on the needs of others, we often succumb to a vague wish to be taken care of, thus losing sight of our personal responsibility for our own welfare.

There are specific, although not unique, stresses related to HIV work. The life-and-death nature of the work brings an urgency to our responses to clients' needs. Many clients are coping with multiple hardships in addition to HIV—poverty, mental illness, drug use, and discrimination. The saturation of losses within certain families and friendship networks can be overwhelming. Many of those who die are young, and the illness itself can be ravaging. In addition, many HIV professionals are personally affected by the HIV epidemic. This can make it hard to separate work and personal life. The following quotes—and those interspersed throughout the chapter—have been taken directly from workshop participants who are HIV providers in a wide range of settings throughout the country:

- The repeated exposure to loss is very hard on me. It is agonizing to watch the disfiguring deteriortation toward death.
- A constant state of grief is completely familiar to me.

527

- I think I'm in control, but at night I have dreams of being overwhelmed by the needs of client's.
- I am terrified of becoming ill.

TRAUMA

Trauma is contagious. It is virtually impossible to be untouched by someone in acute distress. We see tragedy in our clients' lives, and we realize that we, too, are vulnerable. In witnessing a client's struggle, we anticipate our own encounter with a similar disaster. Some HIV providers describe compelling dreams of having AIDS. Others are distressed by repeated worries about crime, or their children's health. We translate client's material into our own areas of vulnerability. This effect is called *vicarious traumatization*.[1] Like emergency workers, we need support, debriefing, and a chance to recover from the onslaught of traumatic material.

The constant stresses of HIV work evoke a wide range of reactions, both for an individual over time and for groups. These differences can be disconcerting because we want our experiences to be shared by others. Tensions can result from what appear to be conflicting reactions; thus, understanding the roots of the differences is important.

Our cultural experience forms the backdrop for our perception and reactions to illness, death, and loss. Our family's style of coping, our personalities, and our history of resolved and unresolved losses all shape our reactions to HIV work. Stresses in our present lives are often an invisible influence on our response to workplace problems.

A trauma model is helpful for understanding the impact of HIV caregiving. Trauma means "wound" or "shock." Trauma is overwhelming. Our psyches tackle pieces of the traumatic experience one at a time. We may experience strong feelings without a clear sense of what evoked them. "Sometimes I weep when driving home, but I don't really know why." Or, we may respond to client's devastating experience with little feeling at all. "I can listen to a client describe a litany of horrid oppotunistic infections and I don't feel a thing. I worry that I don't really care." Compartmentalization of experience can help us function in immediate crisis, and it allows us to integrate the experience with time. Problems can develop, however, when we get stuck in any one way of coping.

Responses to Trauma

Stress, bereavement overload, and vicarious traumatization lead to several common responses in HIV providers:

Flooding and Numbing

Responses to trauma swing between adaptive numbing and flooding of feelings. Either end of this continuum of responses can be disconcerting to a professional. Someone flooding with feelings may feel ashamed that they can not control his or her emotions. Those in adaptive numbing may worry that they do not care enough. In the workplace, this frequently leads to tensions between those at opposing ends of the spectrum and to accusations that some are "overinvolved" while others are "jaded" and "burned out." This can become the basis for many other conflicts and tensions between new and old staff, HIV-positive and seronegative staff, between staff and management, or between direct and indirect service providers.

Anger and Irritability

These symptoms have a variety of causes. Irritability is a result of feeling depleted. We may be enraged at the faceless virus that wreaks havoc on our clients (and loved ones), as well as at our helplessness to change the ultimate outcome. These feelings can easily be displaced to co-workers, friends, and loved ones. "I take the stress out on co-workers." "I am alarmed at how angry I am at home. I seem to be picking fights."

Resistance to Change and Need for Control

Change is a constant in HIV work. Our clients' needs change rapidly, often our workplaces are unstable, and we are overwhelmed by losses. There is an understandable impulse to resist further change. In compensation for the helplessness we often experience with clients, we may try to seize control in other arenas—and find ourselves insistent about relatively minor matters, or furiously attending to small, "do-able" tasks (such as cleaning!).

Avoidance

"I am afraid to meet new people." "I don't answer the phone when I go home." "I avoid friends because I don't have the energy . . . and I do not want to grieve for any more people." "Sometimes I use substances or food to deal with my feelings." In moderation, avoidance provides much-needed shelter and relief from the onslaught of demands and traumatic material. "There is no shame in avoiding elephants" (Vietnamese proverb). In avoiding rest, intimacy, and fun, we are often avoiding the flooding of feelings that can come with slowing down and connecting with ourselves and others. Taken to extremes, it results in the isolation of the professional caregiver—and that can take a toll on our sense of self, our relationships, and our personal interests. Overworking is a disguised form of avoidance. The overworked provider does not have time to let down.

Survivor Guilt

Neglecting our own limits, needs, and interests can also be a symptom of survivor guilt. The most extreme example of survivor guilt is blatantly self-destructive behavior. Survivor guilt functions as an undertow pulling against the tide of self-care. It is difficult for caregivers to reconcile personal well-being with the dire circumstances others face. The "caring" inclination is to level the playing field and join the other in distress. The urge to make a more equitable balance makes it difficult for some individuals to take adequate care of themselves. The result is a state of sympathetic "dis-ease." It takes a concentrated effort to continue to focus on life-affirming, positive activities and goals.

STRATEGIES FOR SELF-CARE

Stress Management

As with so many other conditions, prevention is the most effective approach. There is no way to avoid stress and overload in this work, but the trick is to know your own warning signs and recognize early the need to make adjustments in your work and personal care strategies.

Effective stress management needs to be a daily way of life. Our bodies and emotions need regular breaks from the onslaught of demands as well as opportunities to rejuvenate. Take the time to attend a stress management course or to review one of many stress management workbooks[2] to identify your strengths and weaknesses in coping with stress. Develop a plan which outlines things that may help you when you see your particular "warning signs" of overload.

Other Techniques

In addition to traditional stress management techniques, HIV work requires addressing some specific areas, including the following:

Loss Acknowledgment

Acknowledging loss reminds us that there are external sources of distress and minimizes the tendency to blame ourselves or others for our distress. It is important to acknowledge both immediate losses and the ongoing toll of such losses. Keeping a journal, scrapbook, or other tangible reflection of the losses experienced at work can be helpful. Attending memorials periodically can offer a chance to grieve the accumulation of client losses. Develop rituals to acknowledge losses using music or by taking a special walk.

Trauma Debriefing

People who have witnessed or survived trauma need to tell their story . . . and so will you. Identify ways that you can unload some of the images and emotions that accumulate in working with clients' suffering. Find coworkers to talk to after an upsetting experience. Use case conferences as opportunities to discuss challenging cases. You can also tell the stories through written word, music, or drawings. Find a caregiver support group or start one! Individual counseling can provide a regular opportunity to unload and gain perspective. Beware of feeling that there is no point in talking, or that you do not want to "burden" others. These thoughts are often the result of shutting down emotionally or avoiding the flood of feelings.

Rest and Relaxation

It is important to have regular (many times during a week) opportunities to relax. You need a break from the onslaught of demands. Your body needs frequent opportunities to recuperate; otherwise, stress can lead to more serious physical and emotional problems, including anxiety and depression. Try to find places and people that help you relax from the realities of HIV and work.

Inspiration

What keeps you going—relationships, wilderness, adventure, or spiritual activities? Do them! Go to these wells often and fill up.[3]

Keeping on Track

Plan ways for maintaining and reevaluating your coping strategies. Use your anniversary date at work, your birthday, or the new year as your time to reevaluate your relationship to the work. Ask a trusted friend or colleague for comments on your ways of responding to stress. Write yourself a letter now and put it in your datebook six months from now. What do you want to remind yourself of?

Burnout directly affects patient care. Staff who are emotionally and physically depleted are often more irritable, rigid, and unavailable to the needs of clients and co-workers. Or when overwhelmed, we can lose our perspective and become overinvolved. Some periods of burnout are probably unavoidable in this work, but it is important to heed warning signs early. Otherwise, burnout can lead to serious workplace and personal probems.

POLICY IMPLICATIONS AND RELATED ACTIONS

In response to the question, "How does the wear and tear of HIV work effect your work group," HIV service providers responded with these comments:

- The stress of repeated loss is acted out through splitting and divisive behaviors. The tension between disciplines is destructive and group morale is low—a result of minimum validation of the work we do.
- So many deaths—the group begins to numb their feelings. We act out pain in negative ways—anger, dehumanizing clients, isolating. Death is so normalized, we minimize how work is affecting us.
- We tend to do a lot of complaining, which is in itself stressful.
- I work with an amazing group. We are all very supportive of each other. There is much longevity in the staff. I am amazed.

Although individual commitment to effective self-care is essential, it is often not enough. An effective approach to a productive and positive work environment requires a collaborative effort of individual staff members and the organization as a whole. Health and human service organizations providing HIV services would do well to look to the example of the hospice movement where the commitment to staff support is a part of the bylaws. Certified hospices must have a specific plan to address staff support needs. Staff, management, and supervisors alike must recognize the value of a healthy work environment and its relevance to the quality, effectiveness, and efficiency of client services.

Organizations experience symptoms of overload that parallel the effects on individuals: increased polarization between groups of staff or between staff and management; increased conflict, anger, and scapegoating; inflexibility and rigidity, poor communication, lowered productivity, and increased absenteeism. Survivor guilt can result in a tendency to work in a constant crisis mode or in difficulty setting appropriate limits. These symptoms can cause a variety of problems both internally and in the services to clients. Although the symptoms listed in this chapter can be caused by a variety of organizational problems, they are often inflamed by the stresses of providing HIV care.

Any genuine effort to create a healthy work environment must begin with an assessment of salient organizational issues. If significant change is happening, or if workloads are unrealistically high or unclear, these issues must be addressed first. Otherwise, efforts at establishing staff support mechanisms will be undermined.

Supervisors and managers often have concerns about developing a comprehensive plan for minimizing HIV-related burnout. Common concerns include the amount of time and money involved and whether the process will unleash an endless stream of complaints. A study of a large HIV organization found that "burnout" resulted in significant cost in to the agency in excess absenteeism, increased worker compensation benefits, excess job turnover, and lower productivity.[4] Many of the most meaningful staff support strategies are ones that can be incorporated into existing activities and policies at minimal expense.

The very process of involving staff in the planning process helps clarify employee's expectations of the workplace. One manager reported she was relieved to find how practical her employee's suggestions were. The process of developing specific strategies can counteract vague and therefore often unmet expectations of the organization. Supervisors and managers appreciate having concrete ways to offer support.

Line staff have their own concerns when the focus is on the difficult aspects of HIV work. Some worry that they will be required to be personally revealing at work. This may be personally or culturally repugnant; thus, differences in style must be respected. (This is one reason why support groups alone as a staff support measure are not always effective.)

Staff may also worry that their grieving or coping will be evaluated by supervisors. Indeed, supervisors may need special training to effectively separate their supportive and supervisory roles. It is important not to label or characterize an employee's coping. If asked for feedback, refering to observable behaviors is best. Staff and supervisors can prevent misunderstandings by clarifying when a discussion is for support needs, problem solving, or performance problems.

Workplaces often begin addressing staff support needs at a crisis point, when staff morale is poor, or when internal conflict is high. The solutions sought are either too specific (typically a support group) or too short-lived (a retreat). Just as in individual stress management, organizational vitality depends on the practice of regular and frequent support activities.

The following discusses areas that are important to address in creating and maintaining a healthy work environment in a variety of settings.

Assess the Organizational Culture

Organizational culture refers to the climate, norms, and practices of any given workplace. Leadership can positively influence the organizational culture by evaluating and making changes in the policies, practices, and rewards of the organization. The following values are commonly thought to contribute to a safe and supportive work environment and to minimizing burnout. Determine what the official and actual messages conveyed in your workplace are on the value of the following

- a healthy workplace
- balancing work and personal life
- team work
- autonomy
- setting apropriate limits
- innovation
- quality patient care
- diversity
- open communication
- permission to be emotionally affected by work and
- permission to make mistakes

Assess Personnel Policies and Benefits

Changes in personnel policies and benefits are valuable not only in their tangibility, but also because they reflect organizational commitment to staff support. Personnel policies can address issues very significant in preventing burnout by giving staff more control over their work and the ability to balance work and personal lives:

- Bereavement leave and dependent care policies can be broadened to include nontraditional family members.
- Flex time provides "reasonable accomodation" to periods of acute stress or grief, and gives staff more control over the conditions of work—an important factor in job satisfaction.
- "Mental health" or planned sick days give staff the opportunity to take time off when feeling overwhelmed and allow employers to plan for coverage.

Formalize Staff Appreciation

Individuals and organizations need to balance the constant drain of service provision by creating opportunities for positive interactions. Staff need regular opportunities to talk about their accomplishments and receive feedback from supervisors and co-workers. Some organizations have developed "Bravo" cards so that staff convey their appreciation of each other or pass on client's compliments, with copies going to personnel files. Informal gatherings, lunches, or outings help build trust and good-will. Without these efforts, the internal life of the organization can become bleak.

Acknowledge Loss

Develop ways to acknowledge immediate and cumulative loss. The acknowledgement of losses helps remind staff of the external sources of distress and minimizes the tendency to personalize or blame others for the distress often associated with grief.

Information about a death needs to be conveyed sensitively and consistently to all involved staff members. Some workplaces distribute paper hearts with the names and dates of client deaths to all involved team members. Scrapbooks are used in a wide range of settings to record patient's deaths, with staff adding photos and notes of remembrance. Writing bereavement notes to survivors offers a sense of completion. Simple rituals developed by staff can be held on a semiannual or yearly basis to acknowledge client deaths.

Provide Support

Support strategies provide opportunities for staff to "debrief," to review the details of upsetting cases and to express emotions. Different coping styles require various kinds of support. Time can be set aside at case conferences or at monthly staff meetings to talk about the personal impact of the work. Isolated caregivers need time to attend meetings or conferences with other HIV providers.

Support groups can be helpful when carefully facilitated to keep the focus on the impact of service provision and away from organizational issues. Otherwise, support groups too easily become "gripe" sessions.

Some agencies have had success with monthly team-building sessions or half-day meetings a few times each year. Other agencies offer staff a paid hour off each week to pursue their own stress management routine such as psychotherapy or tai chi.

Provide Staff Development and Diversify Job Duties

For frontline service providers, it is especially important to have opportunities to do different functions—to give talks, to write, to represent the agency, or to do prevention work or research. This is comparable to combat leave—giving staff a break from the front. Staff involved in indirect service may appreciate opportunities to provide some direct service. New learning helps balance the chronic pressures of work and widen one's perspective.

Once a staff support plan is developed, distribute a description of the strategies to new employees and to old staff at annual reviews. Do not be disappointed when the best of plans falls apart. Form a staff support committee to review and revise staff support efforts.

In virtually all areas of psychosocial research, individuals cope best with stress when they feel supported. A supportive workplace is a great boon for the HIV provider.

CONCLUSION

HIV work can be very compelling and rewarding—which is both a blessing and a curse. HIV work can offer a sense of meaning and purpose, intimacy and connection, and accomplishment . . . but sometimes providers find themselves neglecting these needs in their personal lives. We can become acclimated to the intensity of the work, and thus we can find it difficult to pull back. It is important to make a conscious effort to tend to the quality of our own lives as well as to try to enhance our client's lives. We need to practice what we encourage our clients to do: to ask for and accept support, to grieve, and to replenish ourselves physically and emotionally.

NOTES

1. Vicarious Traumatization: A Framework for Understanding the Psychological Effects of Working with Victims. McCann, L., and Pearlman, L.A. (1990). *Journal of Traumatic Stress 3*(1): 131-149.

2. One recommended book is *The Relaxation and Stress Reduction Workbook* by Davis, M., Eshelman, E.R., and McKay, M (1990), New Harbinger Publications, Oakland, CA.

3. A great book for getting back to the activities you love is *The Artist Way*, Cameron, J. (1992), Putnam' Sons, New York.

4. The Cost of Burn Out. Soos J. (1992). *Focus: A Guide to AIDS Research and Counseling 7*(6): 7-8.

REFERENCES

Macks, J. (1992). Sustaining Professional AIDS Caregivers and Their Organizations. In H. Land (Ed.), *AIDS Intervention and Response from the Human Services*. Milwaukee, WI: Family Service America Press.

Schoen, K. (1992). Managing Grief in AIDS Organizations. *Focus: A Guide to AIDS Research and Counseling 7*(6): 1-4.

Meeting the Emotional Needs of Health Care Providers

Jay R. Warren

WHY DO THIS?
STATEMENT OF THE PROBLEM AND ISSUES

As noted in the previous chapter, direct work with people living with HIV can elicit a range of emotional responses in social workers that warrant attention to help prevent worker burnout and ensure quality of care. The same emotional responses are commonly found among physicians, nurses, psychiatrists, case managers, and support staff who care for large numbers of people living with HIV. It is clear that caring for large numbers of persons living with HIV (PLWH) puts intense emotional demands on staff, yet health care settings have been slow to address the needs of providers to attend to these demands.

Social workers in the health care setting are well-situated to help providers address the emotional sequelae that caring for seriously ill individuals evokes. We can also play a key role in fostering a climate in which dealing with the emotionally compelling aspects of the work is integrated into health care delivery. This section will outline some of the emotional challenges providers may face in their work with people living with HIV and will offer suggestions regarding how social workers can act to help address these challenges.

EMOTIONAL CHALLENGES

Perhaps the most obvious and compelling challenge facing health care providers in HIV health care settings is the fact that in spite of our best efforts, many of our patients will get progressively ill and some will die. Integrating multiple losses and dealing with the grief that accompanies them is a task essential to our work but generally is not a component of professional training (Friedland, 1989).

Another potential challenge arises when providers feel a strong identification with their patients. Often, providers will share an HIV risk history or social demographic factor with their patients. Other providers may have had

537

close friends or family members infected with HIV. HIV treatment centers often draw gay male providers or providers in recovery, for example, who approach the work with a strong commitment due to their personal connection with the epidemic. These providers may be particularly affected by cumulative loss due to their stronger identification with their patients. In addition to having an opportunity to integrate the losses, these providers need help negotiating and maintaining professional boundaries between their personal and professional relationships with their patients.

Health care providers who are themselves living with HIV often find providing care to others with HIV to be an empowering way of coping with their own seropositivity. They can present themselves as role models and bring a unique sensitivity and passion to their work. At the same time, they may be increasingly vulnerable to the physical decline of patients with whom they work—especially if their medical histories are similar. For example, an HIV-positive case manager reported that it was chillingly difficult to deal with a client who had a comparatively higher T-cell count than he did yet who died from a rapidly progressive case of PML (primary multifocal leukoencephalopathy).

One unique challenge facing health care providers working in HIV is related to the underlying disease process itself. HIV is a difficult illness to manage, and staff must come to terms with the frustration inherent in this. HIV disease can manifest in virtually any organ system, and its unpredictability can confound providers in their efforts to help their patients. For example, one woman being treated for HIV lymphoma developed bacterial pneumonia as she was nearing the end of her chemotherapy regimen. The chemotherapy had to be stopped in order to treat the underlying pneumonia, which left her providers feeling helpless and frustrated—affects that most providers do not handle with facility.

Another challenge for the medical staff stems from the fact that the person living with HIV (PLWH) may develop a dependent relationship on his or her health care providers. This dependence is likely to be more intense when the PLWH is symptomatic or in emotional distress. The PLWH may make frequent phone calls or begin to demand a lot of the provider's time. Providers can feel torn between their desire to be helpful to patients on the one hand, and the multiple other demands on their time on the other. Patients can feel devalued when providers are not able to respond to specific needs and may become angry or devaluing in return. This can leave the provider feeling guilty, angry, or humiliated.

If left unchecked, the emotions and interpersonal dynamics that providers experience in their work with PLWHs can lead to personal or professional burnout. Low morale, poor job satisfaction, and substandard care can result. Signs of burnout are often subtle and may include aversion to contacts with particularly ill or emotionally challenging patients, avoidance of affectively loaded discussions, or secretly feeling relieved when certain patients fail to show up for appointments.

INTERVENTION STRATEGIES

Social workers who are part of an interdisciplinary team will notice that their mere presence can help others feel some relief from the stress of caring for PLWHs. Our colleagues often express relief that we are able to address the psychosocial aspects of care because this can ease a portion of the burden of their work.

A significant role for social workers on the medical team is assessing the key forces that shape patient behavior and psychological responses to stress. By sharing this perspective at team meetings, we can help health care providers understand the coping styles that our clients utilize. Our awareness of cultural, developmental, and dynamic factors can help staff to contextualize their client's behavior and attitudes and to better manage their responses to such behavior.

The helplessness and frustration that providers feel can result in the unconscious displacement of their feelings onto the PLWH or other staff members. The social worker may notice irritation and anger in providers who usually are more even-tempered. We might try to engage our colleagues in discussion to help them step back from the situation and identify the true source of their anger. Open discussion can help normalize the inherent disappointments of the work and may avert conflicts between staff and the PLWH.

Interdisciplinary team meetings are another potential arena in which to address the needs of our colleagues. Social workers can make sure that the team takes the time to reflect on time-intensive or emotionally stirring cases. Strategies can be developed to help providers involve other team members so as to distribute patient care needs appropriately.

Informal means of intervention, such as personal conversations or "curbside consultations," are quick, nonthreatening ways to allow colleagues to talk about a troubling situation or to reflect on their mood. As social workers, we are usually adept as using our one-to-one collegial relationships to help colleagues vent feelings and to normalize the difficult experiences with which they may be dealing.

Social workers can also help medical staff develop a formalized way of reflecting on recent losses. Some teams devise rituals to help mark the deaths of patients, such as keeping a scrapbook or taking time to memorialize them. Such ventures can be valuable in airing not only the sad feelings, but also the less-sanctioned feelings of anger, despair, and relief.

Formal support groups can be another valuable tool in addressing emotional needs of staff (Makadon, Delbanco, and Delbanco, 1990). Such groups can be hard to actualize in many health care settings. Staff members are often reluctant to acknowledge their need for emotional support so they may elect not to participate. Health care providers can also feel pulled in many directions and may therefore place participants in such groups at a low priority. Agencies may not recognize the value of such groups and may be reluctant to offer them on agency time.

One model of a support group that has met with some success in health care settings is a case-focused interdisciplinary group to discuss cases from a "big picture" view (Frost et al., 1991). In this way, the group need not be designated as a support group per se, which might appeal more to medical staff. Social workers can offer a strong presence at these meetings, making sure that other providers take the time to explore the emotional dimension of the work.

Time-limited support groups offer another alternative, especially if health care providers themselves demonstrate some interest in having a support group. They can be especially useful when a team is developing, as they can create a culture of collegial sharing about the feelings engendered in doing their jobs.

In thinking about the emotional needs of staff, it is important to conclude with the reminder that there are many rewards in the work with PLWH and that the PLWH him or herself can supply much to sustain staff. Small medical victories or warm interchanges can go a long way in keeping morale up. Nevertheless, the need to attend to the emotional aspects of the work are clear, and the social work role in this process can be pivotal.

REFERENCES

Friedland, Gerald H. Clinical care in the AIDS epidemic. *Deadalus.* 1989: 59-83.

Frost JC, Makdon H, Judd D, Lee S, O'Neill S, Paulsen R. (1991) Care for caregiviers: A support group for staff caring for AIDS patients in a hospital-based primary care practice. *Journal of General Internal Medicine 6:* 162-167.

Makadon HJ, Delbanco S, Delbanco T. (1990). Caring for people with AIDS and HIV infection in hospital-based primary care practice. *Journal of General Internal Medicine 5:* 446-450.

Changing the System:
Don't Mourn . . . Organize!

Thomas F. Sheridan

WHY DO THIS?
STATEMENT OF THE PROBLEM AND ISSUES

I wore a button with the slogan "Don't Mourn . . . Organize!" during my graduate work at Catholic University in 1983. At the time, it seemed an appropriate response to the Reagan budget cuts and social policy revolution we were experiencing. I did not know then how deadly the human immunodeficiency (HIV) virus would be for many friends and colleagues, nor did I envision the devastating impact acquired immune deficiency syndrome (AIDS) would have around the world. The uncanny inspiration of this sample slogan has guided my professional life—as a social worker and an advocate.

The AIDS epidemic exemplifies the critical requirement for a social worker to develop the skills to navigate effectively all systems of government. When these federal, local, and state systems of government pose impediments to addressing the needs of a client, the social worker must be ready to advocate for changes within these systems. Additionally, the social worker must be prepared to incur the costs associated with success or failure of advocacy. In the 1980s, the significant barriers experienced by people living with HIV/AIDS in securing adequate health care and support services made it imperative for us to become effective advocates.

Many times, our professional experiences are dominated by systems that we did not set up or design. Therefore, we may not necessarily believe these systems are best suited for the needs of our clients. Despite this dynamic, as a member of the social service network, the social worker has a role in the operation of these systems. The case worker, administrator, clinician, and advocate each have a distinct, specific function within the overall system. The advocate's role is to examine all systems with a critical eye in order to strengthen successful operations and to develop alternatives for flawed practices. Once this examination is concluded, the real work of advocacy must begin—the campaign for

541

change. As an advocate, the social worker must be clearly focused on his or her role as "an agent for change." This chapter is intended to assist the social worker in understanding the tasks and skills necessary to undertake such a campaign.

In the context of AIDS, our ability to successfully create change remains the critical component in our efforts to halt the epidemic. Advocacy dedicated and focused on bringing that change has achieved remarkable success—changes in Medicaid and Medicare, the Ryan White CARE Act, the Housing Opportunities for People With AIDS Act (HOPWA), the San Francisco needle-exchange program, and the repeal of the mandatory HIV testing requirements for a marriage license in Illinois, to name a few. These successes have sustained those affected by the AIDS epidemic, but they have not brought an end to the tragedy of AIDS. Still more work, still more battles must be won before the war will be over.

To approach the issue of "changing the system," a quick review of the "status quo" is essential. AIDS is a deadly worldwide pandemic; HIV is the infectious agent; marginalized and disenfranchised populations are affected; the routes of transmission in the United States are sexual and drug-related; and AIDS is concentrated in urban areas and third world countries. These factors are challenging in and of themselves. They are also politically insolvent and volatile.

Frequently, experts have said that the AIDS epidemic exposes the best and worst in U.S. social and health policy. Perhaps the best exposition is our continued reliance on thousands who volunteer to support communities and families in crisis. The partnerships that have been established between citizens and their government to respond to the AIDS emergency have been exemplary. The worst examples of our national response to the HIV virus include too many callous, indifferent congressional leaders and slow, immovable bureaucracies that do not pretend to understand the urgency of AIDS.

The day-to-day needs of people living with HIV/AIDS challenge our systems of health care and social support services until those systems are stretched to the limit. For some HIV-infected Americans, AIDS brings an end to productive employment that has maintained their basic needs, such as health insurance, rent and nutritional expenses. For others, those basic needs have never been met, and their poverty will worsen as the disease progresses. Perhaps the only assumption one can make in this vast and complex world of AIDS policy is that poverty is "the great leveler." Whether the client starts out poor or is delivered there, reliance upon our public health care system is common. Therefore, the policy challenges at local, state, and federal levels are profound and complex. Similarly, the strategies needed to change existing systems and to create new ones are equally as challenging.

As you read this chapter, it is important to remember that individual social workers and individual clients can engage in any aspect of advocacy. Often, advocacy is perceived as something only massive numbers of people can do, and that only those who "know the ropes" can be successful. *This is false.* The most dramatic changes in the nation's response to AIDS began with the activities of *individuals.* Indeed, the most profound changes in the world frequently begin with the action of an individual. In words of the ancient Chinese philosopher, Lao-Tse, "A journey of a thousand miles must begin with a single step."

HOW TO DEVELOP A LEGISLATIVE GOAL AND ADVOCATE FOR IT

Using the example of the Ryan White Comprehensive AIDS Resources Emergency (CARE) Act of 1990, I will describe the assumptions, strategies, and tactics that were utilized in the successful passage of federal legislation to address a specific problem encountered in the AIDS epidemic—little or no health care and social support for people living with HIV/AIDS.

The Problem and Its Presentation

In 1989, only 5 percent of all federal funds being spent on HIV/AIDS were dedicated to assisting in the coordination and delivery of health care and social support services for people living with HIV/AIDS. Most of the funds were allocated to the important and necessary tasks of research ($473,285,000) and prevention ($304,942,000).[1] Medicaid was available only for people who were *both* poor *and* disabled; Medicare required a twenty-four-month waiting period after an AIDS diagnosis. There was no reliable system to finance health care and social support services for people living with HIV/AIDS. Investments in biomedical research had recently yielded not only a reliable test for the HIV virus, but the promise of a new drug—called AZT—which could slow the progress of disease. However, with little or no public or private health care infrastructure and a social service system largely dependent on volunteer "buddy programs," the need to develop systems of care and mechanisms to fund those systems was becoming increasingly urgent. Hospital stays were frequent and long because there was little or no "early intervention" for people living with HIV/AIDS. The most urgent care needs were tended to—usually for those who were dying.

The federal government and several private charitable foundations had allotted some money in a small number of communities to create service demonstration programs. The most successful of these models became the renowned "San Francisco model." In this model, public health resources, AIDS-specific community-based organizations, and the resources of philanthropic groups were pooled to create a coordinated system of care. Largely dependent on good relationships and the cooperation of the city's public health department, San Francisco demonstrated that a system of services could be built that was both cost-effective and compassionate.

AIDS service organizations were rapidly emerging as the central point for services and support, thereby finding themselves with less resources to meet expanding needs. At the centers of the successful models in San Francisco, Atlanta, and New York were alliances of local interests—public and private—that could prioritize need and organize resources. However, the need was not just money, but the combination of money and community dialogue. A clear message emerged from these initial demonstrations of cooperation—use all existing resources in a community toward AIDS services before creating something new or separate. The urban centers needed the additional resources and a specialized impetus for a community-based response to the AIDS epidemic.

A Plan to Address the Problem

The process for change is complicated, but if well-organized and focused, a campaign for change can be managed. The following six-point program may be helpful in designing strategies to achieve your policy goal.

1. Create a solution.
2. Document the problem.
3. Form a coalition.
4. Master the process.
5. Identify a champion.
6. Assess the political practicality.

Each of these basics has been the subject of entire books! For our purposes, I have tried to simplify these concepts by applying them to the process that was used in the passage of the Ryan White CARE Act.

Create a Solution

The advice of AIDS experts, the perspective of federal bureaucrats, foundation studies, and a few pieces of drafted legislation became the cornerstones for our solution. Joining these perspectives, findings, opinions, and precepts required the skill of dedicated and knowledgeable people who believed it was important to at least try to develop a blueprint for a coordinated federal response to the AIDS epidemic. The legislation was crafted with four tenets in mind—ultimately resulting in the four titles of the Ryan White CARE Act:

I. Cities hardest hit required "disaster relief." These monies would be provided rapidly, controlled by local decision makers and targeted for services that would assist in saving money and lives.

II. States needed to begin comprehensive planning efforts aimed at establishing local planning for health care delivery as the epidemic emerged beyond the large cities. In addition, states had already been given some federal money to help people living with HIV/AIDS purchase medication (most of which were very expensive and not reimbursed by insurance companies). This existing program needed to continue without interruption.

III. As new therapies were being developed to treat people living with HIV/AIDS to prevent opportunistic infections, a closer link between HIV testing programs and treatment programs was needed. The notion of HIV testing linked directly to early intervention required the merger of two traditionally separate public health "camps"—prevention and clinical treatment. In addition, the community-based health clinics most likely to provide health care to populations at high risk for HIV disease required incentives to test clients and establish better treatment programs. By fortifying these existing infrastructures, resources could be maximized and capacity could be increased to address the expected influx of new AIDS cases.

IV. "Special populations" would need continued federal support and security in an overall schematic of funding—services for children, women, adolescents, and Native Americans were particularly important.

With these tenets in mind, legislation began to take form. In the urban areas, the San Francisco model—now the Title I program—was well known, highly publicized, and well respected. For the states, existing federal demonstration grants, the use of the drug assistance program, and the support of state public health experts to provide planning assistance resulted in Title II. Media attention regarding the success of AZT and the federal government's interest in creating incentives for testing helped establish a basis of support for the third title. Existing federal grants and growing political pressure to respond to special populations—particularly children—were ample reason to create the fourth title. Each title has a specific set of goals and objectives, but each was crafted carefully to fully integrate the four titles as a larger system of care. For most of these solutions, there was some existing evidence that the concept would work.

Document the Problem

Although previously described in detail, the problem of AIDS care was articulated to lawmakers as the following: "If we don't act now, we are likely to bankrupt the overall public health system of this country." The disaster of AIDS had clearly unfolded and everyone—save the most dedicated homophobe—recognized that AIDS required an emergency response. Such a response was needed not only so that people living with HIV/AIDS would receive adequate care, but also so that the public health systems could continue to address the needs of other populations.

In the second half of 1989, Hurricane Hugo and the San Francisco earthquake brought the devastation of natural disasters to the forefront of the American consciousness. The policy director for the San Francisco AIDS Foundation, Pat Christen, was the first to seize upon the disaster analogy inherent in AIDS. Using the politically popular and familiar "disaster relief" model was believed to be helpful in removing stigma and focusing helpful media attention. Mainstream America needed to believe in the inevitable conclusion that disasters happen—including AIDS—and thereby demand rapid—and generous—responses.

Form a Coalition

The most important component of our success was our ability to develop a cohesive coalition. To create change, consistent pressure is required from a core group of concerned parties. Whether the change is within a family, a community-based organization, a city council, a state government, or the United States Congress, there is always a need to have a critical mass demanding the change and applying the necessary political pressure to create that change.

To advocate for the Ryan White CARE Act, the coalition was constituted by many national organizations concerned about the health and social service needs of people living with HIV/AIDS. Support from respected public health and medical groups was intrinsic to the process. The leaders in this coalition effort to pass the CARE Act included representatives from the American Nurses Association, the American Public

Health Association, the National Association of Counties, and the U.S. Conference of Mayors. Assistance and support was provided from more than 150 organizations, including the National Association of Social Workers. These groups, speaking in unison, convinced Congress that AIDS legislation was necessary and politically important as well.

Coalitions require the collective efforts of many, and although some participants contribute more than others, everyone must have reason to be "at the table" and to stay there. Managing a coalition requires an enormous amount of dedication, time, and resources, as well as a willingness to compromise, but coalitions are incredibly powerful. To the federal, state, and local audience, coalitions with a singular message can make a small core group of individuals appear to be a large, diverse, and cohesive unit.

Develop a Strategy

This is the "road map" to successful advocacy. You cannot begin change, particularly at a legislative level, unless you know the specific process by which change is accepted or rejected. For example, whether the change requires special funding, regulatory modifications, or new legislators will direct your advocacy. In the case of the Ryan White CARE Act, we had to negotiate within the U.S. Congress's established processes. A pictorial description of the federal legislative process (see Figure 1) provides the "nuts and bolts" by which the CARE Act and other federal legislation are passed. Theoretical knowledge of the formal process is vital, but practical experience with the intricacies of congressional action is essential as well. When planning a strategy, a coalition must include individuals who understand both the theoretical and the practical aspects of legislative process. You as the social worker do not need to be an expert, but you must have one available for advice. Legislative novices should not be dissuaded from engaging in advocacy; fresh ideas and perspectives are valuable parts of any campaign for change.

Some very specific strategic decisions we made included (1) focusing on a single chamber of Congress first, (2) garnering congressional support through grassroots support, and (3) introducing bipartisan legislation. Thousands of bills are introduced in Congress each year; less than 10 percent ever make it all the way to the President for signature. We had to be careful not to squander any political capital or resources. Our coalition focused on the Senate first and the House of Representatives second to focus energy and maintain momentum. In order to avoid polarizing AIDS care as a one-party political issue, our strategy also involved a concerted grassroots effort to introduce a bipartisan bill—supported equally by Demo-

FIGURE 1. How a Bill Becomes Law

This graphic shows the most typical way in which proposed legislation is enacted into law. There are more complicated, as well as similar, routes, and most bills fall by the wayside and never become law. The process is illustrated with two hypothetical bills, House bill No. 1 (HR 1) and Senate bill No. 2 (S 2). Each bill must be passed by both houses of Congress in identical form before it can become law. The path of HR 1 is traced by a solid line, that of S 2 by a broken line. However, in practice most legislation begins as similar proposals in both houses.

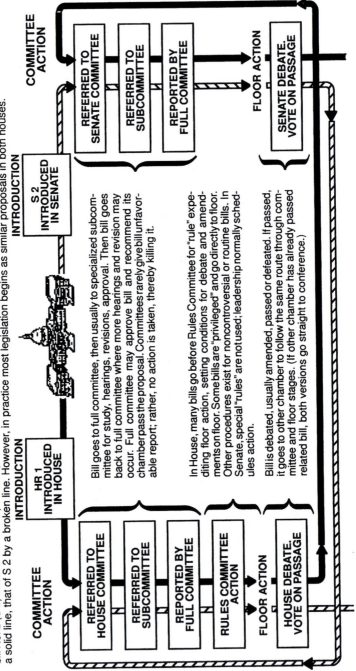

INTRODUCTION

HR 1 INTRODUCED IN HOUSE

INTRODUCTION

S 2 INTRODUCED IN SENATE

COMMITTEE ACTION

REFERRED TO HOUSE COMMITTEE

REFERRED TO SUBCOMMITTEE

REPORTED BY FULL COMMITTEE

RULES COMMITTEE ACTION

FLOOR ACTION

HOUSE DEBATE. VOTE ON PASSAGE

COMMITTEE ACTION

REFERRED TO SENATE COMMITTEE

REFERRED TO SUBCOMMITTEE

REPORTED BY FULL COMMITTEE

FLOOR ACTION

SENATE DEBATE. VOTE ON PASSAGE

Bill goes to full committee, then usually to specialized subcommittee for study, hearings, revisions, approval. Then bill goes back to full committee where more hearings and revision may occur. Full committee may approve bill and recommend its chamber pass the proposal. Committees rarely give bill unfavorable report; rather, no action is taken, thereby killing it.

In House, many bills go before Rules Committee for "rule" expediting floor action, setting conditions for debate and amendments on floor. Some bills are "privileged" and go directly to floor. Other procedures exist for noncontroversial or routine bills. In Senate, special "rules" are not used; leadership normally schedules action.

Bill is debated, usually amended, passed or defeated. If passed, it goes to other chamber to follow the same route through committee and floor stages. (If other chamber has already passed related bill, both versions go straight to conference.)

548

CONFERENCE ACTION

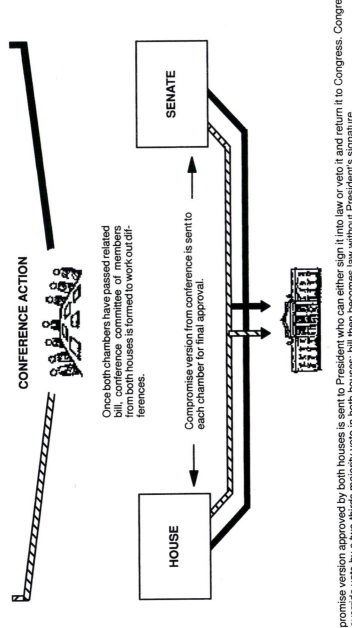

Once both chambers have passed related bill, conference committee of members from both houses is formed to work out differences.

Compromise version from conference is sent to each chamber for final approval.

SENATE

HOUSE

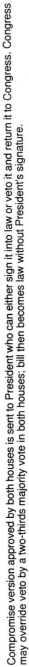

Compromise version approved by both houses is sent to President who can either sign it into law or veto it and return it to Congress. Congress may override veto by a two-thirds majority vote in both houses; bill then becomes law without President's signature.

crats and Republicans. We used grassroots advocacy to develop support from members of both parties. This bipartisan cooperation resulted in a bill that was passed in the Senate and the House with nearly unanimous votes.

The bill was not without critics and detractors. Very powerful forces within the Bush Administration as well as Congress, and even members of the AIDS community thought the CARE Act may be unnecessary or a distraction from other AIDS priorities, such as research and prevention. Assessment of this negativity and neutralization through grassroots advocacy and bipartisan support was pivotal to our success. Clearly, a road map that does not include support from constituents will never succeed. There is probably nothing more important to a politician than being re-elected—his or her constituents usually speak the loudest and have the most influence on a member of Congress.

Identify a Champion

For most social workers and advocates, elective office is rarely part of the career path. But elected officials are the public policy decision makers. Therefore, an advocate is likely to be as successful as the elected official to whom he or she as entrusted with an issue. If you seek legislative change, you must find sympathetic legislators with the ability and the commitment to help you succeed. Indeed, all aspects of great legislation can be in place, but for lack of a champion, you will most certainly be stalled. Enlisting a champion who is the chairperson of the committee is, of course, a wonderful boost to your chances of success.

In our case example, Senator Edward Kennedy, a longtime champion of progressive social and health concerns, not only had a commitment and interest in moving forward on a piece of AIDS legislation, he was also Chairman of the powerful Senate Labor and Human Resources Committee. Of course, an AIDS bill sponsored by Senator Kennedy caught very few by surprise—he had been our leader and champion since the epidemic began. It was Senator Orrin Hatch, the conservative Utah Republican who cosponsored the bill with Senator Kennedy, who really astonished political pundits. Senator Hatch wholeheartedly endorsed the bill, suggesting that it be named after Ryan White—a gesture of genuine support and compassion and a politically savvy decision.

In the House, longtime AIDS champion Representative Henry Waxman, a California Democrat, chaired the Energy and Commerce Subcommittee on Health and the Environment. Representative Waxman, like Senator Kennedy, had long understood the needs of people living with HIV/AIDS and was the leading Democrat on health care programs. Being from Los Angeles, Representative Waxman did not waste time recognizing the disaster unfolding in his community and the need to boldly respond.

Members of Congress are quite busy and rely heavily upon their staff members for advice, assistance, legislative drafting, and specific positions on particular issues. Your champion must have a dedicated staff. Regarding Ryan White, two principal Kennedy staff members worked diligently to craft the CARE Act, which Senator Hatch indicated "Often . . . provides for models of HIV service delivery that are considered to be some of the most successful health care delivery models in history." Michael Iskowitz, a former Head Start teacher, activist, and lawyer was the principal staff leader. Terry Beirn, an AIDS-diagnosed staff member provide spirit, message, and heavy doses of the reality faced by people living with HIV/AIDS. Tim Westmoreland, a congressional aide for over a decade, played a pivotal role in steering the bill through a difficult political process in the House of Representatives.

Assess the Political Realities

This is the break point—the piece of the puzzle that is hardest to articulate and even harder to negotiate. Political realties change in time frames of less than a few hours. What is politically hot and unstoppable one moment can become a political pariah the next. Reading political "tea leaves" is a talent you may not possess, but an informed judgment regarding the political practicalities of your efforts is critical. The same objective analysis a social worker uses to work with a client in a clinical capacity needs to be utilized in making political judgments. No matter how badly we want change or how right we believe our position to be, if the political winds are blowing the wrong way, there is little hope of prevailing.

Political timing is a must when seeking success in the legislature. I have often told audiences that the Ryan White CARE Act could not have occurred if attempted two years earlier. The crisis had not yet hit home for enough mainstream Americans. Public health officials had not yet decided that the crisis was in fact mushrooming beyond their traditional capacity to control it effects. Our coalitions had not yet been formed and our solutions had not yet taken shape. Sometimes, premature action in politics and policy can be more harmful than helpful.

How does an advocate know when the political timing is right? I have struggled with the appropriate answer. I would like to give you a checklist, but that would not be accurate. It is fair to say the 50 percent is based on knowledge and experience and 50 percent is pure seat-of-the-pants good instinct and good luck. The latter is gained over years of advocacy work. I strongly encourage social workers who wish to pursue politics as practice to do two things in order to gain the "gut instinct": (1) practice in a public welfare program for a few years learning how ill-formed policy can harm clients and cripple effective social work practice, and (2) volunteer in a political campaign and/or work in a legislature for at least one year. Politicians are motivated and survive by politics; any policy proposal must fit comfortably into a "political paradigm" for a majority of legislators if it is to be successful.

This is not to suggest a diminished emphasis on the substance of your proposal, nor should you be dissuaded from attempting a long-shot effort for any given change. Indeed, the CARE Act was considered a political longshot by many; it succeeded *despite* the pessimism. Finally, remember the difference between a great idea and an enacted law is purely politics.

The six-point program outlined is not by any means comprehensive. However, it can assist the social worker in seeking change. These six points are designed to help in any effort—from school board campaigns for AIDS education to statewide efforts to utilize exchange strategies to efforts to keep our federal response to AIDS adequate and effective.

POTENTIAL BARRIERS TO SUCCESSFUL INTERVENTION

There are numerous political barriers and legislative obstacles that the advocate will undoubtedly encounter. However, paying attention to the six-point plan outlined in this chapter will help you negotiate those waters. Other areas that social workers and nonprofit agencies usually get tripped up by are the Internal Revenue Service (IRS) regulations regarding lobbying and the restrictions regarding the ability of federal employees to engage in political activities. There are numerous publications on this topic, but a brief review of the rules may be useful:

1. A private charity registered with the IRS as a 501 (c)(3) may use between 5 percent and 20 percent of its budget to directly lobby legislators. The law distinguishes between "direct lobbying," which is permitted generally at 20 percent, and "grassroots lobbying," which is permitted at 5 percent. The differences between direct lobbying and other activities are the direct relationship your agency has to the legislation and the exact request you make of a legislator or your grassroots network. There have been recent modifications to regulations relating to nonprofit lobbying; it is best to make sure that you review the most recent regulations when undertaking a legislative campaign.

2. Nonprofit organizations whose primary mission involves advocacy or lobbying activities (i.e., labor unions) are afforded another category of IRS registration known as a 501 (c)(4). The rules under this classification are different than those for (c)(3) organizations, specifically allowing more direct lobbying, advocacy, and activities in government affairs.

3. Political action committees (PACs) are the most regulated of all political undertakings, and nonprofit organizations face particularly stringent limitations for these activities. PACs are a powerful and effective vehicle for influencing public policy, despite the "black eye" they receive in many forums. PACs can be particularly helpful for small donors who, as individuals will not make much of an impact on issues in the "big money" politics, but collectively can compete with the richest of PACs. For example, National Association of Social Workers (NASW) has a PAC to advance the interest of social workers. There are relatively few social workers who could donate $5,000.00 (maximum allowed by law) to a candidate for Congress. But one thousand social workers donating $5 can equal that amount and give collectively through a PAC. If you choose to establish a PAC, enlist the assistance of a competent expert to guide you through the process.

4. If you are employed by the federal government, you are limited in the kinds of political activities that you may undertake—generally subject to the Hatch Act. Most federal employees understand these rules, but I believe that many social workers do not understand that not all "public agencies" are bound by these rules. Generally speaking, the rules of the Hatch Act prohibit a federal employee from using his or her role as a government official to influence voters. The law does not prohibit anyone from exercising his or her constitution right to be involved in electoral activities. If you are not a *federal* employee, the Hatch Act does not apply to your political activities. You should check with your agency to assess your status under the Hatch Act regulations.

INFORMATION THE CLIENT SHOULD KNOW
BEFORE TAKING ACTION

Clients can be the most powerful advocates for change. There is no substitute for the actual experience of an individual to lend credibility to a social worker's articulation of a problem and the rationale for a solution to that problem. Most successful campaigns for change involve individuals on whose behalf the campaign is waged. Examples of powerful client advocates include the following: welfare mothers during the height of the welfare rights movement; people with disabilities as leaders and spokespeople for passage of the Americans with Disabilities Act; and people living with HIV/AIDS in the formation and passage of the Ryan White CARE Act.

Prior to enlisting the support of clients in a campaign to change or pass a law, it is important to know that politics and legislation are games of "hardball." Clients engaged in this process can be treated poorly. Although this sort of treatment is unusual, it does happen. A client may be called to testify before a legislative committee, and an unsupportive legislator may give a client a rough "third degree"—with intrusive questions and inappropriate comments. There is little you can do to prevent this sort of behavior. However, you must ensure that your client is prepared for any scenario that may present itself. Similarly, client confidentiality must be understood and respected in the political process. Therefore, even though I bring client witnesses to testify in front of Congress with the promise of confidentiality, I always warn the client that this thin veil of protection is easily pierced because actions taken in pursuit of public policy are usually part of a public record.

Your clients and your agency should be forewarned of the prospect of a backlash. If you are successful in winning a campaign for change, there is little doubt that along the way someone was or will be unhappy about your work. You must be aware that the "spotlight" brought on by political work can have significant consequences—both positive and negative. Expect the worst, hope for the best, and plan for both. Controversy may generate terrific awareness of your issue and assist in the campaign for change. Make sure your own professional standards and ethics are flawless. Pay attention to the formalities of laws and regulations. Prepare your supervisors and Board of Directors for the negative press or community reaction by keeping everyone informed, supportive, and *supported* along the way.

How to Organize a Demonstration

Political demonstration can be an extremely effective tool in working for change. A well-timed, well-organized demonstration can instantly create the real—or imagined—pressure for change that frequently moves a politician from neutral to supportive. For a demonstration to be effective, it must be well planned, and every possible scenario should be explored. There are unproductive demonstrations; in these cases, you can lose more than you gain.

Organizing a demonstration takes essentially three things: (1) a network of activists who can respond quickly; (2) underwriting to help defray the cost of organizing, travel, and meals for volunteers and demonstrators; and (3) access to savvy media assistance to ensure that your demonstration will be noticed.

During the effort to pass the Ryan White Care Act, the legislation was set to move forward in the Senate. However, when the bill emerged from the Labor Committee, the floor's legislative calendar was very full. We held a vigil in the Senate gallery until the bill was brought to the floor for consideration. Prior to beginning the vigil each day, we held a rally and press conference in front of the U.S. Capitol Building. This helped us to spread our message wide and far. Senator Kennedy let his colleagues know that Jeanne White and fifty other mothers of people living with HIV/AIDS were in a vigil awaiting the Ryan White CARE Act. Telephone calls were made to key staff personnel and all offices informing members of the Senate that a demonstration was taking place. Our demonstration lasted two days.

How to Work with the Media

Media relations are the venue for getting a wider audience interested in your issues and capturing the attention of political leaders. Media is a whole profession in itself, and I do not claim to be an expert. I do know that positive interest by the media can be a very powerful part of succeeding in your efforts to bring about change. Similarly, not all media is good media. There are times when individuals or organizations attract media interest, but are unprepared for what could be a negative "spin" on the issues. Here are a few basic rules I suggest for working with the media:

1. *Define your message first.* You must tell the media what you want them to know up front. In the case of the CARE Act, we wanted the media to cover the fact that people living with HIV/AIDS were without adequate health care and the public health consequences could bring a disaster upon the nation's largest cities. Simply put, AIDS is a disaster—relief is needed. We always led with that message.
2. *Choose a credible spokesperson.* This individual must combine media interest and the ability to deliver your message. For the CARE Act, Jeanne White, Ryan's mother, was the perfect choice. She freely admitted to being no expert in politics or health care policy, but she brought the message of caring for people living with HIV/AIDS home in a unique and powerful way. For technical information on the bill, strategy, and the Congressional progress, I served as the "background" spokesperson. This combination of media interest and medical informant was effective.

We had one additional advantage—Elizabeth Taylor had chosen AIDS as her issue. Elizabeth Taylor came to Washington, DC in March of 1990 to introduce the original bill with Senators Kennedy and Hatch. This big boost in media attention was incredibly helpful as our efforts progressed throughout the year.

3. *Work with local newspapers' editorial boards.* Every newspaper in the country has an editorial board. These individuals choose the issues that a newspaper will editorialize each day. I have never met a member of Congress nor anyone interested in policy and politics who does not read the editorial page of the local newspaper daily. Often, the barometer of political priority is the editorial page of a newspaper from home. While the big national newspapers (*The New York Times, The Washington Post,* and *The Los Angeles Times,* to name a few) may be difficult to access, it may be quite easy to get an appointment with your local newspaper's editorial board. More than forty editorials in papers from across the nation called for the passage of the Ryan White CARE Act. These editorial boards helped create media pressure that helped pass the CARE bill.

4. *Do not give up.* Reporters and publishers are very busy. They may not respond to your first press release, or even your second. Calls, letters, appointments, and general tenaciousness can be very productive. You are competing for the attention of the general community and often issues like AIDS can be difficult to garner new interest. Be creative. Sometimes media attention has more to do with show than substance. Creating a show that highlights your issue can help get attention. For example, when Jeanne White came to the demonstration to sit in the Senate gallery and wait for the bill to considered, it created a media opportunity.

How to Work with the Grassroots Community and Activists Groups

If there is one unique aspect of creating change in AIDS that stands out above all others, the involvement of the grassroots community and activists groups is the hallmark. Without a doubt, the grassroots groups and activists have facilitated the political response to AIDS thus far. These same grassroots groups and activists will sustain the AIDS movement until a cure is found. For political organizing, grassroots groups are the single ingredient that cannot be skimped on or ignored when seeking change. If you do not have interested voters, you do not have an issue that will win.

That said, working with the grassroots community and activist groups can be a difficult balancing act. When asked about the balance between the practicalities of legislation and the demands of the activists, I often suggest people look at the analogy of an airplane—you need a left wing and a right wing in order to fly. For the social worker concerned with making change, a healthy respect for your activists is essential. They frequently not only define the plane, but usually allow you to take the pilot's seat.

Your grassroots community is your political fuel. You must have a lot of it, constantly monitor how much is left, how much you are expending for various aspects of your campaign for change, and how you can get more when you are running out. For many first-time organizers, the grassroots component sounds like the easiest and the cheapest aspect of the effort. For the veteran organizer, the grassroots community is always the hardest and frequently the most expensive part of the effort.

Grassroots organizing requires dedicated people in key local areas. These individuals will become your infrastructure. The production of letter, phone calls, faxes, editorial board meetings will depend on these principal players. You must choose them well, train them well, and feed them with information and resources constantly.

Every campaign will not require mobilization of the full grassroots network. Targeting is a very important aspect of your grassroots relations—deciding what state or district should be influencing a member at what time. Good targeting not only economizes the time of volunteers, but saves vast sums of money, particularly for efforts that are national in scope. Knowing which members of Congress need pressure and at what time that pressure is needed is key. If you are working with your state legislature and the committee that is considering your bill has twelve members, your efforts should be focused on those districts represented by the twelve members of the committee. Do not waste time and stamps on the others—you will need them if the bill makes it to the full legislature.

Your grass roots cannot respond to everything, every time. My rule of thumb is that a maximum of only 10 percent respond to a mailing alert at any given time. That figure drops if you are alerting people all the time for all kinds of issues. There is a difference—and there should be a distinction between—an action alert and communications/education. I advise clients to have different letterhead or formats for different types of grassroots communication. For example, your alerts should be serious and urgent. Use red ink, boldface type, and italics. Keep it short and simple. Give clear directions and the necessary information to get the job done (i.e., a list of committee members with phone numbers). Your newsletter or update information should be "kinder and gentler" in design and style. You may write with education as your goal, not action.

Activist groups are different from the general grassroots community. Activists are frequently either your loyal lieutenants in the field or your most troubling nemeses. Remember to think of the airplane analogy when you need to cope with difficult situations. *You need your activists.* They keep passion, attention, honesty, and action on the radar screen. Essentially, activism is usually the first step toward change. Examine any political movement: civil rights; women's rights; antiwar efforts; pro-choice activism; and AIDS activism. You will find the same patterns. Activism first—it grabs attention and demands a revolution. Change second—it comes more slowly and through some mediating process.

At the time of passage of the Ryan White CARE Act, the AIDS Coalition To Unleash Power, ACT UP, was considered the activist community. Did everyone agree with the tactics and strategy of ACT UP? Certainly not. Did everyone hear their message? They certainly did. Similarly, the kind of radical extremism demonstrated by people such as Senator Jesse Helms from North Carolina effectively completed the right wing of the same political airplane. In many cases, truth and reality are defined by the middle—the same is true for politics. It was useful in passing the CARE Act to have the left wing (ACT UP) and the right wing (Jesse Helms). Most members of Congress wanted a reasonable way to be in the middle, and the CARE Act was a perfect alternative.

It is difficult to establish relationships between your activists and the mediating change agents. It is appropriate for political roles to be different and for tactics to be different. There were days when I wanted to put on my military boots and jeans shorts and scream in front of the U.S. Capitol Building, but it would not have helped. My role was to wear the suit, walk past the activists and into the U.S. Capitol Building, and attempt to seize the opportunity created by the activists outside. The activists did not get all that they demanded; they would be disappointed and even angry with me. But, the right wing did not get all that they wanted either. There were days when frustration with the activists on my side would rise to the boiling point; however, respecting the strategic requirement to have a vocal—and sometimes angry—activist community provided the perspective to keep moving toward the middle. I have a sign in my office that has the following inscribed on it: "I know I'm being fair when both sides accuse me of unfairness."

Your sympathies, allegiances, friends, and heart may be on the activist side, but your talent may be to steer toward the sometimes unrecognizable middle ground. During the process, there may be few outlets for the social worker in this position. When the process is over, hopefully, you will have the satisfaction of winning and knowing you were part of the process that brought it into reality.

CONCLUSION

Evaluating the prospects for change within the systems that assist or oppress your clients is a vital and necessary role for the social worker. I believe there is a professional and ethical responsibility to seek changes in structures that ameliorate individual suffering so that long-term and significant differences are achieved.

I do not know how many thousands of social workers have been involved—and are still involved—in meeting the challenges imparted by the AIDS epidemic. What I do know is that social workers were a remarkable, yet somewhat invisible part of the success of the Ryan White CARE Act, and they are part of the creation of solutions that are yet unfinished. For people living with HIV/AIDS, the social worker's job is not over. Many more hurdles lie ahead for social workers to confront with a commitment to revolutionize a change. Be it through congressional letter-writing campaigns, excellent program management, aggressive case work, or even volunteer work in a political campaign, each social worker can do something that becomes part of changing the system. This is my experience as a social worker, my pleasure as a professional, and indeed my perception of being human.

"Don't mourn . . . ORGANIZE."

RECOMMENDED READINGS

Meredith, Judith, and Meyer, Linda. (1982). "Lobbying on a Shoestring." Massachusetts Poverty Law Center.

Rodman, Eric. (1993). *The Dance of Legislation.* New York: Simon and Schuster.

Wallach, Lawrence (1993). *Media Advocacy and Public Health: Power for Prevention.* Newbury Park, CA: Sage Publications.

Index

Page numbers followed by the letter "i" indicate illustrations; those followed by the letter "t" indicate tables.

Order Your Own Copy of
This Important Book for Your Personal Library!

HIV AND SOCIAL WORK
A Practitioner's Guide

_____ in hardbound at $69.95 (ISBN: 0-7890-0180-2)

_____ in softbound at $24.95 (ISBN: 1-56023-906-9)

COST OF BOOKS_____

OUTSIDE USA/CANADA/
MEXICO: ADD 20%_____

POSTAGE & HANDLING_____
(US: $3.00 for first book & $1.25
for each additional book)
Outside US: $4.75 for first book
& $1.75 for each additional book)

SUBTOTAL_____

IN CANADA: ADD 7% GST_____

STATE TAX_____
(NY, OH & MN residents, please
add appropriate local sales tax)

FINAL TOTAL_____
(If paying in Canadian funds,
convert using the current
exchange rate. UNESCO
coupons welcome.)

Prices in US dollars and subject to change without notice.

☐ **BILL ME LATER:** ($5 service charge will be added)
(Bill-me option is good on US/Canada/Mexico orders only;
not good to jobbers, wholesalers, or subscription agencies.)

☐ Check here if billing address is different from
shipping address and attach purchase order and
billing address information.

Signature_____

☐ **PAYMENT ENCLOSED: $**_____

☐ **PLEASE CHARGE TO MY CREDIT CARD.**

☐ Visa   ☐ MasterCard   ☐ AmEx   ☐ Discover
☐ Diner's Club

Account #_____

Exp. Date_____

Signature_____

NAME _____

INSTITUTION _____

ADDRESS _____

CITY _____

STATE/ZIP _____

COUNTRY _____ COUNTY (NY residents only) _____

TEL _____ FAX _____

E-MAIL_____
May we use your e-mail address for confirmations and other types of information? ☐ Yes   ☐ No

Order From Your Local Bookstore or Directly From
The Haworth Press, Inc.
10 Alice Street, Binghamton, New York 13904-1580 • USA
TELEPHONE: 1-800-HAWORTH (1-800-429-6784) / Outside US/Canada: (607) 722-5857
FAX: 1-800-895-0582 / Outside US/Canada: (607) 772-6362
E-mail: getinfo@haworth.com
PLEASE PHOTOCOPY THIS FORM FOR YOUR PERSONAL USE.

BOF96